Color Atlas of Ophthalmology

The Manhattan Eye, Ear, & Throat Hospital Pocket Guide

Color Atlas of Ophthalmology

The Manhattan Eye, Ear, & Throat Hospital Pocket Guide

Suresh Mandava, M.D.
Tara Sweeney, M.D.
David Guyer, M.D.

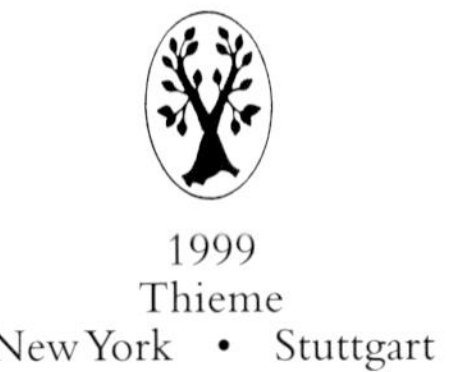

1999
Thieme
New York • Stuttgart

Thieme New York
333 Seventh Avenue
New York, NY 10001

Editor: Andrea Seils
Editorial Assistant: Jinnie Kim
Editorial Director: Ave McCracken
Director, Production & Manufacturing: Maxine Langweil
Production Editor: Michele Mulligan
Marketing Director: Phyllis Gold
Sales Manager: David Bertelsen
Chief Financial Officer: Seth S. Fishman
President: Brian D. Scanlan
Cover Designer: Kevin Kall
Compositor: Compset, Inc.
Printer: G. Canale SC.

Suresh Mandava, M.D.
Tara Sweeney, M.D.
David Guyer, M.D.

Library of Congress Cataloging-in-Publication Data
Color Atlas of Ophthalmology: The MEETH Pocket Guide / edited by Suresh Mandava, Tara Sweeney, David Guyer.
p. cm.
Compiled in conjunction with the Dept. of Ophthalmology, Manhattan Eye, Ear, & Throat Hospital (MEETH).
Includes index.
ISBN 3-13-107941-X. — ISBN 0-86577-685-7
1. Eye—Diseases—Atlases. 2. Eye—Diseases—Handbooks, manuals, etc. 3. Ophthalmology—Atlases. 4. Ophthalmology—Handbooks, manuals, etc. I. Mandava, Suresh. II. Sweeney, Tara. III. Guyer, David R. IV. Manhattan Eye, Ear, and Throat Hospital. Dept. of Ophthalmology.
[DNLM: 1. Eye Diseases atlases. 2. Ophthalmology handbooks. WW 17 M495 1998]
RE71.M44 1998
617.7′0022′2—dc21
DNLM/DLC
for Library of Congress 98-25048
CIP

Important note: Medical knowledge is ever-changing. As new research and clinical experience broaden our knowledge, changes in treatment and drug therapy may be required. The authors and editors of the material herein have consulted sources believed to be reliable in their efforts to provide information that is complete and in accord with the standards accepted at the time of publication. However, in view of the possibility of human error by the authors, editors, or publisher of the work herein, or changes in medical knowledge, neither the authors, editors, publisher, nor any other party who has been involved in the preparation of this work, warrants that the information contained herein is in every respect accurate to complete, and they are not responsible for any errors or omissions or for the results obtained from use of such information. Readers are encouraged to confirm the information contained herein with other sources. For example, readers are advised to check the product information sheet included in the package of each drug they plan to administer to be certain that the information contained in this publication is accurate and that changes have not been made in the recommended dose or in the contraindications for administration. This recommendation is of particular importance in connection with new or infrequently used drugs.

5 4 3 2 1

TNY 0-86577-685-7
GTV 3-13-107941-X

CONTENTS

EXTENDED CONTENTS

LIST OF CONTRIBUTORS

David H. Abramson, M.D.
Clinical Professor of Ophthalmology
New York Hospital-Cornell
Medical Center
Department of Ophthalmology
Manhattan Eye, Ear and
Throat Hospital
New York, New York

Scott Anagnoste, M.D.
Department of Ophthalmology
Manhattan Eye, Ear and
Throat Hospital
New York, New York

Gavin Bahadur, M.D.
Department of Ophthalmology
Manhattan Eye, Ear and
Throat Hospital
New York, New York

Paul E. Beade, M.D.
Department of Ophthalmology
Manhattan Eye, Ear and
Throat Hospital
New York, New York

Brian Brazzo, M.D.
Department of Ophthalmology
Manhattan Eye, Ear and
Throat Hospital
New York, New York

Stephen Brown, M.D.
Department of Ophthalmology
Manhattan Eye, Ear and
Throat Hospital
New York, New York

Benjamin Chang, M.D.
Ophthalmologist
Eye Associates
Department of Ophthalmology
Manhattan Eye, Ear and
Throat Hospital
New York, New York

Jack M. Dodick, M.D.
Clinical Professor
Columbia University College of
Physicians and Surgeons
Chairman, Department
of Ophthalmology
Manhattan Eye, Ear and
Throat Hospital
New York, New York

Eric E. Donnenfeld, M.D.
Associate Professor
of Ophthalmology
New York University School
of Medicine
Co-Chairman, External Disease
Manhattan Eye, Ear and
Throat Hospital
New York, New York

Vadim Filatov, M.D.
Department of Ophthalmology
Manhattan Eye, Ear and
Throat Hospital
New York, New York

Yale L. Fisher, M.D.
Clinical Assistant Professor
of Ophthalmology
Cornell Medical Center

Department of Ophthalmology
Manhattan Eye, Ear and
Throat Hospital
New York, New York

Thomas Flynn, M.D.
Columbia Ophthalmology
Consultants
Columbia University
Department of Ophthalmology
Manhattan Eye, Ear and
Throat Hospital
New York, New York

Dawn Jackson Fyler, M.D.
Department of Ophthalmology
Manhattan Eye, Ear and
Throat Hospital
New York, New York

Richard P. Gibraltar, M.D.
Department of Ophthalmology
Manhattan Eye, Ear and
Throat Hospital
Lenox Hill Hospital
Mt. Sinai Hospital
New York, New York

David Guyer, M.D.
Clinical Associate Professor
of Ophthalmology
Cornell University Medical Center
Director of Residency Training
Manhattan Eye, Ear and
Throat Hospital
New York, New York

David H. Haight, M.D.
Corneal and Refractive Specialist
Department of Ophthalmology
Manhattan Eye, Ear and
Throat Hospital
New York, New York

Raymond Harrison, M.D.
Surgeon, Director, and Chief,
Glaucoma Service, Emeritus
Manhattan Eye, Ear and
Throat Hospital
New York, New York

Evan Held, M.D.
Department of Ophthalmology
Manhattan Eye, Ear and
Throat Hospital
New York, New York

Albert Hornblass, M.D.
Clinical Professor of Ophthalmology
State University of New York–
College of Medicine
Surgeon Director
Chief of Oculoplastic Surgery
Manhattan Eye, Ear and
Throat Hospital
Director of Oculoplastics
Lenox Hill Hospital
New York, New York

Julia Hsu, M.D.
Department of Ophthalmology
Manhattan Eye, Ear and
Throat Hospital
New York, New York

James Kelly, M.D.
Department of Ophthalmology
Manhattan Eye, Ear and
Throat Hospital
New York, New York

Jessica Lattman, M.D.
Department of Ophthalmology
Manhattan Eye, Ear and
Throat Hospital
New York, New York

Mary Gilbert Lawrence, M.D., M.P.H.
Associate Professor of Ophthalmology
University of Minnesota Medical
School
Minneapolis, Minnesota

Carolyn Lederman, M.D.
Department of Ophthalmology
Manhattan Eye, Ear and
Throat Hospital
New York, New York

David Leventer, M.D.
Department of Ophthalmology
Manhattan Eye, Ear and
Throat Hospital
New York, New York

Michael Levine, M.D.
Department of Ophthalmology
Manhattan Eye, Ear and
Throat Hospital
New York, New York

Richard D. Lisman, M.D., F.A.C.S.
Clinical Professor of Ophthalmology
New York University School
of Medicine
Department of Ophthalmology
Manhattan Eye, Ear and
Throat Hospital
New York, New York

Maurice Luntz, M.D.
Department of Ophthalmology
Manhattan Eye, Ear and
Throat Hospital
New York, New York

Alfred E. Mamelok, M.D.
Associate Clinical Professor
of Ophthalmology
Cornell Medical College
Attending Ophthalmologist
New York Hospital
Attending Surgeon and Co-Chief
Uveitis Service
Manhattan Eye, Ear and
Throat Hospital
Section Chief of Ophthalmology
Beth Israel North Hospital
New York, New York

Naresh Mandava, M.D.
Department of Ophthalmology
Manhattan Eye, Ear and
Throat Hospital
New York, New York

Suresh Mandava, M.D.
Department of Ophthalmology
Manhattan Eye, Ear and
Throat Hospital
New York, New York

Norman B. Medow, M.D.
Attending Ophthalmologist
Cornea and Cataract Service
Manhattan Eye, Ear and
Throat Hospital
Assistant Adjunct
Department of Ophthalmology
Lenox Hill Hospital
New York, New York

Michael Nejat, M.D.
Department of Ophthalmology
Manhattan Eye, Ear and
Throat Hospital
New York, New York

Jeffrey Odel, M.D.
Associate Clinical Professor
of Ophthalmology
Columbia Presbyterian
Medical Center
Department of Ophthalmology
Manhattan Eye, Ear and
Throat Hospital
New York, New York

Kristin Pisacano, M.D.
Department of Ophthalmology
Manhattan Eye, Ear and
Throat Hospital
New York, New York

Renée Richards, M.D.
Department of Ophthalmology

Manhattan Eye, Ear and
Throat Hospital
New York, New York

René Rodriguez-Sains, M.D.
Clinical Assistant Professor
Department of Ophthalmology
New York University School of
Medicine
Attending Surgeon & Chief, Ocular
Tumor and Orbital Clinic
Attending Surgeon, Ophthalmic
Plastic & Reconstructive
Surgery Clinic
Manhattan Eye, Ear and
Throat Hospital
Attending Surgeon, Ophthalmic
Plastic Surgery Service
Bellevue Hospital-NYU
New York, New York

Steven Rosenberg, M.D.
Department of Ophthalmology
Manhattan Eye, Ear and
Throat Hospital
New York, New York

Abraham Schlossman, M.D.
Adjunct Associate Clinical Professor
Department of Ophthalmology
Mt. Sinai School of Medicine
Attending Surgeon, Emeritus
Department of Ophthalmology
Manhattan Eye, Ear and
Throat Hospital
New York, New York

Amelia Schrier, M.D.
Department of Ophthalmology
Manhattan Eye, Ear and
Throat Hospital
New York, New York

Belinda Shirkey, M.D.
Department of Ophthalmology
Manhattan Eye, Ear and
Throat Hospital
New York, New York

Jason S. Slakter, M.D.
Assistant Clinical Professor
of Ophthalmology
Columbia University College of
Physicians and Surgeons
Attending Surgeon
Vitreoretinal Service
Manhattan Eye, Ear and
Throat Hospital
New York, New York

Michael B. Starr, M.D.
Department of Ophthalmology
Manhattan Eye, Ear and
Throat Hospital
New York, New York

Tara Sweeney, M.D.
Department of Ophthalmology
Manhattan Eye, Ear and
Throat Hospital
New York, New York

John Talamo, M.D.
Director of Refractive Surgery
Massachusetts Eye and Ear
Infirmary
Boston, Massachusetts

Lawrence Yannuzzi, M.D.
Vice Chairman, Department of
Ophthalmology
Director of Retinal Services
Manhattan Eye, Ear and
Throat Hospital
New York, New York

PREFACE

The beginning of ophthalmology residency was one of the most challenging periods of our professional careers. It seemed years of medical training had suddenly failed us, as we found ourselves scrambling through textbooks and atlases for a picture to match the unknown images that were staring at us through our slit-lamps and ophthalmoscopes. Then we would consult other texts to learn how to manage the disease. In a field where we learn, teach, and diagnose visually, we were surprised that no one, compact text satisfied our daily needs.

We later realized that the need for a quick, comprehensive reference was not limited to residents alone; a concise, orderly reference with pictures would be invaluable for optometrists, ophthalmic technicians, primary care practitioners, and even experienced ophthalmologists. For example, a rare finding, such as a Lisch iris nodule, may be seen only a few times in a career, but can aid in the important diagnosis of neurofibromatosis. An unfamiliar corneal dystrophy may stump a busy retinal specialist. A primary care or emergency room physician may need a reference to ascertain that an unusual optic nerve was caused by benign optic disc drusen, not life-threatening papilledema. Finally, ophthalmic personnel, nurses and even patients may better understand a condition after seeing a photograph in a text rather than listening to a clinician's description alone.

During residency at Manhattan Eye, Ear & Throat Hospital (MEETH), we had an unusual opportunity to tap into a large source of high-quality photographs. The volunteer faculty at MEETH number over one hundred—many have large slide collections. Knowing that this wealth of resources existed, the ophthalmology residents, in conjunction with the faculty of the Department of Ophthalmology, undertook the challenge of compiling this pocket atlas.

Although over forty physicians contributed to this book, a few people deserve special recognition. First, Dr. Frederick H. Theodore painstakingly photographed and catalogued hundreds of ophthalmic conditions throughout his career. His family donated his exquisitely preserved slide collection to the resident's library, and then allowed us to use the slides in this text. His dear friend, Dr. Abraham Schlossman, uncovered these photographs to us and encouraged every resident throughout the preparation of this book. Dr. Eric Donnenfeld graciously gave us access to an enormous slide collection that he compiled during his own residency at MEETH. Without the generosity of these donors and the rest of the faculty at MEETH, this book would not exist.

Finally, the editors acknowledge the generosity of several collegues who loaned us slides for inclusion in this book: Mark Duffy (Chapter 4); Edward Holland, Jay Krachmer, and Michael Newton (Chapter 5); Gary Glickman (Chapter 9); and Jane Beeman, Tim Comstock, Hugo Siguenza, Sylvie Sulaiman, and Brian Weaver (Chapter 16).

We hope that this pocket atlas aids everyone from the ophthalmic specialist to the primary care physician in providing patients with the best care possible.

Suresh Mandava
Tara Sweeney
David Guyer

Chapter 1
OCULAR TRAUMA

James Kelly, Amelia Schrier,
Benjamin Chang

1.1 Anterior Segment Trauma

1.1.1 Eyelid Laceration—blunt or penetrating trauma to eyelid resulting in partial or full-thickness tear(s).

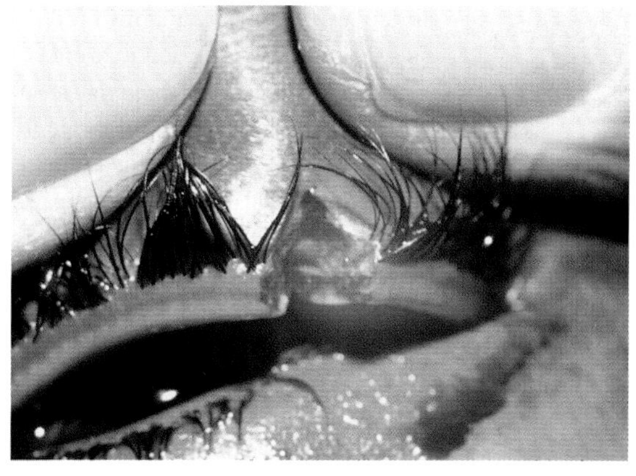

FIGURE 1.1.1 Full-thickness eyelid laceration.

Presentation eyelid ecchymosis, edema, variable ptosis, usually visible laceration. Patients may complain of pain, decreased visual acuity, and epiphora.

Management complete history and ophthalmic examination. Determine depth and location of injury and whether a foreign body or orbital fracture exists. May need CT scan or B-scan to rule out ruptured globe and associated trauma.

- Superficial lacerations: sterilize and irrigate the area, debride necrotic tissue, and search for and remove foreign bodies. Very superficial wounds may be closed with steri strips applied with antibiotic ointment. Otherwise, skin-orbicular sutures (6-0 silk or nylon) may be needed with systemic antibiotics (e.g., Keflex, 500 mg PO bid).
- Deeper lacerations not involving the lid margin: deep closure of tarsus with 6-0 vicryl, followed by the skin-orbicular closure as above. If the septum has been violated and orbital fat is seen, ptosis may result secondary to levator damage. Follow this ptosis for up to 6 months for spontaneous improvement.
- Lid-margin lacerations: the margin is carefully closed with three, 6-0 interrupted, silk sutures: one at the gray line, one at the tarsus, and one for the subcutaneous tissue. Tie suture ends to skin to avoid corneal irritation.
- Canalicular/nasolacrimal system lacerations: Repair these in the OR. May require oculoplastic service for the intubation and reconstruction of the medical canthal and canalicular system.
- Skin sutures should be removed at 5 days, but lid-margin sutures should remain for 12 days.

1.1.2 Subconjunctival Hemorrhage—blood located under the conjunctiva or Tenon's capsule.

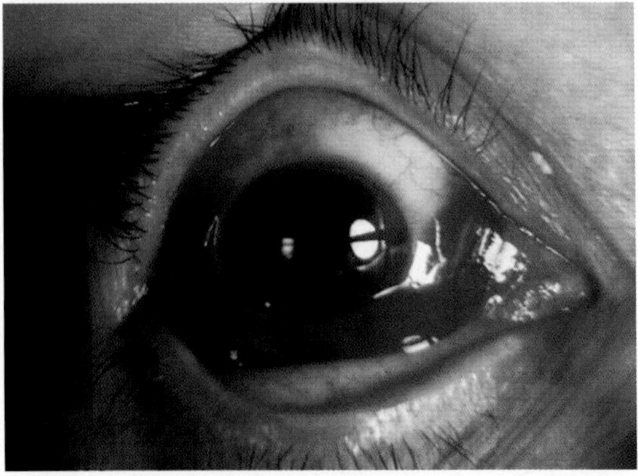

FIGURE 1.1.2 Subconjunctival hemorrhage.

Presentation blood usually located under a portion of the conjunctiva. Patients are usually concerned but asymptomatic.

Differential Diagnosis conjunctivitis, conjunctival laceration, conjunctival foreign body, conjunctival tumor.

Management history of trauma, Valsalva's maneuver, anticoagulant use, hypertension, bleeding diatheses. Rule out a ruptured globe and check the IOP. Check the patient's blood pressure. Treat with artificial tears if symptomatic and reassure that blood will clear within 2 weeks with possible color changes similar to a bruise. In cases of recurrent hemorrhage, advise a medical consultation.

1.1.3 Conjunctival Laceration—a tear in the conjunctiva, and possibly Tenon's capsule, with no underlying scleral involvement.

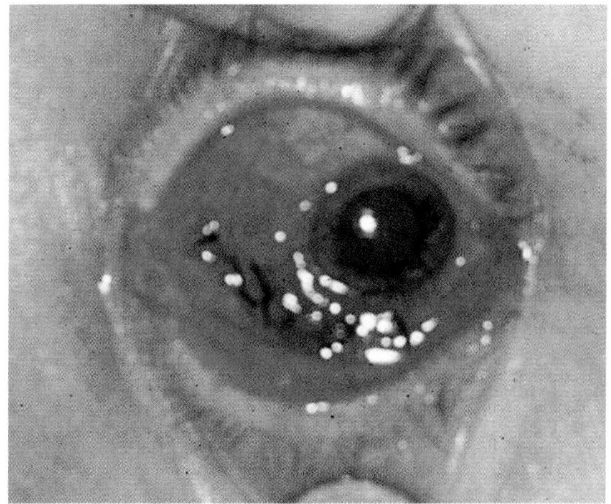

FIGURE 1.1.3 Sutured conjunctival laceration.

Presentation red eye with mild irritation. The patient may have a history of trauma or foreign-body exposure.

Management take a careful history of any possible foreign body and carefully inspect the globe and check the dilated funduscopic examination to rule out an embedded particle or a scleral laceration, constituting a ruptured globe.

- Small lacerations (<1.5 cm): treat with topical ointment or antibiotics.
- Large lacerations (>1.5 cm): if there is any question of a ruptured globe, B-scan, CT scan, and/or surgical exploration may be indicated. If not, consider surgical closure with vicryl or plain suture in addition to topical ointment or antibiotics.

1.1.4 Chemical Exposure

1.1.4 Chemical Exposure—exposure of the eye to any chemical such as solid, liquid, gaseous, or aerosol agents. Household cleaning supplies and cosmetics are common offenders.

Presentation pain, tearing, photophobia, decreased visual acuity.

- Mild to moderate exposure: eyelid edema, chemosis, conjunctival injection, corneal abrasion, anterior uveitis.
- Severe exposure: conjunctival and episcleral whitening, corneal edema, and opacification with corneoscleral melting, severe iritis, secondary glaucoma, posterior segment destruction.

Differential Diagnosis corneal abrasion or foreign body, dry eye syndrome, infectious keratitis.

Management test the conjunctival pH, place topical anesthesia, and begin irrigation immediately. After 30 minutes, recheck the conjunctival pH and double evert the lids to remove any particulate matter. Continue to irrigate until the pH is 7.0. Take a thorough history of the type of chemical and duration and volume of exposure and complete the ophthalmic examination.

- Mild to moderate exposure: the mainstays of treatment include topical antibiotics, aggressive lubrication, cycloplegia, and pain medication. Doxycycline (100 mg PO

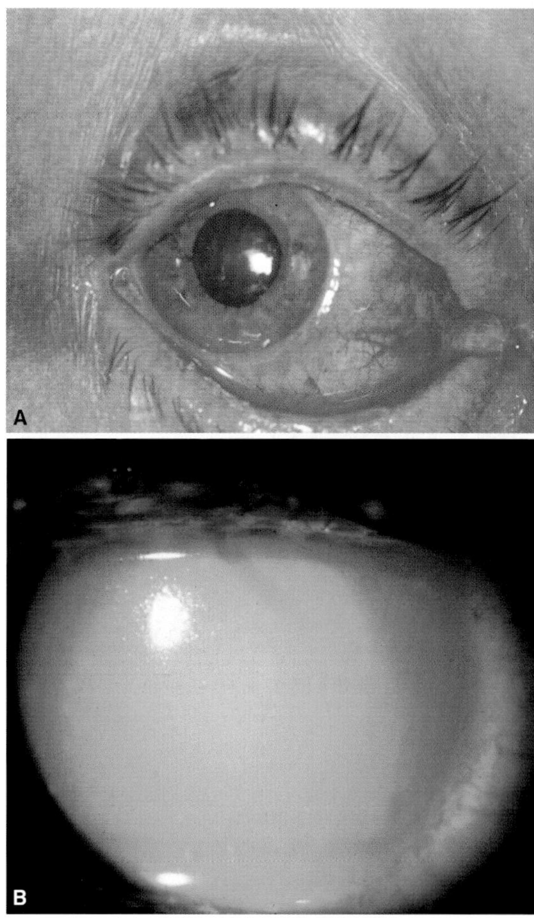

FIGURE 1.1.4a Mild chemical exposure.
FIGURE 1.1.4b Severe alkali burn with corneal edema and opacification.

bid) may help to promote collagen synthesis, topical steroids may help to reduce inflammation, and oral acetazolamide (Diamox) or topical β-blockers may be needed to treat elevated IOP.

- Severe exposure: consider debridement of necrotic tissue and glass-rod lysis of symblepharon. In addition,

tarsorrhaphy, cyanoacrylate tissue adhesive, limbal conjunctival autograft transplants, and even penetrating keratoplasty may be needed.
- Follow-up according to severity and every day until stabilization.

1.1.5 Corneal Abrasion—corneal epithelial defect.

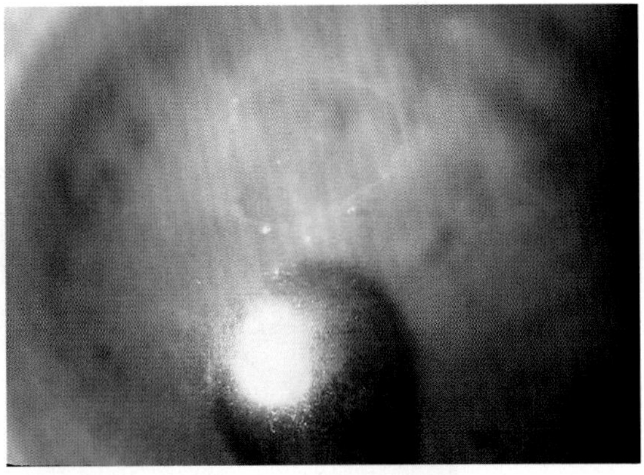

FIGURE 1.1.5 Corneal erosion.

Presentation pain, eyelid edema, tearing, photophobia. Fluorescein will stain the epithelial defect, and chemosis and conjunctival injection may be seen.

Differential Diagnosis recurrent erosion with corneal dystrophy, keratitis, infectious corneal ulcer, neurotrophic or shield ulcer.

Management history of contact lens wear, dry eye syndrome or corneal dystrophies, trauma, foreign body, or other exposure. Measure size and location of defect. Double evert the lids to check for a foreign body. Be sure to rule out a corneal ulcer and do not patch lens wearers.

- Small defects: options range from antibiotic ointments (erythromycin or bacitracin) and drops (Polytrim, Ciloxan, Ocuflox) to nonsteroidals (Acular, Voltaren).

- Large defects: consider cycloplegia and ointment with pressure patch if the patient is not a contact lens wearer. If the patient is a contact lens wearer, consider topical antibiotics and nonsteroidals, bandage contact lens, or collagen shield
- Follow-up daily until the epithelial defect is healed. Warn patients about recurrent erosion syndrome.

1.1.6 Corneal Foreign Body—traumatically induced foreign body in cornea with a suggestive history.

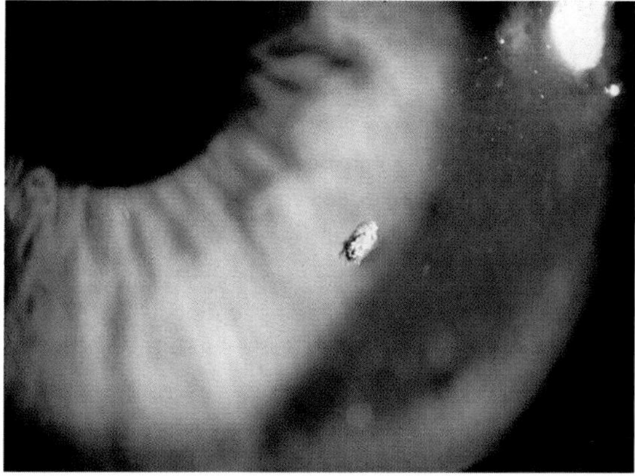

FIGURE 1.1.6 Metallic corneal foreign body under high-power magnification.

Presentation decreased visual acuity in a swollen painful red eye with tearing and photophobia. Corneal foreign body is usually embedded superficially; metallic foreign bodies containing iron may have an accompanying rust ring. There may also be a corneal ulcer, a stromal immune ring, and mild anterior uveitis.

Management is there a history of foreign-body exposure? In hammering or power-tool injuries, do a careful ocular examination, especially looking for transillumination defects of the iris and the anterior lens capsule, in addition to gonioscopy and dilated funduscopic examination to rule out penetrating or perforating injuries of the globe. Inspect the fornices for other particulate matter. After instilling topical anesthesia, a 25- to 30-gauge needle or a jewellers' forceps may be used to remove the corneal foreign body. Full-thickness foreign bodies should be removed in the OR. A burr may be helpful for rust ring removal. If rust remains in the visual axis, wait for it to migrate to the surface rather than inducing stromal scarring. Prescribe cycloplegics and topical antibiotics and consider pressure patching or a soft bandage lens. Follow-up daily until resolution of epithelial defect.

1.1.7 Corneal Laceration—a traumatic corneal tear ranging from partial to full thickness, constituting a ruptured globe.

Presentation pain, decreased visual acuity, photophobia, tearing. Full-thickness defects are Seidel (+), and there may be prolapsed uveal tissue.

Management a complete history and ocular examination, especially in the case of a full-thickness laceration.

- Partial-thickness lacerations: if truly Seidel negative and the anterior chamber has not been entered, cycloplegia,

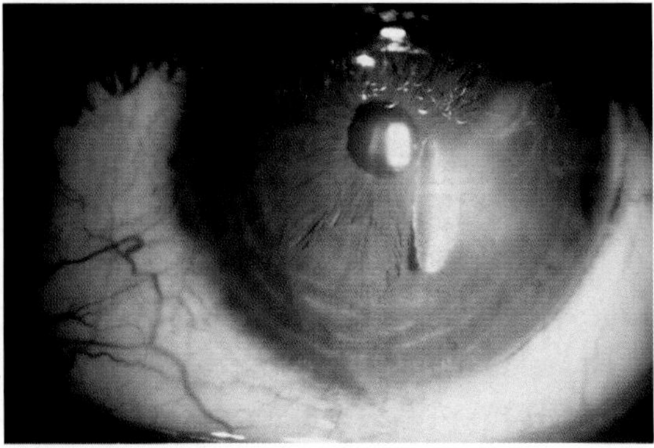

FIGURE 1.1.7a Small corneal laceration.

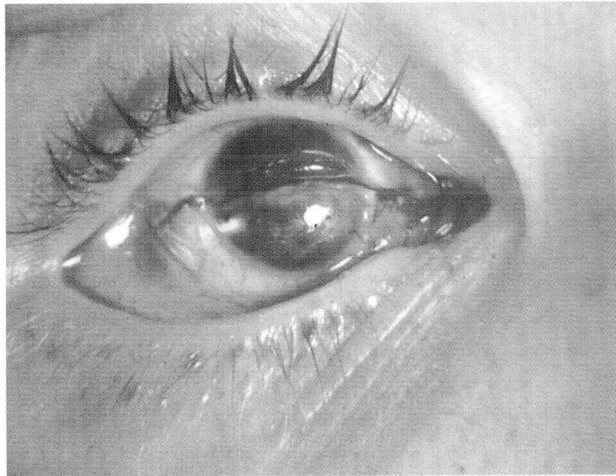

FIGURE 1.1.7b Extensive corneal laceration with hyphema.

antibiotics, and bandage lens or pressure patching are the mainstays of treatment.

- Full-thickness lacerations: immediately shield the eye, keep the patient NPO, and administer IV antibiotics. Consider B-scan and/or CT scan to rule out an orbital or intraocular foreign body. Explore and repair surgically with the patient under general anesthesia.

1.1.8 Traumatic Iritis—inflammation of the iris and ciliary body secondary to any type of trauma.

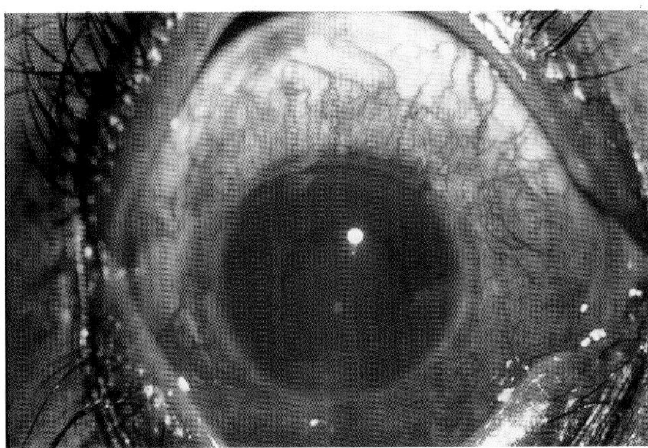

FIGURE 1.1.8 Traumatic iritis with ciliary flush.

Presentation photophobia, pain and tearing, decreased vision after blunt trauma; anterior chamber white cells and flare with ciliary flush. The IOP may be low or high in relation to the other eye.

Management a dilated funduscopic examination looking for other signs of ocular trauma. Cycloplegia is recommended for 1 week. Gonioscopy is recommended to rule out angle recession glaucoma. If inflammation persists, topical steroids are then recommended. If IOP is elevated, treat accordingly.

1.1.9 Iris Sphincter Tear—a defect in the constrictor muscle of the iris, usually resulting from blunt trauma.

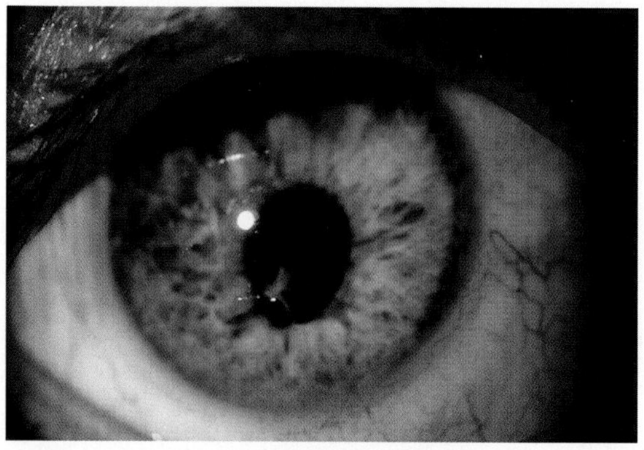

FIGURE 1.1.9 Multiple iris sphincter tears inferiorly.

Presentation possible complaint of photophobia, depending on the extent of mydriasis.

Differential Diagnosis pharmacological mydriasis, iris atrophy.

Management full ocular examination. In the absence of trauma sequelae, such as uveitis and hyphema, no intervention is necessary.

1.1.10 Iridodialysis—separation of the iris base from the ciliary body due to blunt trauma or surgery.

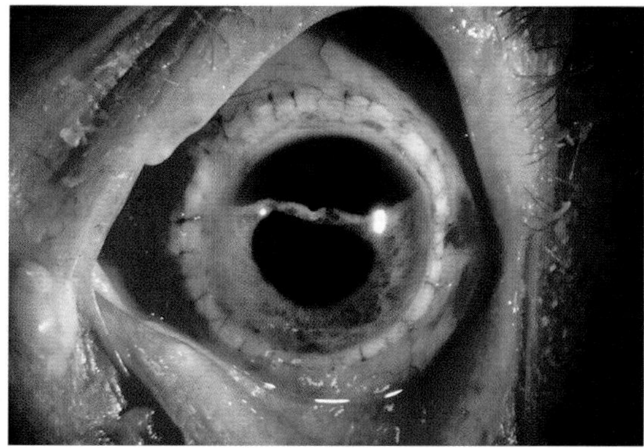

FIGURE 1.1.10 Iridodialysis from the 9-o'clock to the 2-o'clock position.

Presentation possible complaint of monocular diplopia or glare due to corectopia or polycoria. The dehiscence may be small or involve the iris root for 360°. Iridodialysis is often associated with hyphema and other trauma sequelae.

Management
- Small dialyses: no treatment.
- Large dialyses: may require surgical intervention, such as the McCannel suturing technique, to remedy visual problems and to prevent formation of synechiae.

1.1.11 Lens Dislocation/subluxation—zonular rupture with lens subluxation (portion within pupil) or dislocation (no portion within pupil) as a result of blunt or penetrating trauma.

Presentation decreased visual acuity, monocular diplopia, high degrees of astigmatism, impaired accommodation. Iridodonesis,

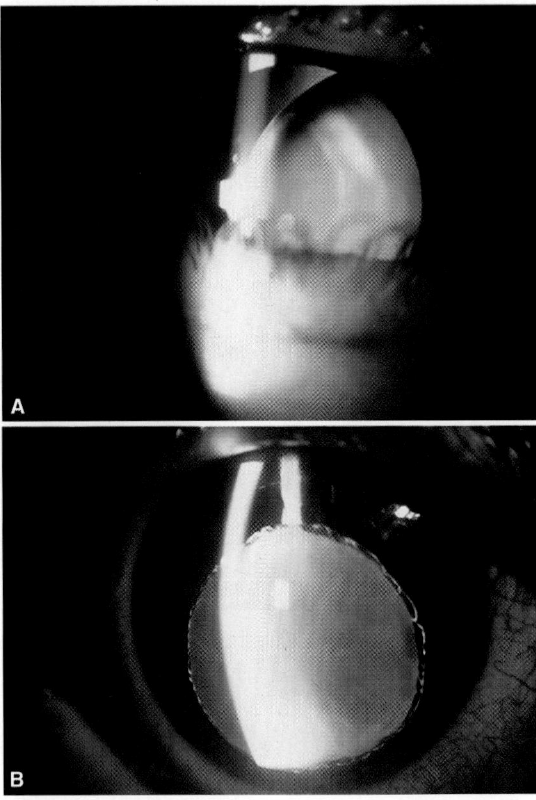

FIGURE 1.1.11a Subluxated lens.
FIGURE 1.1.11b Anteriorly dislocated lens.

phacodonesis, and the ectopic lens position may be seen at the slit lamp. Other signs of trauma may be noted such as vitreous in the anterior chamber, Vossius' ring, and posterior synechiae formation. Any type of cataract may develop, with cortical changes being the most common. Emergent complications are pupillary block and phacoantigenic glaucoma.

Differential Diagnosis

Marfan syndrome, homocystinuria.

Management assess the position of the lens, the visual acuity, and the IOP to determine proper treatment and timing of intervention.

- Lens in posterior chamber: if ophthalmic examination is otherwise normal and the IOP is controlled, observation is warranted. If vision is suboptimal, consider cataract extraction at a later time. If the examination reveals a lens, with an intact capsule, dislocated into the vitreous, examine the patient carefully for other trauma sequelae. Eventual visual rehabilitation is possible with a contact lens or secondary intraocular lens, either sutured, posterior chamber lens, or anterior chamber intraocular lens.
- Lens in anterior chamber: an ocular emergency due to possible damage to the corneal endothelium and to a rise in intraocular pressure. If the lens is not cataractous and the IOP is normal, one can try to maximally dilate the pupil and lay the patient in the supine position. The lens may migrate posteriorly to the iris plane and then pilocarpine may be instilled. However, if the lens becomes cataractous and intumescent, manage the patient with topical antiinflammatory and antiglaucoma medications until a definitive surgical procedure may be performed.

1.1.12 Microhyphema/hyphema—anterior chamber hemorrhage ranging from suspended RBCs (microhyphema) to layering of different levels to total (eight-ball) filling of anterior chamber.

Presentation pain, photophobia, decreased visual acuity with RBCs suspended or layered in anterior chamber.

Differential Diagnosis HSV infection, rubeosis iridis, tumor, or postsurgical complication. In children, consider retinoblastoma, leukemia, bleeding diathesis, child abuse, or juvenile xanthogranuloma.

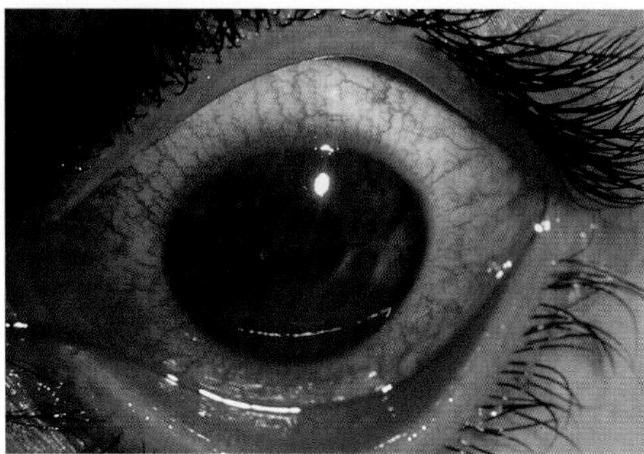

FIGURE 1.1.12 Hyphema.

Management

rule out ruptured globe and associated trauma. In the initial evaluation, do not perform scleral depression or gonioscopy. Consider B-scan or CT scan, and a sickle cell prep if indicated. Document percentage of anterior chamber filled with blood, the IOP, and whether there is corneal blood staining.

- Normal IOP: admit children to the hospital and strictly warn adults to refrain from all physical activity and to sleep with the head of the bed elevated. Prescribe cycloplegics (atropine) and topical steroids. Shield the eye at all times and avoid aspirin and oral nonsteroidals. See the patient daily to monitor the IOP and for signs of rebleed. Due to the 5 to 10% rebleed rate, usually between days 3 and 5, some centers advocate the use of aminocaproic acid (50 mg/kg IV q4h) to decrease the rebleed rate. The complication rate is not necessarily related to initial hyphema size. At 1 month after injury, the patient may undergo scleral depression and gonioscopy to rule out angle recession. If present, the patient needs to be checked for future development of glaucoma.
- Elevated IOP: treat as above and be sure to avoid carbonic anhydrase inhibitors in patients with sickle cell disease. If treating a rise in IOP secondary to a rebleed, it may be more difficult to control and may more likely

result in corneal blood staining. If the IOP remains at 50 mm Hg for 5 days, 35 mm Hg for 7 days, or 25 mm Hg for 1 to 2 days in the presence of optic neuropathy or sickle cell disease/trait, or if there is early corneal bloodstaining, consider an anterior chamber washout. In cases of pupillary block, a laser or surgical iridotomy is indicated, and a trabeculectomy may be needed in cases of uncontrolled glaucoma. These patients need a lifetime of follow-up.

1.1.13 Ruptured Globe—any full-thickness laceration of the cornea or sclera.

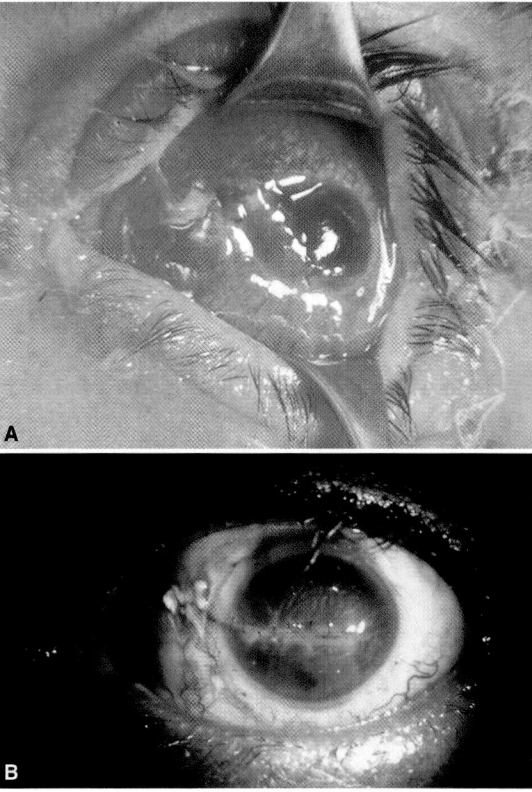

FIGURE 1.1.13a Surgical exploration of ruptured globe.
FIGURE 1.1.13b Repaired ruptured globe with hyphema.

Presentation vision intact or severely decreased. There is usually a subconjunctival hemorrhage. Corneal lacerations will be Seidel (+) and may have incarcerated uveal tissue, a shallow anterior chamber, and a hyphema. Scleral lacerations may present with incarcerated uveal tissue or foreign bodies. IOP is usually decreased, and other trauma sequelae, such as iris, ciliary body, and zonular disruption, as well as vitreous, retinal, and choroidal hemorrhages, may be present.

Differential Diagnosis partial-thickness laceration.

Management question previous ocular history, especially extracapsular cataract extraction or corneal surgery, such as PK or RK. Examine the globe for possible rupture sites and previous surgical wounds. Consider gentle B-scan or CT scan if the diagnosis is unclear or if there is a history of a possible intraocular foreign body. Remember that the globe may also be ruptured posteriorly. Do not remove large, imbedded foreign bodies at the slit lamp. Once a diagnosis is made, shield the eye, keep the patient NPO, and administer broad-spectrum systemic antibiotics. Exploration and repair of all ruptured globes is done in the OR with the patient under general anesthesia. The primary objective is to restore the integrity of the globe. A vitreoretinal surgeon should be involved if posterior segment involvement, including posteriorly located intraocular foreign body, is suspected. Interventions such as intraocular lens placement or evacuation of persistent or vitreous hemorrhage may be performed at a later date. Consider enucleation for extensive trauma if the vision is clearly unsalvageable.

1.2 Posterior Trauma

1.2.1 Cyclodialysis—rupture of the scleral insertion of the longitudinal muscle fibers of the ciliary body, resulting in cleft formation.

Presentation bare sclera visible at the site of the cleft. On gonioscopy, there is a deep angle recess. Hypotony is often present secondary to ciliary process hyposecretion and increased uveoscleral outflow. If the dialysis and hypotony are chronic, choroidals and macular edema may be present.

Management first line of therapy is cycloplegia. If this fails, consider the reapposition of the ciliary body to the sclera through photocoagulation, cryotherapy, or suturing. Closure of a cyclodialysis cleft may result in glaucoma if concomitant trabecular meshwork damage exists.

1.2.2 Commotio Retinae—Berlin's edema. Outer retinal edema usually induced as a result of blunt trauma causing a disruption of the photoreceptor segments.

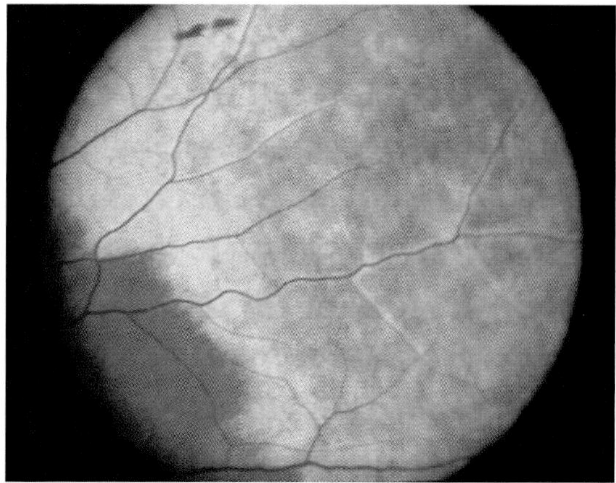

FIGURE 1.2.2 Retinal whitening of commotio retinae.

Presentation asymptomatic or markedly reduced visual acuity. On DFE, deep retinal opacification (usually gray-white) with or without scattered retinal hemorrhages. May be located anywhere in the retina.

Differential Diagnosis retinal detachment, branch retinal artery occlusion, white without pressure.

Management there is no treatment for commotio except to treat other related trauma. Follow-up weekly with full DFE and retinal detachment warnings. Visual recovery is typically good and usually occurs within 1 month. However, there are poor outcomes secondary to RPE disturbances and macular hole development.

1.2.3 Choroidal Rupture—break in Bruch's membrane and the overlying RPE and the underlying choriocapillaris.

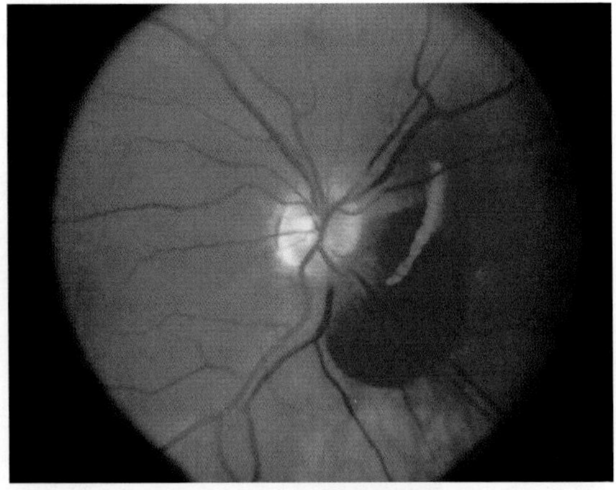

FIGURE 1.2.3 Choroidal rupture with subretinal hemorrhage.

Presentation decreased visual acuity if rupture in the foveal area. Initially, the presence of a choroidal rupture may be obscured by overlying subretinal hemorrhage. Following resolution of any hemorrhage, there is a white, crescentic lesion deep to the retina that is often concentric to the optic disc. Lesions may be single or multiple.

Differential Diagnosis angioid streaks or lacquer cracks.

Management after complete ophthalmic examination, there is no treatment. Close follow-up is warranted if the fovea is involved or heme obscures a part of the retina. Give the patients retinal detachment warnings and instruct them to use an Amsler grid to detect the early or late complication of choroidal neovascularization, which may or may not be amenable to photocoagulation.

1.2.4 Giant Retinal Tear—retinal break >90°.

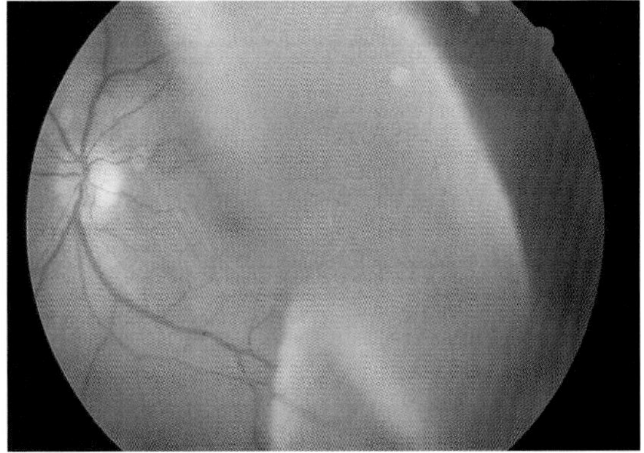

FIGURE 1.2.4 Giant retinal tear.

Presentation decreased visual acuity, visual field deficits, flashes and floaters, with a suggestive history. There is usually a visual field defect, decreased IOP, tobacco dust, and a large retinal break parallel to the posterior margin of the vitreous base. There may also be a vitreous base avulsion and/or a vitreous hemorrhage associated with the giant retinal tear. In chronic cases, there may be signs of PVR.

Differential Diagnosis retinal dialysis, retinoschisis, choroidal detachment, Marfan syndrome.

Management identify all retinal pathology with scleral depression. Surgical management consists of a variety of retinal procedures: TPPV, TPPL, scleral buckling, and the use of perfluorocarbon liquids, gas–fluid exchanges, and endolaser. There is a high incidence of PVR and redetachment. The fellow eye must be thoroughly evaluated.

1.2.5 Intraocular Foreign Body—metallic, wood, or other foreign substance that has penetrated the globe, usually lying in the vitreous cavity or on the retina.

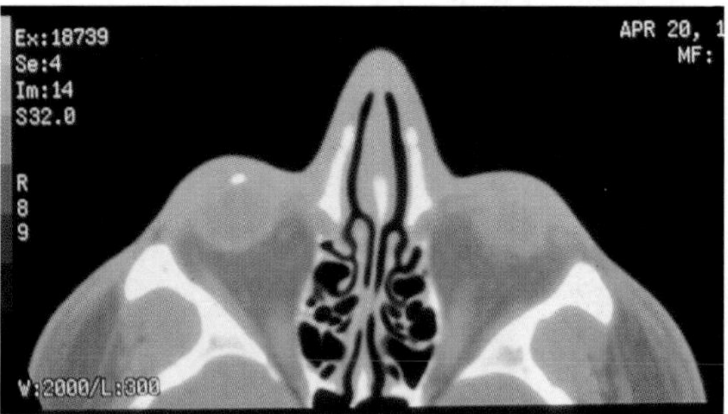

FIGURE 1.2.5 CT scan of metallic foreign body.

Presentation vision decreased or intact; varying degrees of inflammation, and other trauma sequelae. The patient technically has a globe rupture, but the full-thickness opening may have sealed by the time of presentation.

Management history is extremely important in trying to determine the composition and trajectory of the object. If the globe is obviously ruptured, shield the eye and treat accordingly. The object may be removed at the time of globe repair. If the integrity of the globe appears intact, examine the cornea, the iris, and the anterior lens capsule for entrance site clues. In addition, perform gentle gonioscopy and DFE. Consider B-scan and/or CT scan. Some foreign bodies, such as glass and lead, are relatively inert and may generally be left in the eye if not impeding the visual axis, whereas iron and steel produce aggressive inflammatory reactions and must be removed. If a foreign body is left in the eye, serial ERGs should be performed to detect early signs of retinal toxicity.

1.2.6 Traumatic Optic Neuropathy—blunt, shearing, compression, or penetrating forces resulting in damage of varying degrees to the optic nerve.

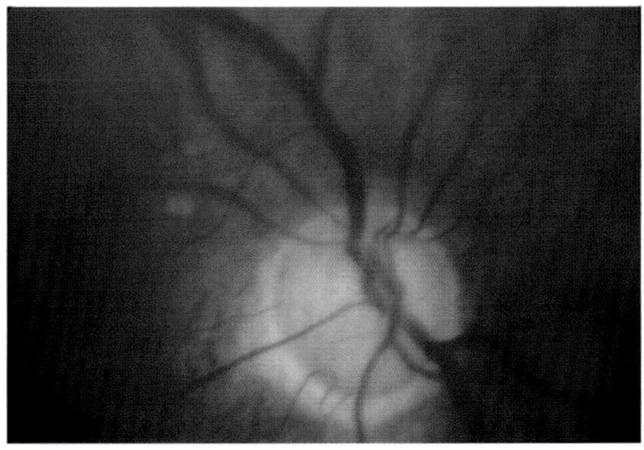

FIGURE 1.2.6 Late optic atrophy.

Presentation decreased visual acuity and color vision and a visual field defect with a trauma history. Initially, an afferent pupillary defect is often present, but optic nerve head pallor will take weeks to develop. Depending on the extent of the injury, there may be partial or complete avulsion of the optic nerve. The underlying nerve damage may be difficult to assess in the presence of a large hyphema or extensive vitreous and retinal hemorrhage.

Differential Diagnosis intracranial mass or hemorrhage, anterior ischemic optic neuropathy, central retinal artery occlusion, fracture of bony walls of orbital apex.

Management do a full neuro-ophthalmic examination and rule-out a ruptured globe. Consider B-scan and or CT scan especially if a foreign body or fracture is suspected. Although it is controversial, high-dose IV steroids (Solumedrol, 250 mg IV, q6h for 2 to 3 days) may be given. If an expanding retrobulbar hemorrhage is also present, orbital decompression surgery is indicated. The patient must be evaluated daily, and the prognosis is exceedingly poor.

1.3 Orbital Trauma

1.3.1 Orbital Contusion—blunt trauma to the eye resulting in a "black eye" with peribulbar and possible retrobulbar swelling.

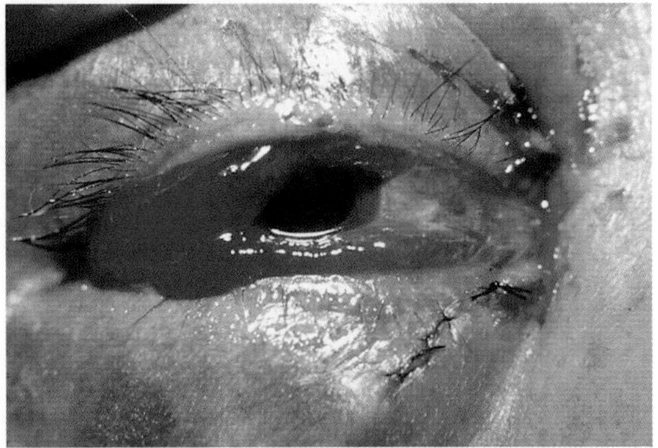

FIGURE 1.3.1 Periorbital edema, chemosis, subconjunctival hemorrhage with lid laceration.

Presentation typically, pain and a mild decrease in visual acuity with eyelid ecchymosis and edema. The eye may be proptotic, with limited EOMs and restriction to retropulsion. Chemosis, subconjunctival hemorrhage, and elevated IOP may be present.

Differential Diagnosis retrobulbar hemorrhage, orbital fracture, orbital cellulitis, arteriovenous abnormality.

Management may need to pry open the lids to complete the ocular examination. A ruptured globe, orbital fracture, foreign body, or cellulitis, as well as other forms of trauma, must be ruled out. Treat simple contusion with ice compresses, oral pain medications, and topical antibiotics for several days. If indicated, lower the IOP.

1.3.2 Orbital Fractures

—disruption of the bony contents of the orbital floor or roof, the medial or lateral walls, or the optic canal.

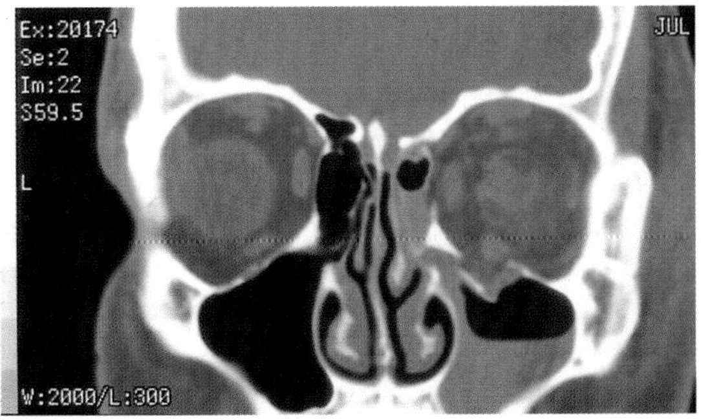

FIGURE 1.3.2 CT scan of orbital floor fracture.

Presentation typically presents with eyelid ecchymosis and edema and variable amounts of subcutaneous emphysema (often after nose-blowing), diplopia, and enophthalmos and ptosis. The vision may be intact or decreased from other trauma sequelae or due to injury to the bony fragments surrounding the optic nerve.

Differential Diagnosis orbital cellulitis.

Management the periorbital area may be too edematous to determine whether there is a step-off fracture. Perform a full ocular examination to determine the extent of the traumatic injury. Be sure to rule out a ruptured globe. Determine whether there is limitation of EOM secondary to muscle entrapment. Measure Hertels to determine whether there is greater than 2 mm of enophthalmos. The globe may be proptotic if there is a coexisting retrobulbar hemorrhage.

If vision is compromised, determine whether there is a fracture of the orbital apex or the presence of a traumatic optic neuropathy. Obtain a CT scan to determine the extent of the injury.

- Floor, roof, or wall injuries: orbital floor and medial wall injuries are most common. Place the patient on oral antibiotics for 7 to 10 days to protect against sinus bacteria and the development of orbital cellulitis, use Afrin nasal spray, and tell the patient to refrain from nose blowing. If there is diplopia, muscle entrapment or enophthalmos of more than 2 mm, surgical intervention is warranted. The goal of surgery is to relieve any muscle entrapment and to restore the orbital contents to their original place by bridging the fracture site. Most ophthalmologists prefer to wait 1 to 2 weeks for a decrease in the periorbital swelling. At some centers, ENT or oral maxillofacial surgeons may intervene within 48 hours of the injury. This is a very controversial issue.
- Optic canal/orbital apex injuries: if the vision is compromised secondary to optic nerve damage or impending injury, intervene immediately. These fractures often require ENT or oral maxillofacial assistance and may have a poor outcome.

1.3.3 Retrobulbar Hemorrhage—bleeding within the orbit with a history of blunt, penetrating, or surgical trauma (e.g., retrobulbar anesthesia).

Presentation acute to subacute development of eye pain and decreased visual acuity and color vision. Eyelid edema, proptosis, resistance to retropulsion, chemosis, subconjunctival heme and injection, increased IOP and restricted EOMs may be found. Depending on severity, there may also be an APD, CRAO, and/or choroidal folds.

Differential Diagnosis orbital contusion, orbital cellulitis, orbital fracture, arteriovenous abnormality.

Management rule out ruptured globe; if time permits, perform B-scan and/or CT scan if vision is not threatened. If vision is decreased, especially in the presence of elevated IOP or the presence of CRA pulsations, institute treatment immediately. Perform a lateral canthotomy and cantholysis. In addition, to decrease IOP rapidly, consider systemic acetazolamide (Diamox), IV mannitol, and/or anterior chamber paracentesis. If symptoms persist and vision and IOP do not respond, emergent orbital decompression surgery is indicated. Patients who present with a coexisting orbital fracture may not require lateral canthotomy or emergent surgery, because the fracture may auto-decompress the orbit.

Chapter 2

EYELIDS AND LACRIMAL SYSTEM

Brian Brazzo, Albert Hornblass,
Richard D. Lisman

2.1 Ectropion

the eyelid margin everts from the globe.

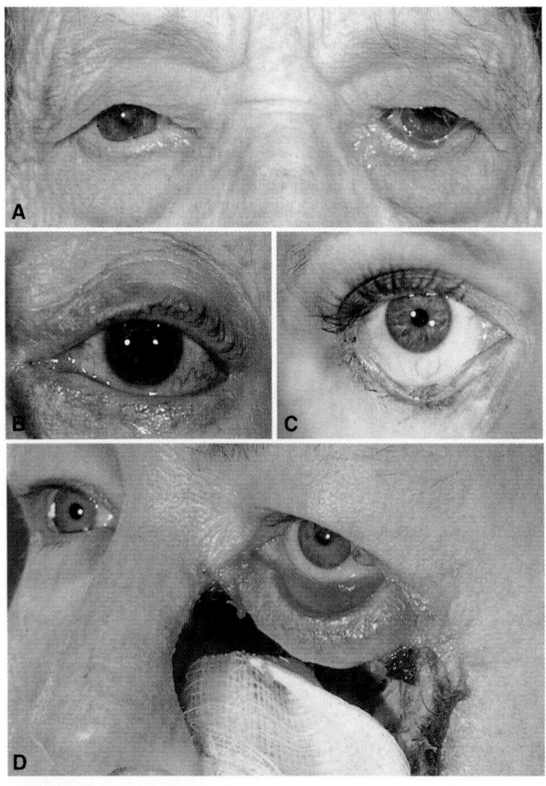

FIGURE 2.1a Acquired ectropion.
FIGURE 2.1b Acquired ectropion.
FIGURE 2.1c Cicatricial ectropion.
FIGURE 2.1d Cicatricial ectropion.

Presentation

tears may collect at an area of lid eversion, causing epiphora. Palpebral conjunctival exposure may cause hyperemia, edema, irritation, and ultimately keratinization. Corneal exposure can lead to pain and visual complications from keratitis or ulceration.

Differential Diagnosis

acquired or involutional (usually a result of medial or lateral canthal tendon laxity), cicatricial changes, paralytic (CN VII nerve palsy), congenital.

Management

eyelid distraction test: evaluate eyelid tension by pulling the lid margin away from the globe and assessing how quickly the lid returns to the normal position. Pull the eyelid laterally to observe medial retroplacement of the punctum. Exposure keratitis should be treated medically with lubricants and possibly antibiotics. Surgical correction of acquired ectropion usually includes horizontal shortening of the eyelid or reattaching it to the lateral canthus, possibly with reinsertion of the lower eyelid retractors. Lateral tarsorrhaphy is often recommended for paralytic ectropion that does not resolve after 6 months. Cicatricial ectropion often requires skin grafting following scar excision. Congenital ectropion may require reconstruction of deficient tissue in the anterior lamella of the eyelid.

2.2 Entropion

the eyelid margin turns inward against the globe.

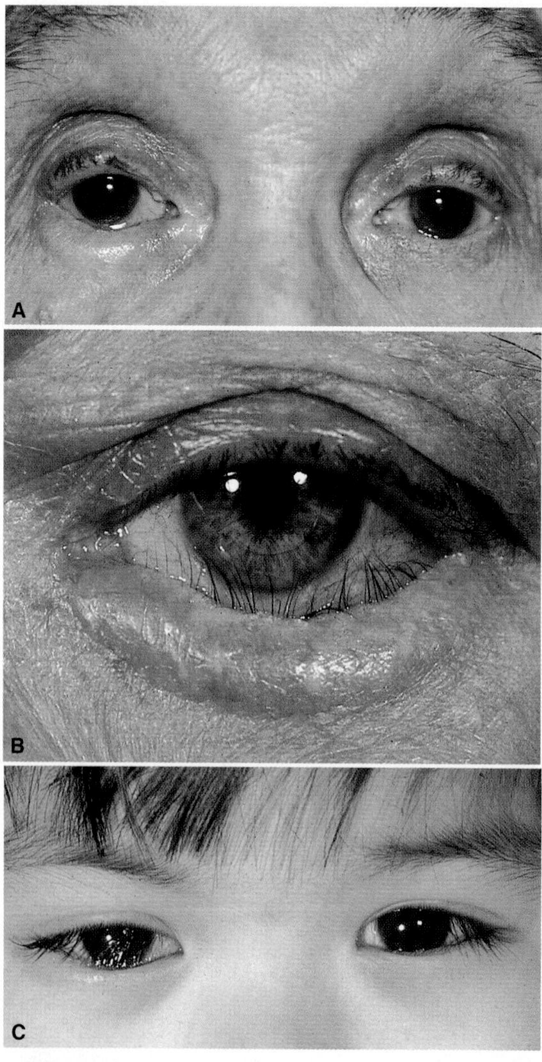

FIGURE 2.2a Acquired entropion.
FIGURE 2.2b Overriding preseptal orbicularis muscle.
FIGURE 2.2c Congenital entropion.

Presentation foreign-body sensation, tearing, recurrent conjunctivitis, and keratitis.

Differential Diagnosis acquired or involutional, cicatricial, congenital.

Management acquired entropion has several contributing factors. Enophthalmos may exacerbate the condition. The preseptal orbicularis muscle may override the lower edge of tarsus during contraction. Disinsertion of the lower eyelid retractors has been demonstrated in entropion in combination with eyelid laxity. Medical treatment is directed toward reducing corneal irritation. Numerous surgical procedures that are described to correct the underlying anatomic defects include Quickert sutures, lateral tarsal strip procedure, and transfer of overriding orbicularis muscle combined with horizontal eyelid shortening.

2.3 Ptosis

a congenital or acquired drooping of the upper eyelid.

Presentation patients complain of a tired appearance and superior field defects. Drooping of eyelids may vary during the day. Patients may use elevation of the chin or contraction of the brow to overcome ptosis. The congenitally ptotic lid is higher in downgaze than the normally functioning lid because of the inability of the fatty, infiltrated levator to relax.

Differential Diagnosis levator muscle disinsertion or dehiscence, neurogenic secondary to congenital Horner's syndrome, CN III nerve palsy, or myasthenia gravis, mechanical secondary to tumor or dermatochalasis.

Management assess levator function to determine etiology and treatment plan. If there is minimal to absent levator function (<4 mm), consider a frontalis suspension procedure. If

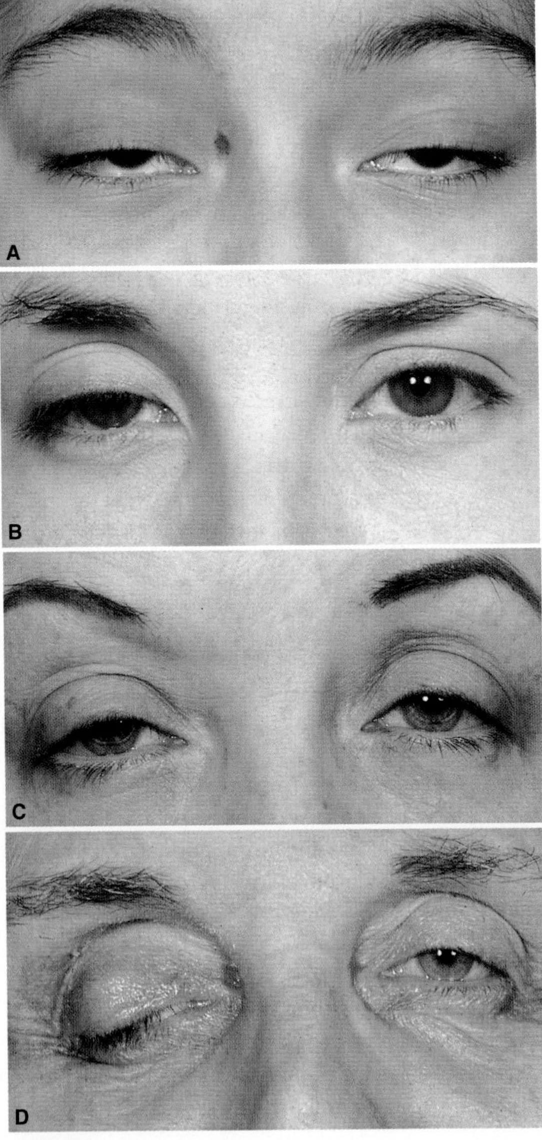

FIGURE 2.3a Congenital ptosis.
FIGURE 2.3b Congenital unilateral ptosis.
FIGURE 2.3c Levator muscle dehiscence.
FIGURE 2.3d Neurogenic ptosis.

there is reasonable levator function, consider a levator aponeurosis advancement or a muscle resection. Minimal ptosis can be corrected by conjunctival mullerectomy or Fasanella-Servat procedure. Schirmer test results for tear function, visual fields, and photographs should be obtained prior to surgery.

2.4 Dermatochalasis

excessive skin due to involutional skin laxity, loss of elasticity secondary to sun exposure, or chronic edema.

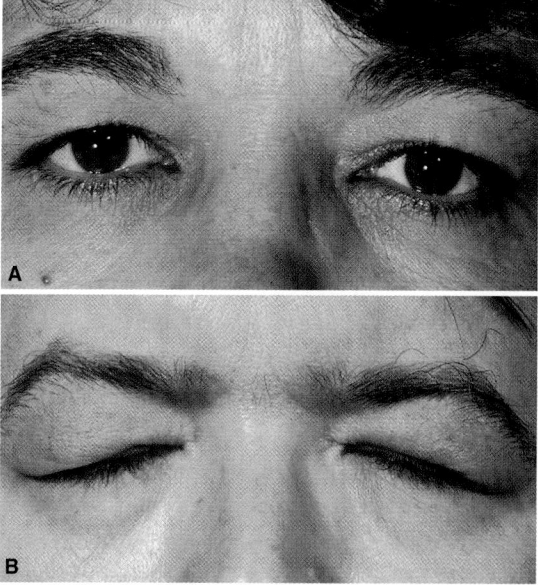

FIGURE 2.4a Dermatochalasis.
FIGURE 2.4b Dermatochalasis.

Presentation

dermatochalasis is often associated with herniated orbital fat. The skin may drape over the lid margin and obscure vision. Desquamated skin may cause keratitis.

Differential Diagnosis eyebrow ptosis or prolapsed lacrimal gland may contribute to fullness of the upper eyelid fold.

Management blepharoplasty includes skin and orbital fat excision, with reconstruction of the upper eyelid crease.

2.5 Eyelid Retraction

a widened palpebral fissure height with excess scleral show.

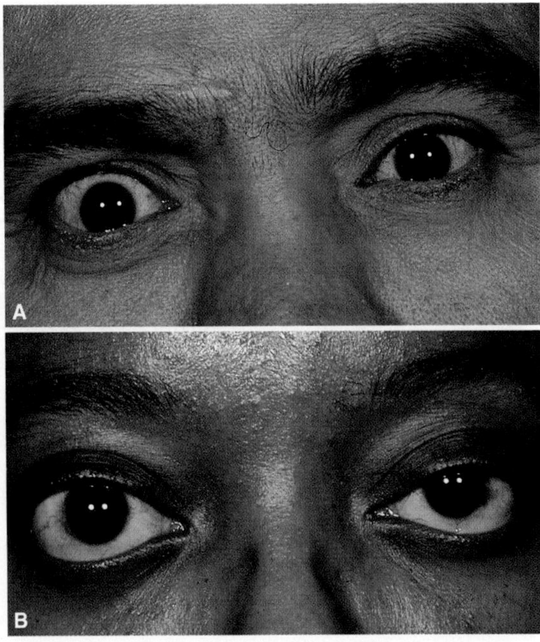

FIGURE 2.5a Eyelid retraction of right eye secondary to thyroid disease.
FIGURE 2.5b Inferior scleral show in retraction.

Presentation the upper eyelid may rest at or above the superior limbus, and the lower eyelid may allow sclera to be seen. Exposure keratopathy and lagophthalmos may be present.

Differential Diagnosis thyroid disease causes contraction of eyelid retractors and adhesions with the orbital septum, complications of vertical strabismus correction, postoperative ptosis repair, Hering's law with contralateral ptosis.

Management for mild retraction, treat medically with artificial tears and lubricating ointments. For more severe cases, surgical options include mullerectomy, levator aponeurosis recession, or a spacer implantation between the aponeurosis and tarsus.

2.6 Floppy Eyelid Syndrome

an easily everted upper eyelid that may spontaneously evert during sleep when the globe retroplaces.

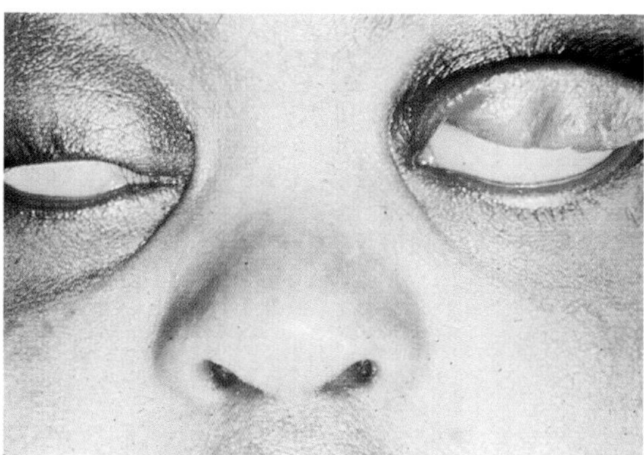

FIGURE 2.6 Spontaneously everted upper eyelid in floppy eyelid syndrome.

Presentation commonly obese people complain of red, irritated eyes secondary to superior tarsal papillary conjunctivitis and foreign-body sensation secondary to SPK.

Differential Diagnosis ectropion, dermatochalasis, giant papillary conjunctivitis, superior limbic keratitis.

Management treat corneal symptoms with lubricants. Tape eyelids shut at night to prevent eversion. If severe, consider eyelid-shortening procedures.

2.7 Chalazion

a chronically enlarged meibomian gland with an obstructed orifice, retained secretory products, and inflammation produces a lipogranuloma. An acute infection of a meibomian gland is an internal hordeolum.

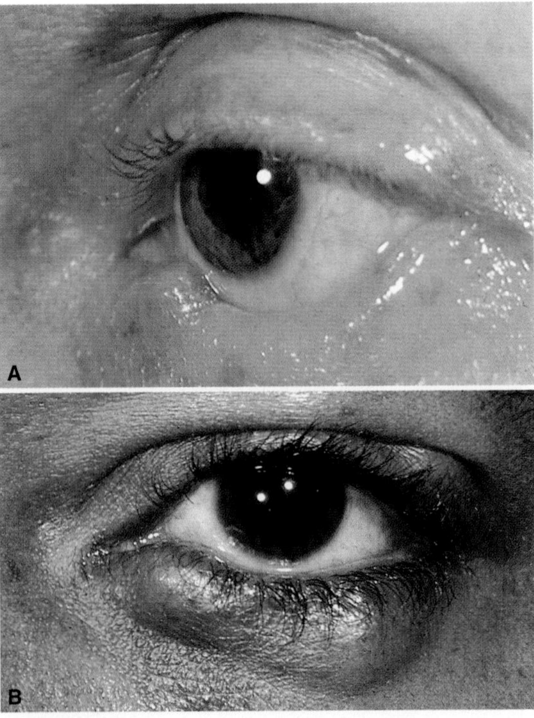

FIGURE 2.7a Blepharitis and lower eyelid chalazion.
FIGURE 2.7b Chronic chalazia of upper and lower eyelids.

Presentation an inflamed or acute chalazion may have a concomitant bacterial infection and appear as a preseptal cellulitis. A chronic chalazion that is no longer inflamed is typically a soft, mobile, nontender subcutaneous mass.

Differential Diagnosis blepharitis, cellulitis, pyogenic granuloma, eyelid tumor (particularly sebaceous carcinoma if chalazion is recurrent).

Management treat with warm compresses of 30 minutes, four times per day, and topical antibiotics, with or without steroids. If the lesion does not subside within a few weeks, subcutaneous or intralesional steroid injection or excision from a posterior eyelid approach may be considered.

2.8 Cysts—Moll/Zeis/Sebaceous

an acute infection of the glands of Moll or Zeis is known as an external hordeolum.

Presentation eyelid swelling and erythema surrounding a cyst or pustule, usually near the eyelid margin.

Differential Diagnosis internal hordeolum, chalazion.

Management warm compresses, topical antibiotics; surgical excision if persistent.

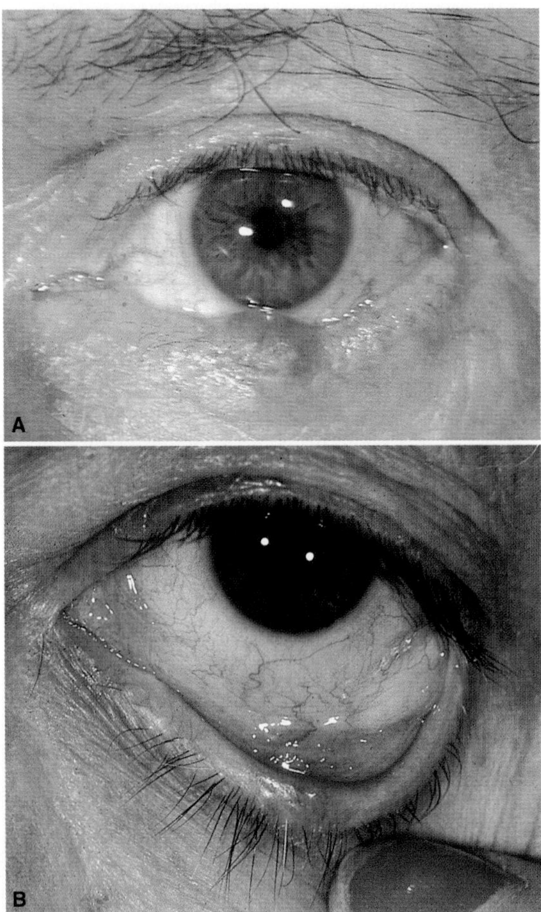

FIGURE 2.8a External hordeolum.
FIGURE 2.8b Cyst of Moll.

2.9 Eyelid Edema

swelling of the eyelids with or without erythema.

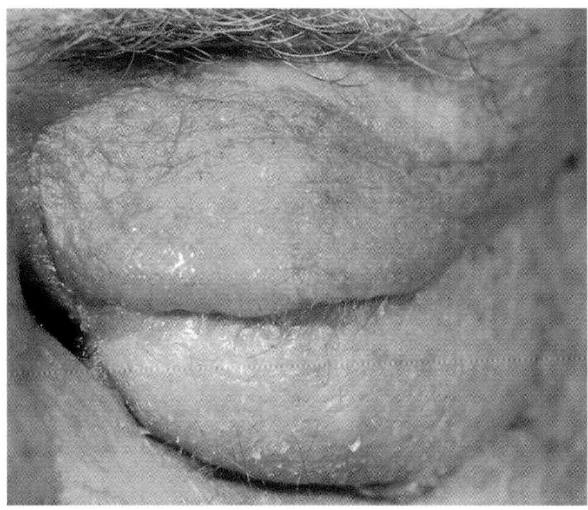

FIGURE 2.9 Eyelid edema.

Presentation eyelid edema is usually minor when associated with inflammation of the globe. Conjunctivitis, keratitis, and corneal ulcers frequently cause mild sympathetic swelling. Orbital processes such as pseudotumor, thyroid ophthalmopathy, and tumors may lead to swelling but often have other signs. Local or diffuse trauma, insect bites, allergic reactions, and chemical injuries are frequent etiologies of edema. Infectious etiologies may include preseptal cellulitis or orbital cellulitis, erysipelas, dacryoadenitis (inflammation of lacrimal gland), or dacryocystitis.

Differential Diagnosis thyroid dysfunction, renal failure, sinusitis and allergies, and other inflammatory and infectious processes of skin, ocular adnexa, eye, and orbit.

Management treatment is directed at the underlying cause of the edema. Systemic diuretics are of temporary help.

2.10 Blepharoptosis and Blepharophimosis Syndrome

this syndrome includes the following:

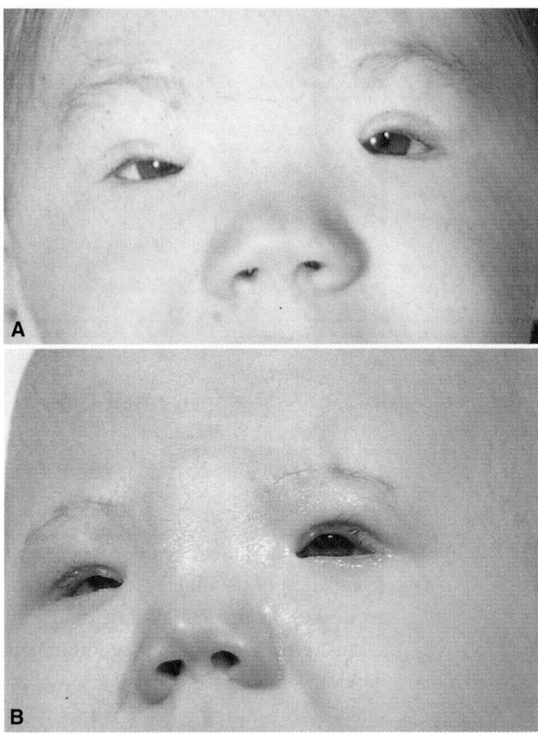

FIGURE 2.10a Blepharophimosis syndrome.
FIGURE 2.10b Blepharophimosis syndrome.

- Blepharoptosis—drooping of the eyelids.
- Blepharophimosis—shortening of the horizontal palpebral fissure to 18 to 22 mm (from normal 25 to 30 mm).

- Epicanthus inversus—skin folds that pass from the lower eyelid upward to cover the medial canthus.
- Telecanthus—increased distance between medial canthi.
- Have lateral ectropion due to skin shortage (25% of patients).

Presentation diagnosis is based on clinical and hereditary characteristics. This syndrome is inherited as an autosomal dominant trait with high penetrance.

Differential Diagnosis congenital or traumatic ptosis, congenital fibrosis syndrome.

Management surgical correction can usually be delayed until preschool years, if ptosis is not causing amblyopia. Medial canthoplasty eliminates epicanthus inversus and telecanthus and reduces blepharophimosis. Ptosis may be corrected by frontalis suspension. Surgery is usually performed in staged procedures.

2.11 Epiblepharon

horizontal redundant medial canthal skin fold that may be present all across the horizontal dimension of the eyelid; this induces vertical orientation of cilia and sometimes a true trichiasis (eyelashes brushing against globe).

Presentation epiblepharon is usually detected as an incidental condition. It may be associated with mild keratitis. Asian children are most commonly affected.

Differential Diagnosis congenital entropion (rare).

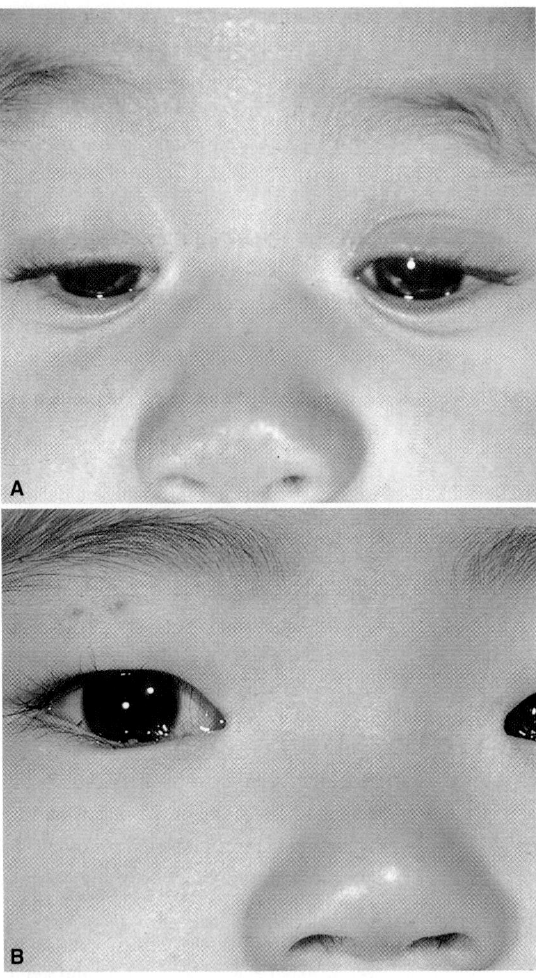

FIGURE 2.11a Epiblepharon in downgaze.
FIGURE 2.11b Vertical orientation of cilia.

Management epiblepharon usually resolves spontaneously by age 3. Surgery is reserved for rare persistent cases and involves resection of a spindle of skin and orbicular muscle to externally rotate the eyelashes during the skin suturing.

2.12 Epicanthus

four types of epicanthus have been described:

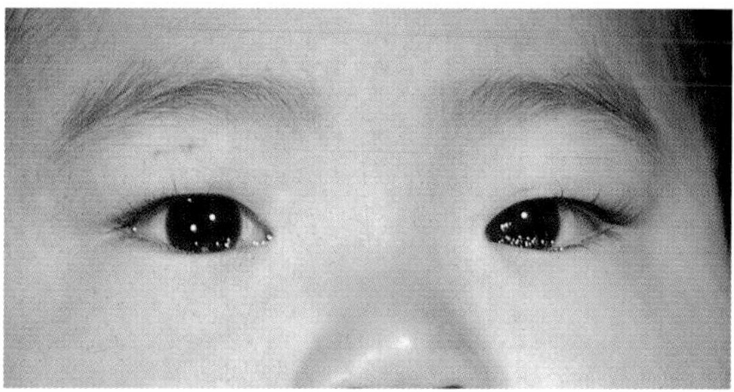

FIGURE 2.12 Epicanthus inversus.

- Epicanthus inversus—small fold of skin arises in lower eyelid and extends upward to partially cover medial canthus.
- Epicanthus tarsalis—skin fold arises in tarsal fold and extends downward to skin around medial canthus.
- Epicanthus palpebralis—skin fold from upper eyelid above tarsus to lower orbital margin.
- Epicanthus supraciliaris—skin fold from eyebrow to lower orbital rim.

Presentation epicanthal folds occur in some children of all races but persist in a significant number of Asians.

Differential Diagnosis epiblepharon, blepharophimosis syndrome, epicanthus inversus.

Management several surgical techniques have been developed to correct nontraumatic ethnic epicanthal folds.

2.13 Eyelid Coloboma

an embryonic cleft usually in the medial, upper eyelid but can be present in any position in either eyelid.

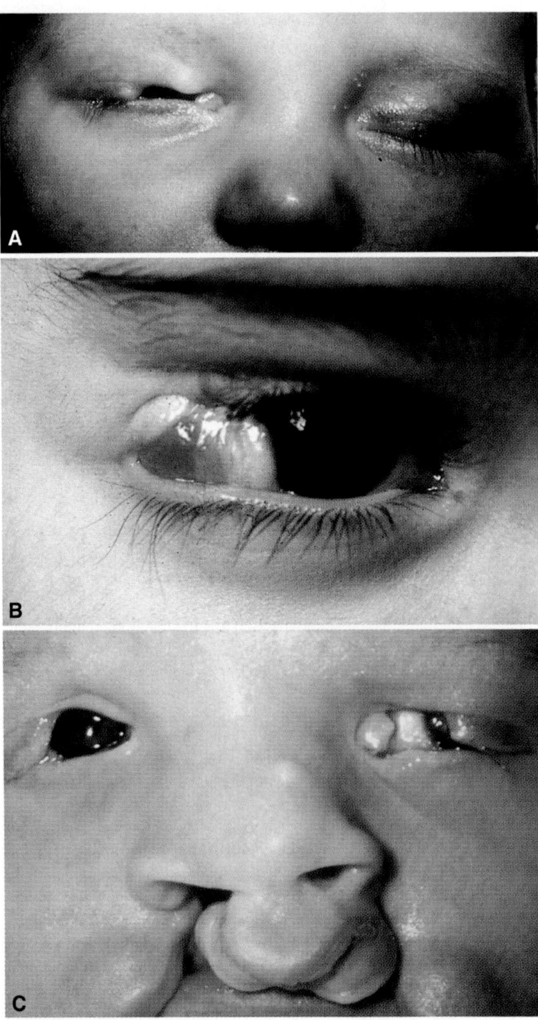

FIGURE 2.13a Upper eyelid coloboma.
FIGURE 2.13b Coloboma in association with dermoid.
FIGURE 2.13c Bilateral coloboma with craniofacial disorder.

Presentation colobomas of the eyelid are usually full-thickness deficits. They may be unilateral or bilateral and involve the upper or lower eyelids. Lower lid colobomas are frequently associated with other anomalies, including soft tissue or bony clefts, lacrimal disorders, dermoids, and dental defects. While most colobomas assume small triangular configurations, some may result in absence of most of the eyelid.

Differential Diagnosis ablepharon (congenital absence of eyelid).

Management medical treatment focuses on prevention of exposure keratopathy. Small colobomas may be surgically converted into a pentagonal deficit and then repaired as a full-thickness wedge resection. Cantholysis or myocutaneous flaps may be necessary to obtain additional tissue for closure.

2.14 Eyelid Tumors

2.14.1 Papilloma—an eyelid growth appearing as a frond with a central vascular pedicle.

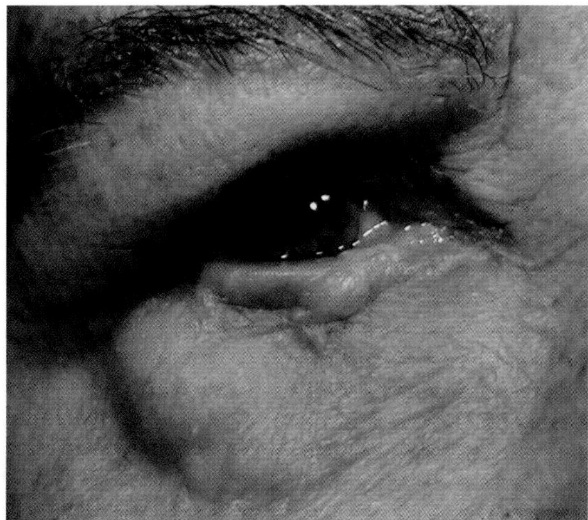

FIGURE 2.14.1 Lower eyelid papilloma.

Presentation may present as verruca vulgaris or a raised "nevus"-like lesion.

Differential Diagnosis verruca vulgaris, molluscum contagiosum, seborrheic keratosis.

Management photodocumentation and observation for small lesions. If diagnosis is uncertain, perform a shave biopsy. Otherwise, surgical excision is the treatment of choice.

2.14.2 Seborrheic Keratosis—a common benign skin tumor of unknown etiology.

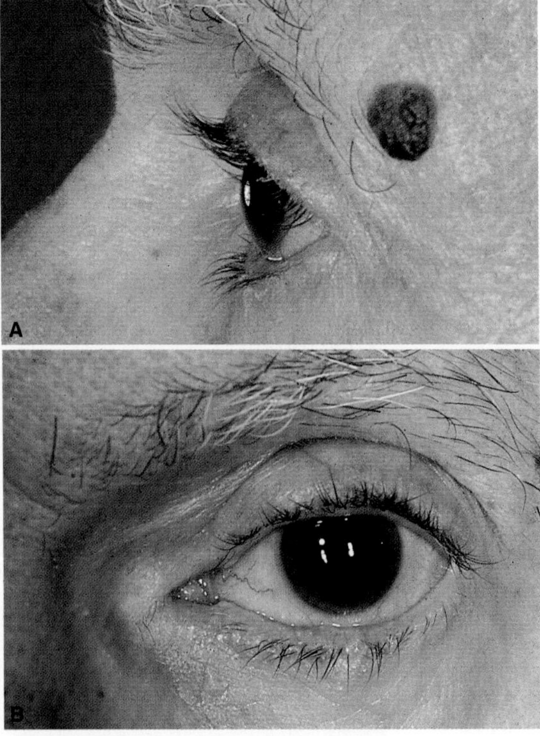

FIGURE 2.14.2a Seborrheic keratosis.
FIGURE 2.14.2b Flat, well-demarcated brown macule.

Presentation lesions commonly begin as flat, well-demarcated brown macules, which become polypoid with an irregular surface and a "stuck-on" appearance.

Differential Diagnosis nevus, acrochordon (skin tag), actinic keratosis, melanoma.

Management light desiccation with curettage or cryotherapy is effective in removing the majority of these lesions. There is no malignant potential.

2.14.3 Actinic Keratosis—the most common epithelial precancerous lesion among light-complexioned individuals.

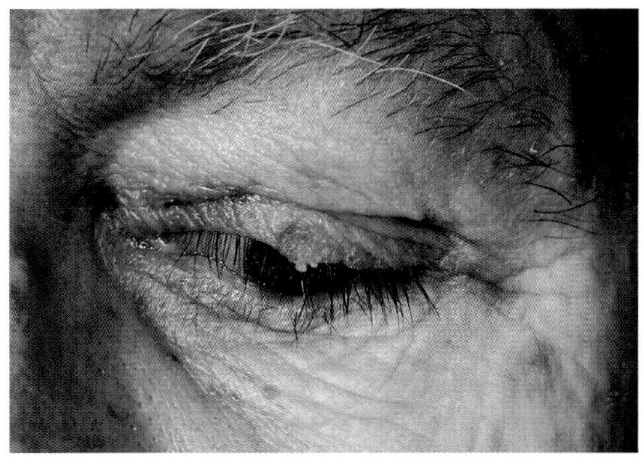

FIGURE 2.14.3 Poorly demarcated papule covered by a dry scale.

Presentation lesions begin as brown or yellow, poorly demarcated macules or papules, covered by a dry scale. They are often asymptomatic and multiple and appear on the sun-exposed areas of the body. An actinic keratosis with profound hyperkeratosis mimics a cutaneous horn.

Differential Diagnosis early seborrheic keratosis, nevus, early basal cell carcinoma, early squamous cell carcinoma, cutaneous horn (if with hyperkeratosis).

Management frequently effective treatments include cryosurgery or electrodesiccation with curettage. Actinic keratosis may evolve into either basal or squamous cell carcinoma.

2.14.4 Keratoacanthoma—a common benign tumor that is believed to arise from hair follicles. It is a form of pseudoepitheliomatous hyperplasia.

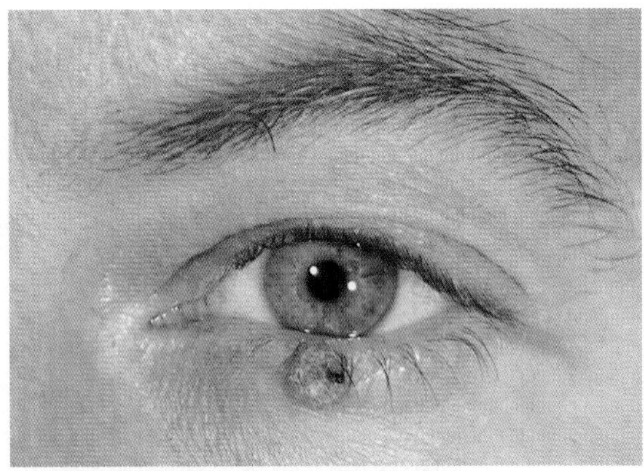

FIGURE 2.14.4 Dome-shaped lesion with a central crater.

Presentation nearly 75% of keratoacanthomas arise from the face and neck. Characteristically, they grow rapidly, often reaching a large size over 6 weeks, and finally involute over the next few months. Lesions are often dome shaped, red and shiny, surrounded by telangiectasias, and often develop a central crater filled with keratin.

Differential Diagnosis squamous cell carcinoma, verruca vulgaris, cutaneous horn, molluscum contagiosum.

Management most keratoacanthomas regress spontaneously but may leave a scar. If the diagnosis is not in doubt, the lesion may be shaved flush with the skin or may be removed with cryotherapy. In most cases, excision of the entire lesion is recommended, especially if the diagnosis is not certain.

2.14.5 Molluscum Contagiosum—a common benign skin and mucous membrane disorder of viral etiology, usually affecting children.

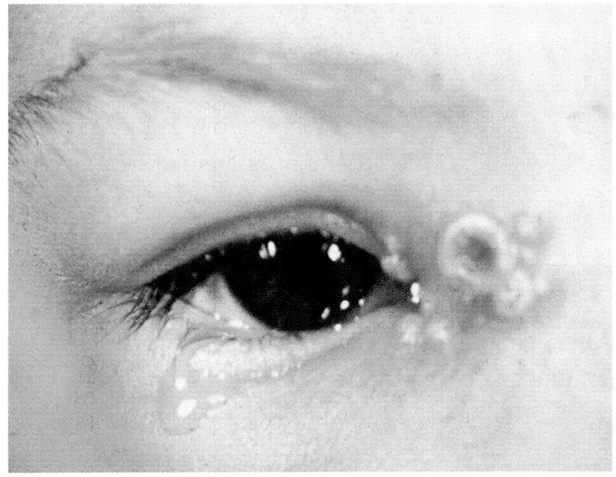

FIGURE 2.14.5 Smooth, pearly papules with a central umbo.

Presentation lesions generally begin as smooth, pearly, discrete, dome-shaped papules, which develop a central umbo. Lesions are usually grouped in one or two regions of the body. They are often asymptomatic but may be associated with chronic conjunctivitis, keratitis, or eczematous dermatitis. There is an increased incidence and severity in AIDS patients.

Differential Diagnosis verruca vulgaris, varicella, papilloma, epithelioma.

Management cryosurgery and curettage are both effective in eliminating molluscum, although lesions frequently recur.

2.14.6.1 Intradermal Nevus—a well-demarcated pigmented lesion entirely within the dermis.

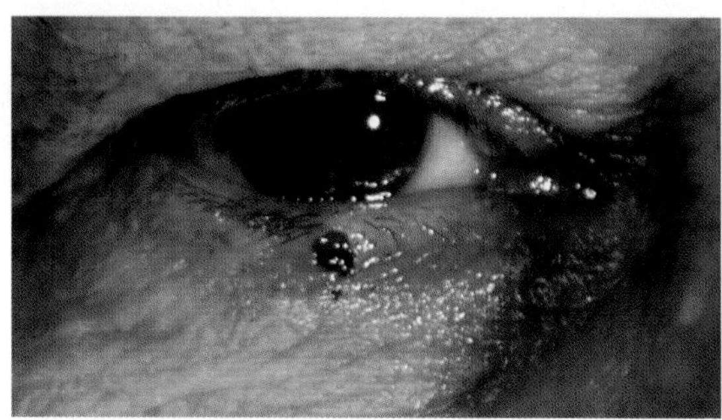

FIGURE 2.14.6.1 Intradermal nevus.

Presentation a painless, flat or elevated, often pigmented eyelid lesion.

Differential Diagnosis blue nevus, compound nevus, nevus of Ota, molluscum contagiosum, malignant melanoma.

Management follow for a change in size and color. If color deepens or tumor enlarges, recommend surgical removal.

2.14.6.2 Compound Nevus—a melanocytic lesion that combines both junctional and intradermal components.

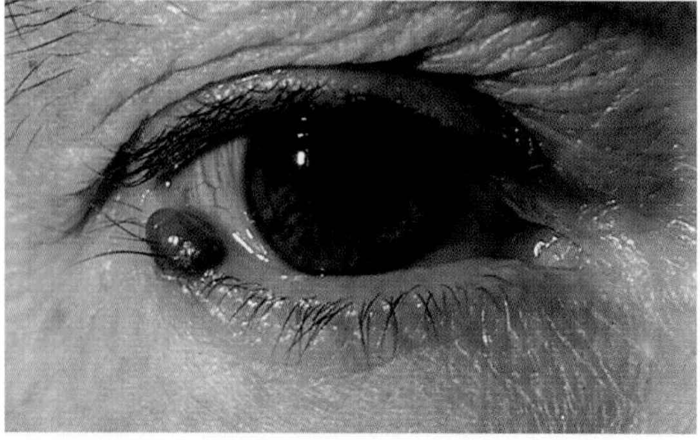

FIGURE 2.14.6.2 Compound nevus.

Presentation a pigmented eyelid lesion.

Differential Diagnosis malignant melanoma.

Management observation with photography. If lesion increases in size, recommend surgical removal.

2.14.6.3 Nevus of Ota

2.14.6.3 Nevus of Ota—congenital oculomelanocytosis or a form of blue nevus associated with an increase of melanocytes in the dermis, episclera, sclera, and uveal tissues.

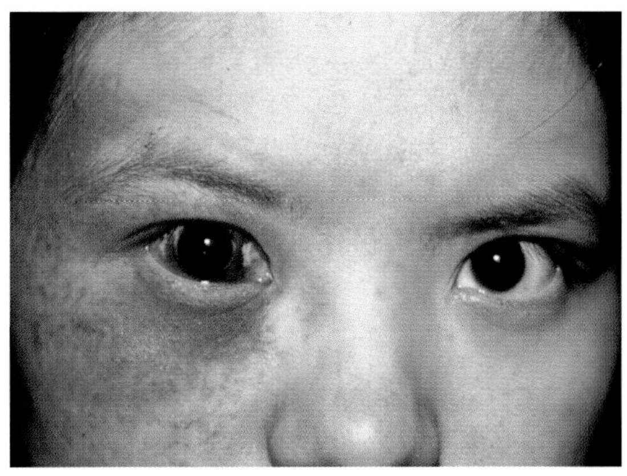

FIGURE 2.14.6.3 Nevus of Ota.

Presentation congenital with an abnormal amount of pigmentation in the ocular structures. There is an association with glaucoma.

Differential Diagnosis malignant melanoma.

Management follow for malignant change and glaucoma.

2.14.7 Xanthelasma

2.14.7 Xanthelasma—infiltrations or tumors of the skin due to an aggregation of lipid material. When xanthomas are flat, they are often referred to as xanthelasma. They arise in individuals who have one of a variety of dyslipoproteinemias, although most patients with xanthelasma are normolipoproteinemic.

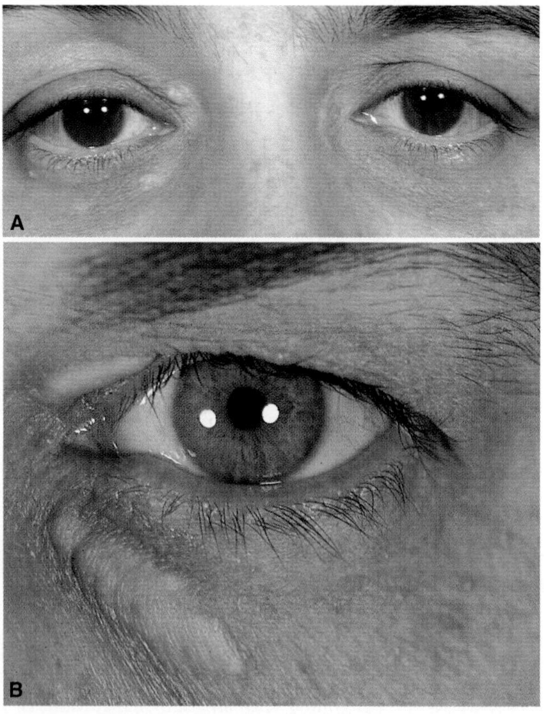

FIGURE 2.14.7a Flat xanthoma.
FIGURE 2.14.7b Yellowish, slightly raised oval plaque.

Presentation yellowish, slightly raised oval plaques on the eyelid skin. They are particularly found in the medial canthal area.

Differential Diagnosis syringoma, eccrine hydrocystoma.

Management elective surgical excision is often unsatisfactory, because lesions tend to recur. Application of trichloroacetic acid, followed by alcohol neutralization, may be attempted. In addition, carbon dioxide laser vaporization may be used. Suggest serum lipid profile in patients younger than age 40.

2.14.8 Trichoepithelioma—skin tumors with a predominance of glycogen and hair differentiation. They are often multiple and inherited but may be solitary and nonhereditary.

Presentation multiple trichoepithelioma begin around puberty, usually on the face. Lesions are slightly pink with telangiectatic vessels on the surface. They seldom ulcerate. Solitary trichoepitheliomas appear as a firm, skin-colored nodule in adults, usually on the face.

Differential Diagnosis verruca, basal cell carcinoma.

Management surgical excision or carbon dioxide laser removal.

2.14.9 Syringoma—a benign tumor of skin appendages, with eccrine differentiation.

Presentation syringomas occur more frequently in women, beginning at puberty, and are often located on the eyelids. They are skin-colored papules, 1 to 2 mm in diameter, which often progress in size and quantity.

Differential Diagnosis verruca, xanthelasma, cylindroma, eccrine spear adenoma.

Management lesions may be removed by surgical excision or by electrodesiccation and curettage. Syringomas may recur.

2.14.10 Neurofibroma—infiltrative nerve cell tumor predominantly composed of Schwann cells (see also Section 15.19.1).

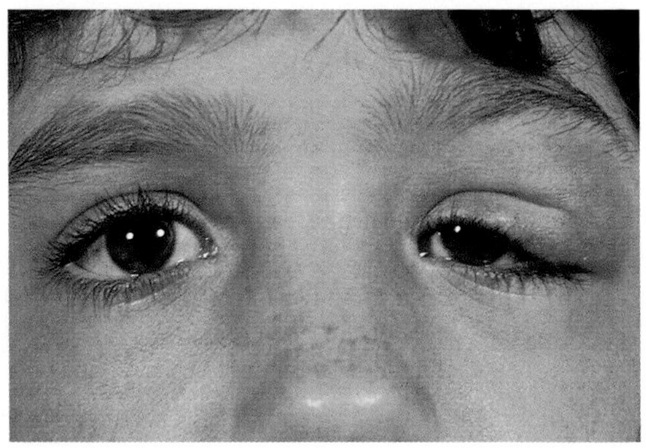

FIGURE 2.14.10 Plexiform neurofibroma.

Presentation may present as a plexiform or a discrete lesion. A plexiform lesion usually presents as a vascularized tumor of the upper, lateral eyelid, which tends to give the eyelid an S-shaped appearance.

Differential Diagnosis capillary hemangioma, lymphoma.

Management surgical excision may be attempted but is less successful in plexiform neurofibromas.

2.15.1 Basal Cell Carcinoma—a malignant epithelial tumor of the skin, arising from the basal cells of the epidermis. It is the most common eyelid malignancy.

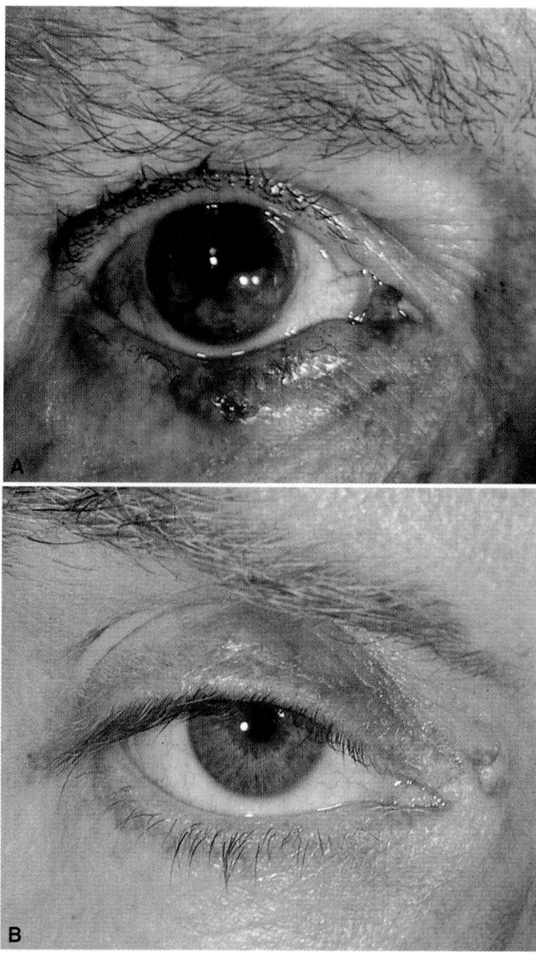

FIGURE 2.15.1a Telangiectatic lesion of lower lid.
FIGURE 2.15.1b Basal cell carcinoma of medial canthal region.

Presentation

these lesions present typically as firm, small, elevated nodules with raised, translucent pearly margins and telangiectatic vessels. They are usually reddish, located on the lower eyelid, with a size less than 10 mm in diameter.

Differential Diagnosis squamous cell carcinoma, sebaceous carcinoma, kerato-acanthoma, nevus, melanoma, trichoepithelioma.

Management cure rates of greater than 90% have been described for the following procedures: surgical excision, cryosurgery, curettage and electrodesiccation, radiotherapy, and Mohs' surgery.

2.15.2 Squamous Cell Carcinoma—a malignant epithelial tumor arising from differentiated cells in the epidermis, which demonstrates maturation toward keratin formation.

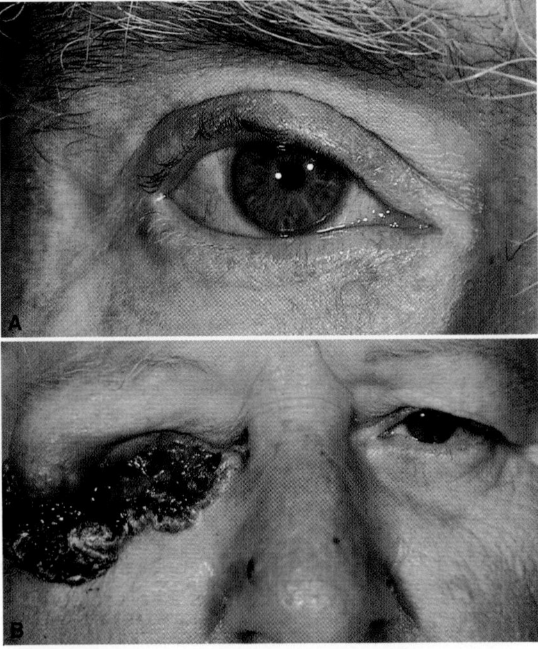

FIGURE 2.15.2a Early squamous cell carcinoma of upper eyelid.
FIGURE 2.15.2b Extensive squamous cell carcinoma.

Presentation often these lesions are diagnosed by observing a scaly, indurated plaque with central ulceration or crusting and indurated edges. They often occur in sun-damaged areas of fair-skinned elderly people and are often detected near other precursor lesions, known as actinic keratoses. Squamous cell carcinoma is much less frequent than basal cell carcinoma on the eyelids, but the growth of squamous carcinoma is much faster.

Differential Diagnosis basal cell carcinoma, actinic keratosis, keratoacanthoma, pseudoepitheliomatous hyperplasia, senile keratosis, inverted follicular keratosis.

Management the same techniques employed to remove basal cell carcinoma may be used for squamous cell carcinoma; however, a wider excision is recommended. Most ophthalmologists prefer surgical excision with frozen-section margins.

2.15.3 Sebaceous Gland Carcinoma

2.15.3 Sebaceous Gland Carcinoma—a malignant cutaneous neoplasm arising from sebaceous glands, which accounts for less than 1% of eyelid carcinomas. They are rarely found elsewhere on the body.

Presentation these cancers typically present in the seventh decade on the upper eyelid, more often in women. The clinical appearance is highly variable, as sebaceous carcinoma may mimic benign conditions such as chalazion and blepharoconjunctivitis or numerous other skin lesions, both benign and malignant. Classically, this lesion is a firm, painless, indurated mass or ulceration associated with localized loss of cilia, in an area that has been treated for "recurrent chalazia."

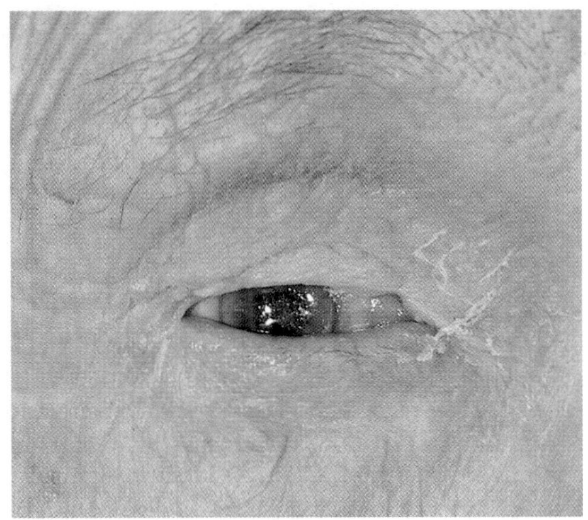

FIGURE 2.15.3 Sebaceous cell carcinoma with loss of cilia.

Differential Diagnosis chalazion, blepharoconjunctivitis, basal cell carcinoma, squamous cell carcinoma.

Management surgical excision with wide surgical margins and fresh-frozen section controls is necessary to delineate the tumor edges. With this method, mortality is near zero. Conjunctival mapping is important to control pagetoid spread. Evaluation of preauricular and cervical lymph nodes is important to evaluate metastasis, and the presence of other internal malignancies should be investigated.

2.15.4 Cutaneous Malignant Melanoma—a rare eyelid lesion arising from the proliferation of atypical epidermal melanocytes. The three most common types include superficial spreading melanoma, lentigo maligna melanoma, and nodular melanoma.

Presentation

- Lentigo maligna is a tan or brown macular lesion with irregular borders and is the premalignant stage of lentigo maligna melanoma. When the purely intraepithelial melanocytes of lentigo maligna invade the der-

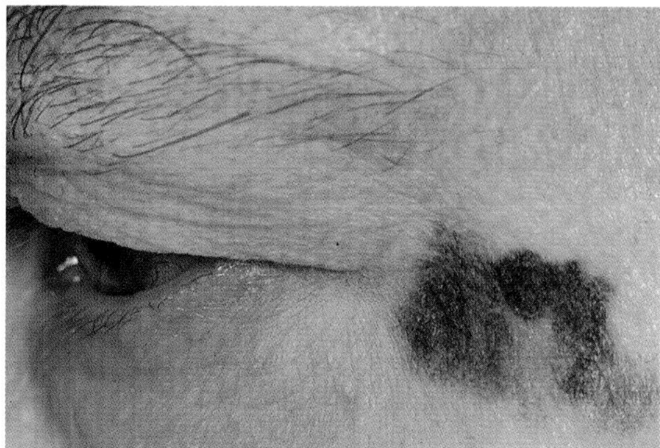

FIGURE 2.15.4 Cutaneous melanoma.

mis, the lesion becomes darker and elevated and is then termed lentigo maligna melanoma. These two lesions usually occur on the faces of elderly patients.

- Superficial spreading melanomas are less common on the face. The clinical scenario involves a middle-aged patient with a brown, irregularly shaped macule.
- Nodular melanomas are typically dark brown or black nodules or plaques, which are rare on the eyelids.

Differential Diagnosis nevus, squamous cell carcinoma, keratoacanthoma, seborrheic keratosis.

Management surgical treatment is recommended for all cutaneous malignant melanomas. The extent of surgical and adjunctive treatment is determined by tumor type, level, and clinical stage of disease.

2.16 Distichiasis and Trichiasis

Distichiasis refers to an eyelid defect in which an accessory row of lashes grows from the meibomian gland orifices on the posterior lid margin. Trichiasis refers to abnormal lashes that are in contact with the globe.

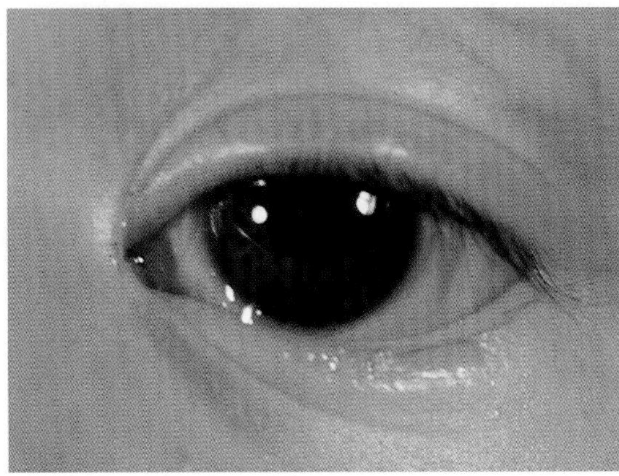

FIGURE 2.16.1 Trichiasis.

Presentation

these two conditions may be asymptomatic or may cause tearing and redness related to the lashes irritating the cornea or conjunctiva. Corneal changes include keratitis, ulceration, vascularization, or scarring.

Differential Diagnosis

distichiasis is usually congenital but may occur in Stevens-Johnson syndrome, ocular cicatricial pemphigoid, and severe chemical injuries. Trichiasis may result from the same processess but is more often secondary to injury or surgery to the lid margin.

Management

numerous procedures have been attempted to remove the aberrant lashes. Epilation gives temporary relief, although new lashes regrow in 6 weeks. Contact lenses provide relief from keratitis. Electrolysis can be attempted if only a few lashes are misdirected. Full-thickness wedge resection may be performed if the abnormal lashes are located in close proximity. Cryotherapy has been attempted for lashes scattered along the posterior lamella. Surgical intervention for distichiasis involves excising the posterior lamella and performing mucous membrane grafting.

2.17 Lacrimal System Disorders

2.17.1 Canaliculitis—infection of the canaliculi of the lacrimal drainage system.

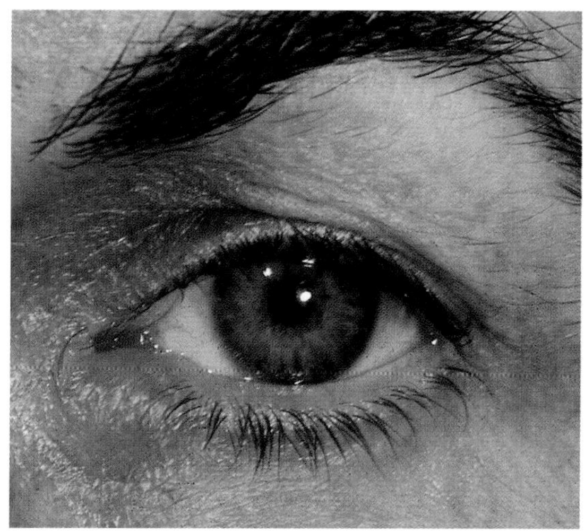

FIGURE 2.17.1 Lower eyelid canaliculitis.

Presentation chronic unilateral conjunctivitis and epiphora (excessive tearing) result from inflammation and obstruction of the canaliculi. One or both puncta may be dilated and inflamed. Direct pressure applied to the skin overlying the canaliculus will produce a white or yellow discharge from the punctum. The medial eyelid skin may be secondarily inflamed.

Differential Diagnosis conjunctivitis, nasolacrimal duct obstruction, dacryocystitis, eyelid or punctal malposition, keratitis.

Management medical treatment with warm compresses and topical antibiotics for gram-positive organisms is usually ineffective. Surgical treatment is directed at identification of canalicular diverticuli or dacryoliths, marsupialization of canaliculi, and removal of the obstructing material from them by curettage.

2.17.2 Dacryocystitis—infection of the nasolacrimal sac.

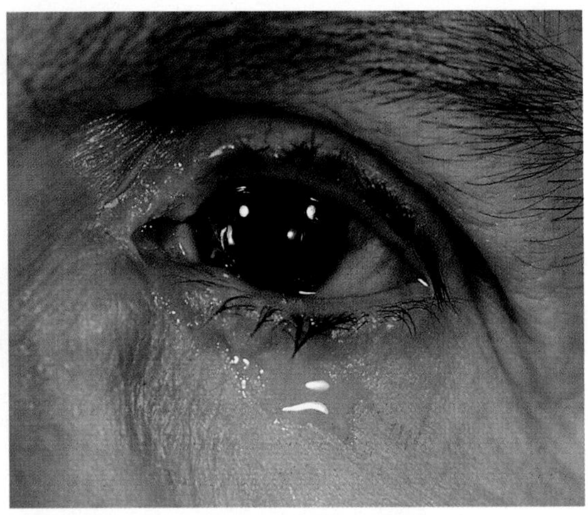

FIGURE 2.17.2 Chronic dacryocystitis with swelling inferior to medial palpebral ligament.

Presentation an acute dacryocystitis presents with pain, redness, tenderness, and pus. Swelling occurs inferior to the medial palpebral ligament. Progression of the process can lead to preseptal cellulitis, orbital cellulitis, or abscess. Chronic infection often produces tearing, sometimes associated with conjunctivitis. Reflux of mucopurulent material from the puncta may occur following pressure over the lacrimal sac.

Differential Diagnosis for acute presentation, consider cellulitis or abscess. In chronic conditions, consider other processes that cause tearing, such as keratitis, eyelid malposition, or occlusion at any point along the drainage system not necessarily caused by infection. Dacryocystitis occurring in infants is frequently secondary to incomplete formation of the nasolacrimal system.

Management irrigation of the drainage system may indicate complete or partial obstruction. Mild acute infections can be treated with warm compresses and topical and oral antibiotics such as Augmentin (amoxicillin and clavulanate potassium) or a cephalosporin. More severe dacryocystitis, in which cellulitis or abscess has formed, may require intravenous antibiotics. Cultures should be taken from any purulent discharge from the puncta. If infection progresses to a fluctuant localized mass, surgical drainage may be attempted. Chronic dacryocystitis seldom responds to medical management, and dacrocystorhinostomy is the recommended treatment.

2.17.3 Nasolacrimal Duct Obstruction

2.17.3 Nasolacrimal Duct Obstruction—obstruction of tear drainage system may be congenital or acquired. This finding occurs in up to 30% of infants at birth, although less than 4% of these children are symptomatic. Acquired obstruction is usually secondary to trauma or infection.

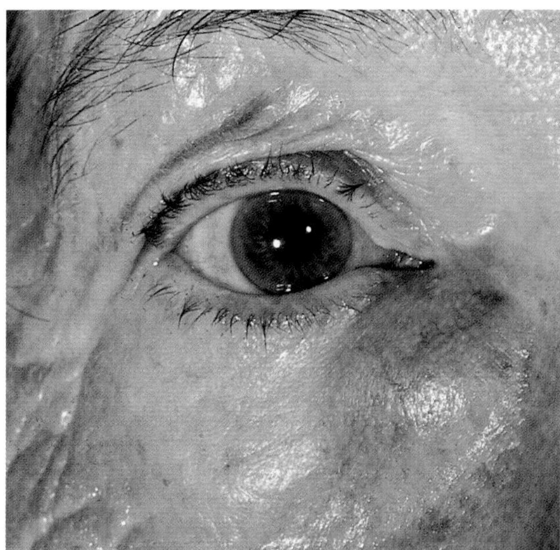

FIGURE 2.17.3 Acquired nasolacrimal duct obstruction secondary to chronic dacryocystitis.

Presentation patients have increased tear meniscus, epiphora (tears running down cheek), or crusting of the lashes. Attention must be given to eyelid and punctal position and contour.

Differential Diagnosis dacryocystitis, keratitis, conjunctivitis, congenital glaucoma.

Management Schirmer's test is routinely performed to rule out tear overproduction. Saccharine test, Jones primary and secondary dye tests, and irrigation of canaliculi may be performed to evaluate patency. Depending on the level of obstruction, various surgical procedures are employed, the most common of which is nasolacrimal duct probing, followed by dacryocystorhinostomy with silicone tube placement. (See Section 12.3 for congenital nasolacrimal duct obstruction.)

Chapter 3

ORBITAL INFECTIONS, INFLAMMATION, AND NEOPLASMS

Dawn Jackson Fyler, Albert Hornblass

3.1 Preseptal Cellulitis

inflammation and infection confined to the eyelids and periorbital structures anterior to the orbital septum. Structures posterior to the orbital septum are not infected but may be secondarily inflamed.

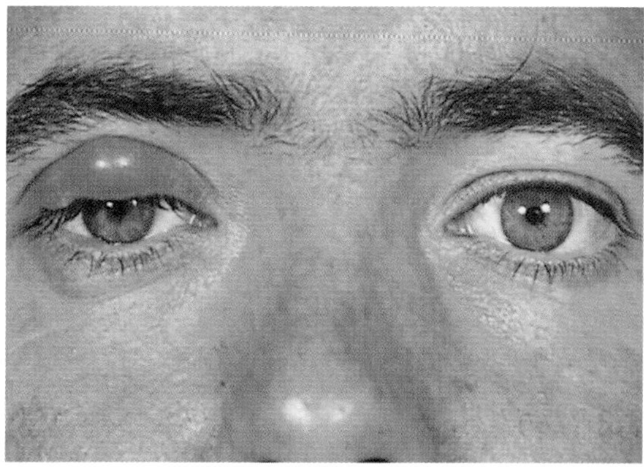

FIGURE 3.1 Preseptal cellulitis due to a chalazion.

Presentation usually results from puncture wounds following trauma, insect bites, chalazion, or skin infection. There may be eyelid edema and erythema. In contradistinction to orbital cellulitus, pupillary reaction, visual acuity, and motility are normal. Pain on eye movement and significant chemosis are extremely rare. Children under the age of 5 years are susceptible to infection from *Haemophilus influenzae,* presenting with a history of upper respiratory infection, fever, irritability, and a characteristic violaceous erythema and marked swelling of the eyelids.

Differential Diagnosis orbital cellulitis, allergic edema, contact dermatitis, conjunctivitis.

Management rule out orbital cellulitus (see Section 3.2.1). Culture any drainage. Preseptal cellulitis in infants and children may be associated with bacteremia, septicemia, and meningitis and should be treated aggressively with hospitalization and IV antibiotics after blood cultures (e.g., ceftriaxone and vancomycin). Treat mild cases cautiously with oral antibiotics and daily follow-up. Obtain a CT scan for any patient not responding to oral antibiotics or if posterior extension is suspected. Teenagers and adults usually respond quickly to oral antibiotics (amoxicillin–clavulanate [Augmentin], 250 to 500 q8h; cefaclor [Ceclor], 250 to 500 q8h; or erythromycin, 250 to 500 q6h). Treat severe or refractory cases with IV antibiotics (e.g., ceftriaxone and vancomycin).

3.2 Orbital Inflammation

3.2.1 Orbital Cellulitis/Subperiosteal Abscess/Cavernous Sinus Syndrome

—infection of the orbital soft tissue posterior to the orbital septum. Common causes are *Staphylococcus* species, *Streptococcus* species, and *H. influenzae.*

Presentation fever, axial proptosis, chemosis, pain increase on eye movement, ocular motility deficits. Severe cases cause decreased visual acuity and visual field defects. There may also be congestion of the veins of the retina and choroid as well as disc edema and periphlebitis. The most common source of infection is the sinuses, although the disease may also develop from contiguous inflammatory dis-

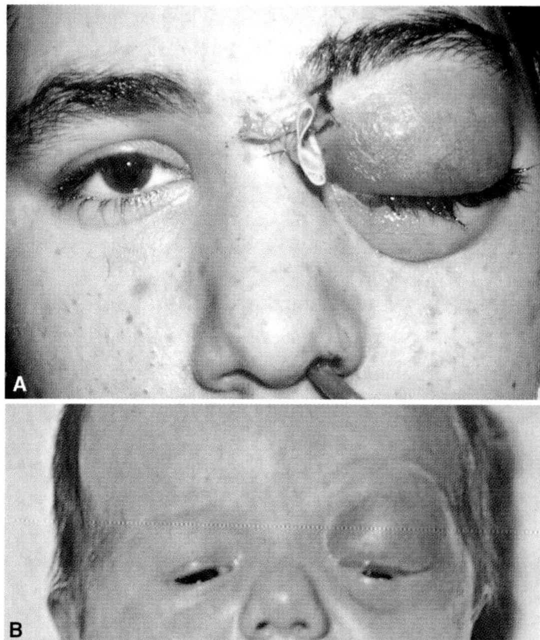

FIGURE 3.2.1a Surgical drainage for orbital cellulitis.
FIGURE 3.2.1b Subperiosteal abscess in an infant.

eases of the face and oropharynx, trauma, foreign bodies, or septicemia.

- Subperiosteal abscess: organization of infection may cause an abscess. These patients usually present with a history of sinusitus, a medial mass, nonaxial proptosis, and local tenderness, which may lead to intraconal or extraconal orbital abscess, increased intraocular pressure, ophthalmoplegia, and visual deficit.
- Cavernous sinus thrombosis: spread of the infection by means of the vascular emissaria to the cavernous sinus. Patients develop diplopia, headache, nausea, vomiting, fever, fluctuations in mental status, bilaterality, and a blue-purple lid. Cranial neuropathy involving CN III,

IV, and VI causes diplopia and dilated pupil. There may be an ipsilateral Horner's syndrome (ptosis, miosis, anhydrosis).

Differential Diagnosis

uveitis, scleritis, orbital inflammation such as orbital pseudotumor, Graves' ophthalmopathy, vasculitis (Wegener's granulomatosis), lymphoma. Subperiosteal abscess can be confused with mucocele and sinusitus. Cavernous sinus thrombosis can be confused with arteriovenous fistula, mucormycosis, and Tolosa-Hunt syndrome (below). In children, there may be rhabdomyosarcoma, ruptured dermoid cyst, metastatic neuroblastoma, capillary hemangioma, neurofibroma, and acute leukemia.

Management

admit patients with orbital cellulitis for IV antibiotics. Culture any drainage. Obtain blood for complete blood count with differential and cultures, and a CT scan to localize the cellulitis and/or abscess. The CT scan is also useful to follow improvement or worsening of the disease.

- Children: nafcillin (150 mg/kg/day IV divided q4h), vancomycin (40 mg/kg/day IV divided q8h or q12h) in addition to ceftazidime (30 to 50 mg/kg divided IV q8h), or ceftriaxone (100 mg/kg/day divided q12h).
- Adults: ceftazidime (1 to 2 g IV q8h), ceftriaxone (1 to 2 g IV q8h), or gentamicin (1.75 mg/kg IV and then 1 mg/kg q8h) in addition to nafcillin (1 to 2 g IV q4h) or vancomycin (1 g IV q12h); add clindamycin (300 mg IV q6h) for adults with chronic orbital cellulitis or if an anerobic infection is suspected.

An ENT consult is also warranted for surgical drainage of the sinuses, if necessary. In the event of abscess formation or progressive deterioration of the vision to below 20/60, surgical drainage is mandatory. When the inflammatory symptoms are clearly improving, change from the IV antibiotics to oral antibiotics to complete a 2-week course. Follow the outpatient's case every few days until the condition resolves.

3.2.2 Graves' Ophthalmopathy or Orbitopathy—this thyroid-related immune orbitopathy is the most common cause of unilateral or bilateral proptosis in adults. An accumulating body of evidence links the orbitopathy and the thyroid disorder to immune mechanisms with both cell-mediated and humoral components.

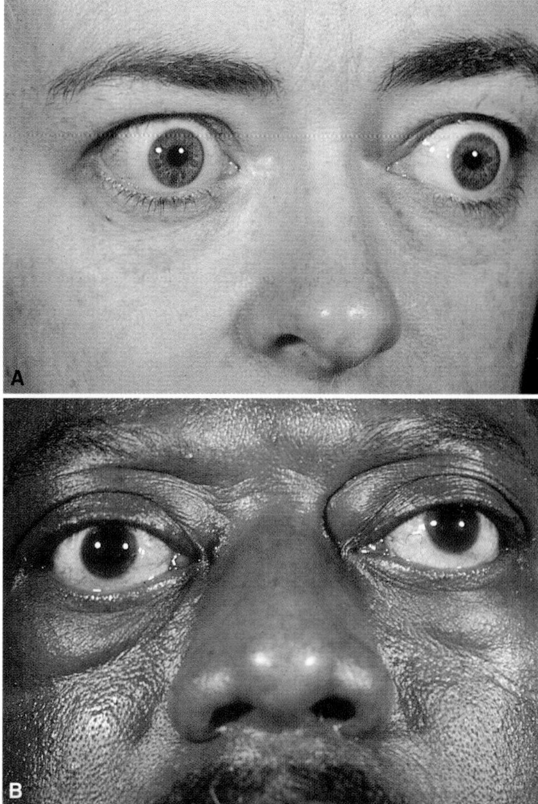

FIGURE 3.2.2a Exophthalmus and lid retraction.
FIGURE 3.2.2b Thyroid orbitopathy.

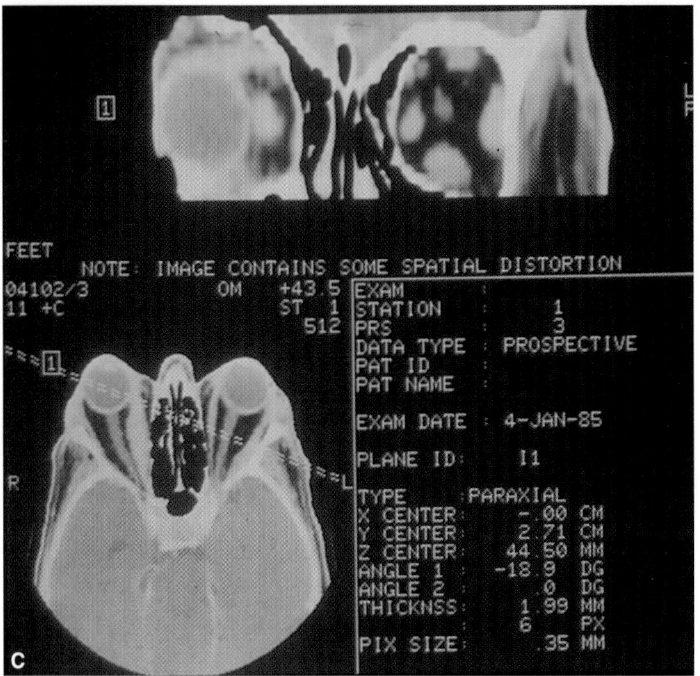

FIGURE 3.2.2c CT scan: thyroid disease (note muscle enlargement with tendon sparing).

Presentation four to five times more frequent in females; usually occurs with hyperthyroidism, but subclinical thyroid abnormalities or even normal thyroid function may be noted. There are two clinical groups:

- Noninfiltrative (mild) orbitopathy: minimal inflammatory reaction leading to mild lid retraction in often younger patients.
- Infiltrative (severe) orbitopathy: a more fulminant course with infiltration, inflammation, and consequent scarring. These patients often have lid swelling and chemosis with corneal exposure, proptosis, and optic neuropathy. Extraocular muscle myositis and enlargement can lead to restriction in ocular motility and diplopia. The inferior and medial rectus are most commonly involved.

A mnemonic for the course of Graves' ophthalmopathy is NOSPECS: *no* ocular signs or symptoms; *s*oft tissue swelling; *p*roptosis; *e*xtraocular muscle involvement; *c*orneal exposure; *s*ight loss due to optic nerve involvement.

Differential Diagnosis

orbital cellulitis, orbital pseudotumor, trauma leading to retrobulbar hemorrhage and intraorbital foreign body, orbital vasculitis, arteriovenous fistula, cavernous sinus thrombosis, cranial nerve palsy, myopia, enophthalmos of the fellow eye.

Management

diagnosis is usually made by CT scan, which shows extraocular muscle enlargement with sparing of muscle tendons (in contrast to orbital pseudotumor). Thyroid function tests are less helpful diagnostically; however, if abnormal, thyroid dysfunction should be treated. Rule out myasthenia gravis, because it is often associated with Graves' ophthalmopathy, and treat corneal exposure with lubricants and ointment.

- Acute: systemic corticosteroids or immunosuppressive agents may limit damage to extraocular muscles and decrease orbital edema and compressive optic neuropathy. High doses in the range of 80 to 100 mg of prednisone daily are administered to adults. External beam radiation applied to the orbital apex may limit inflammation.
- Chronic: when findings stabilize (usually after 6 to 12 months), eyelid recession of the levator aponeurosis or inferior retractor muscle layer reduces corneal exposure. Recession of a restricted muscle is preferable to resection of the contralateral muscle. Adjustable suture

techniques are helpful. Orbital decompression surgery is an effective treatment for compressive optic neuropathy and is also useful to minimize the cosmetic deformity in Graves' ophthalmopathy.

3.2.3 Orbital Pseudotumor

3.2.3 Orbital Pseudotumor—an idiopathic inflammation of almost any orbital tissue, unrelated to Graves' orbitopathy or any other systemic disorder.

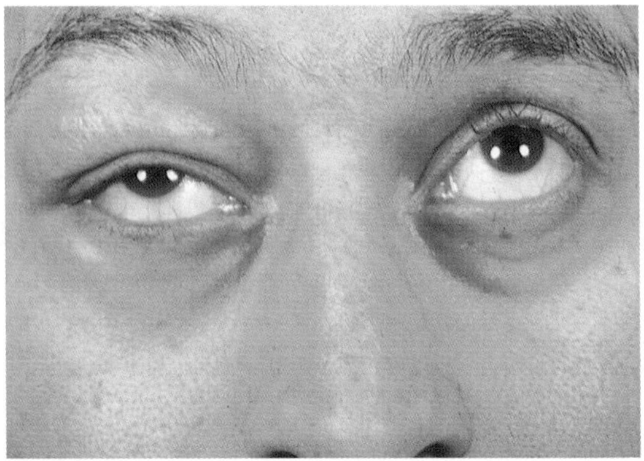

FIGURE 3.2.3 Pseudotumor of the right orbit.

Presentation acute onset of orbital pain and usually unilateral proptosis. Chemosis, lid edema, and erythema are common. Other symptoms depend on which ocular structures are involved; pain on eye movement, diplopia, and visual loss may result. Dacryoadenitis can also occur. Bilateral inflammation is rare in adults and should prompt further workup:

- In children: bilateral findings common (about one-third of the time). Half of all children have headache, fever, vomiting, and lethargy. Uveitis and papillitis are more common.

- Tolosa-Hunt syndrome: a variant causing inflammation of the orbital apex, affecting structures in the vicinity of the superior orbital fissure or anterior cavernous sinus. The syndrome causes painful ophthalmoplegia, minimal proptosis, and decreased visual acuity.
- Sclerosing orbital pseudotumor: characterized by late patient presentation of a scarred lesion within a muscle or retrobulbar fat pad. Proptosis may be absent, and even enophthalmos may occur.

Differential Diagnosis

depends on the location of the inflammation. Graves' ophthalmopathy, lymphoma, lymphoid hyperplasia, orbital cellulitis, scleritis, uveitis; in young persons, rhabdomyosarcomas, metastatic neuroblastomas, or leukemic infiltration of the orbit. Orbital myositis can mimic arteriovenous fistulas, Tolosa-Hunt syndrome, and myasthenia gravis. Orbital apex inflammation can mimic optic neuritis, apical tumors, and cavernous sinus thrombosis. Lacrimal inflammation can be confused with viral and bacterial dacryoadenitis, ruptured dermoid cyst, sarcoid, and Sjögren's disease.

Management

CT scan and B-scan reveal thickening of the extraocular muscles and their tendons (unlike Graves' orbitopathy, where the tendons are spared). Inflammation of the retrobulbar fat pad and contrast enhancement of the sclera due to tenonitis may produce a "ring sign." Treat with systemic steroids in the range of 60 to 80 mg/day and topical corticosteroid drops (prednisolone qid). Rapid response is pathognomonic of orbital pseudotumor. Taper steroids slowly over a period of months to avoid recurrence of symptoms. If inflammation does not respond, perform biopsy before further therapy, which may include addition of IV dexamethasone, orbital irradiation, or cyclophosphamide.

3.2.4 (Benign) Reactive Lymphoid Hyperplasia—a benign lymphoproliferative disease of the orbit.

Presentation an indolent course of painless proptosis without functional deficit. The lesions appear as firm to rubbery, slightly nodular anterior orbital infiltrations. There may be a conjunctival lesion that has a fleshy appearance. This process may be confined to the conjunctiva, in which case the lesions tend to be smaller, fleshy, and multinodular. Patients may also develop systemic involvement with lesions occurring in other areas, such as the gastrointestinal and respiratory tracts.

Differential Diagnosis non-Hodgkin's lymphoma, metastatic disease, limbal dermoid, pyogenic granuloma, lymphangioma, Kaposi's sarcoma.

Management biopsy is required for certain diagnosis. The presence of eosinophils and plasma cells helps to establish the reactive and, thus, benign nature of this process. If there are atypical mononuclear cells mixed in the lesion, it is a borderline lesion bridging benign and malignant. These cases must be carefully followed. These lesions can generally be treated by excision and topical steroid drops. Those who fail to respond or have widespread involvement can be treated with cytotoxic agents such as chlorambucil or with local low-dose radiation.

3.2.5 Orbital Lymphoma—the largest group of lymphoproliferative disorders seen in the orbit, most commonly of the Non-Hodgkin's variety.

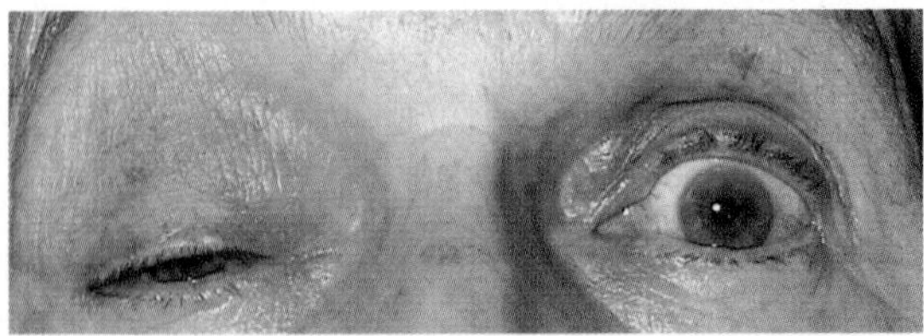

FIGURE 3.2.5 Ptosis secondary to lymphocytic lymphoma.

Presentation onset is usually in the sixth to seventh decades of life; lymphomas occur rarely in children. Most orbital lymphomas are low-grade to intermediate-grade lesions. Malignant lymphoma can produce a painless progressive proptosis accompanied by extraocular motility disturbance, visual loss, and lacrimal gland involvement. If confined to the anterior orbit, the proptosis may not be evident. In addition, lymphoma in the anterior orbit may be associated with a "salmon"-colored conjunctival tumor that molds to the shape of the globe.

Differential Diagnosis orbital pseudotumor, reactive lymphoid hyperplasia, metastasis, sarcoidosis.

Management B-scan and CT scan reveal a solid infiltrating tumor. CT may reveal a characteristic puttylike molding of the tumor to preexisting orbital structures. Bone changes are not usually seen. A biopsy specimen is required to establish the diagnosis. Pathologic studies include electron microscopy and immunopathologic cell marker studies.

Management the treatment for both benign and malignant lymphoid lesions of the orbit is irradiation. Systemic chemotherapy is usually introduced if there is dissemination.

3.3 Other Orbital Neoplasms

3.3.1 Dermoid Cyst/Epidermoid Cyst—choristomas that develop from dermoid and epidermoid elements that get pinched off along bony suture lines in the course of embryonic development. Dermoid cysts are lined by keratinizing epidermis with dermal appendages in the wall, such as hair follicles and sebaceous glands. Epidermoid cysts are lined by epidermis only, are usually filled with keratin, and do not contain dermal appendages.

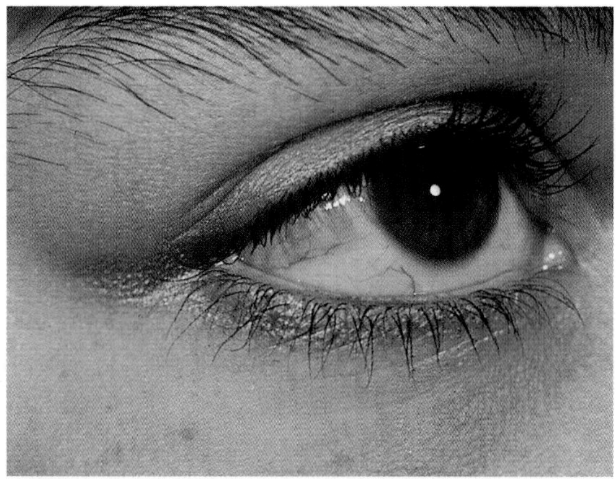

FIGURE 3.3.1 Dermoid cyst (note the superotemporal location).

Presentation both epidermoid and dermoid tumors present similarly and can be superficial or deep.

- Superficial orbit: found in infancy and childhood as palpable, smooth, painless, oval masses that slowly enlarge in the area of the lateral brow and upper lid adjacent to the zygomaticofrontal suture. Rupture of the cyst can lead to an acute inflammatory process if part of the cyst wall or the irritating contents are allowed to remain within the eyelid or orbit.
- Deep orbit: dermoids present as slow-growing masses later in life. They usually arise superotemporally but can

be found medially, laterally, or even apically. Axial or nonaxial proptosis may ensue.

Differential Diagnosis cavernous hemangioma, mucocele, neurofibroma, schwannoma, optic nerve glioma or meningioma, hemangiopericytoma, lymphangioma, lymphoid tumors or orbital pseudotumor, primary and secondary lacrimal tumors (lateral), mucoceles or encephaloceles (medial).

Management obtain a CT scan.

- Superficial dermoids are rounded, clearly defined masses frequently containing a lucent center suggestive of fat. There is no bony erosion, and they may be surgically excised.
- Deep dermoids have relatively well-defined margins with central radiodensity between fat and muscle. Almost invariably there is evidence of a break or full-thickness defect in the orbital bony wall, which has irregular or notched borders and may be enlarged. Calcification at the rim is a useful sign in that most soft tissue masses of the orbit other than mucoceles do not have rim calcification. Treatment of deep dermoids is also surgical excision and can be challenging, depending on location.

3.3.2 Capillary Hemangioma—a primary benign hamartoma of children composed of abnormal growth of blood vessels and endothelial proliferation.

Presentation usually present within the first months of life in the head and neck region, commonly in the orbit. An initial, small, flat lesion undergoes rapid expansion over weeks to months, and then typically involutes. Capillary hemangiomas are divided into superficial, deep, and combined lesions.

- Superficial, cutaneous lesions may resemble a strawberry ("strawberry nevus").

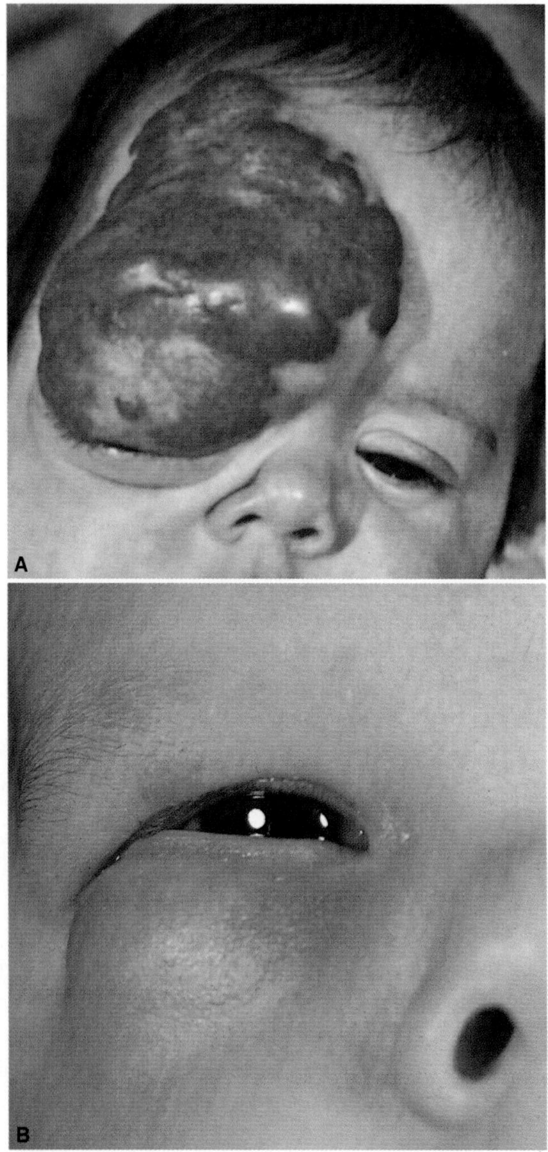

FIGURE 3.3.2a Extensive capillary hemangioma.
FIGURE 3.3.2b Orbital capillary hemangioma.

- Deeper lesions lie posterior to the septum and may cause proptosis and subtle pulsation. There may be obvious dilatation of the overlying lid or facial vessels, and blue-violet discoloration of the lids or conjunctival may be noted. When palpable through the lid, they have a rubbery consistency and a smooth contour. The size and location of these lesions often produce distortion or obstruction of the visual axis, with subsequent amblyopia or strabismus.
- Large visceral lesions may lead to sequestration of thrombocytes and RBCs with thrombocytopenia and bleeding diathesis (Kasbach-Merritt syndrome).

Differential Diagnosis

- Superficial: dermoid cyst, plexiform neurofibroma, lymphangioma.
- Deep: cavernous hemangioma, lymphangioma, rhabdomyosarcoma, dermoid cyst, orbital pseudotumor, metastatic neuroblastoma, neurofibroma, orbital cellulitus, teratoma, optic nerve glioma.

Management on CT scan, the margins of deep and combined hemangiomas vary from well defined to infiltrating. They can show moderate to intense enhancement with IV contrast. On angiography, these lesions frequently have multiple enlarged feeding vessels from both the ophthalmic artery and external carotid branches. The vast majority of these lesions regress spontaneously. A "herald spot" (fine stellate area of pale scarring) indicates resolution. Large lesions causing visual axis obstruction or severe disfigurement may require treatment. Intralesional steroids, dermal laser, cryotherapy, or radiotherapy are options. For deep and combined hemangiomas, systemic and locally injected corticosteroids are favored. Surgical resection is used when steroids fail.

3.3.3 Lymphangioma

3.3.3 Lymphangioma—hamartomas without systemic vascular connections. Histologically, they are large serum-filled spaces lined by flattened, endothelial cells.

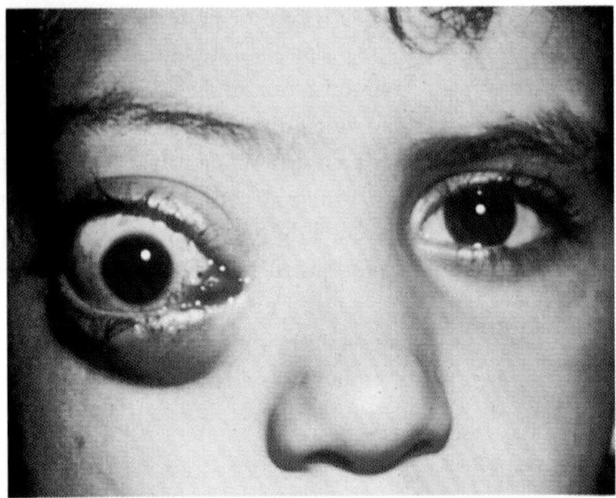

FIGURE 3.3.3 Deep, orbital lymphangioma.

Presentation

generally become apparent in the first decade of life.

- Superficial lymphangiomas: visible lesion of the lid or conjunctiva alone. These can consist of multiple clear cystic spaces, may contain blood-filled cysts, or may simply consist of a transilluminating bluish cyst just underneath the skin. Recurrent conjunctival hemorrhage, periorbital ecchymosis, and swelling may occur.
- Deep lymphangiomas: typically present later in life with sudden proptosis due to spontaneous hemorrhage into what was a previously unrecognized lesion. The blood may become loculated and form "chocolate cysts" containing old, dark blood. The acute orbital hemorrhage may cause optic nerve compression.
- Combined lymphangiomas: Usually recognized within the first year of life. They slowly enlarge over many years.

Differential Diagnosis

enlarging orbital mass in children. Dermoid and epidermoid cyst, rhabdomyosarcoma, optic nerve glioma, leukemia, metastatic neuroblastoma, plexiform neurofibroma, teratoma, capillary hemangioma, orbital cellulitis, orbital pseudotumor.

Management CT scans of combined and deep lymphangiomas show low-density, cystlike masses behind the orbital septum in the intraconal and extraconal spaces that enhance with contrast. The bony orbit may be enlarged. Spontaneous regression often occurs, so surgical intervention should be deferred unless unavoidable; however, superficial lesions may be removed for cosmetic purposes. In the case of acute orbital hemorrhage, aspiration of blood through a needle or by open surgical exploration may be attempted. Surgical debulking is necessary in cases when the optic nerve is compromised or where there is significant cosmetic deformity. Excision of deep and combined lesions is more complex as the lesion does not respect tissue planes, and abnormal tissue left in the orbit causes a high incidence of recurrence. The CO_2 and contact Nd:YAG lasers are useful for hemostasis and obliteration of unresectable areas of tumor.

3.3.4 Rhabdomyosarcoma—the most common primary orbital malignancy in childhood. Microscopically, rhabdomyosarcoma may be grouped into four categories: embryonal, alveolar, pleomorphic, and botryoid.

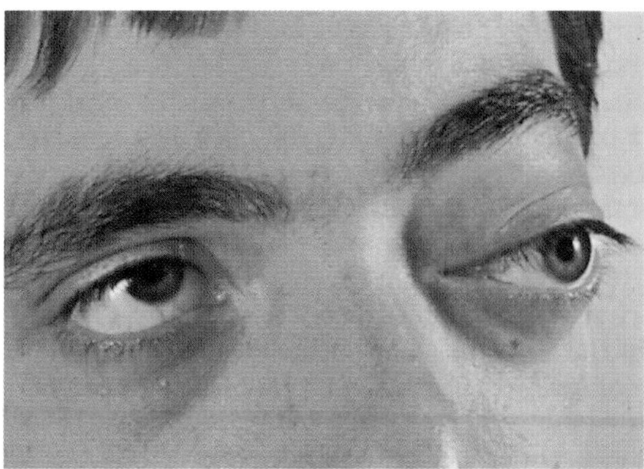

FIGURE 3.3.4 Proptosis due to orbital rhabdomyosarcoma.

Presentation average age of onset is 7 to 8 years, although it has been reported from birth to 70 years of age. The majority present acutely with rapidly developing exophthalmos, injection and swelling of the lids, and a downward and outward displacement of the globe. About half are retrobulbar, with one-quarter above and a smaller fraction below the globe. About one-quarter of the patients have a palpable mass, and one-third have ptosis. Pain and decreased vision are uncommon. Metastases from orbital sites are to lung, bone, and lymph nodes. Local recurrence may extend into the intracranial and nasal cavities.

- Embryonal: most common (accounts for two-thirds of cases); has a predilection for the superior nasal quadrant of the orbit.
- Botryoid: a "grape"-like form that is a rare variant of embryonal rhabdomyosarcoma; it is rarely found in the orbit except as an invader from the sinuses or the conjunctiva.
- Alveolar: poorly differentiated tumor cells arranged in a pattern resembling alveoli of the lung; poorest prognosis; more common in the inferior orbit.
- Pleomorphic: the most rare, most differentiated, and the best prognosis; occurs in older children.

Differential Diagnosis of rapidly developing tumors of childhood: Orbital pseudotumor, acute leukemia, trauma, metastatic neuroblastoma, lymphangioma, capillary hemangioma, dermoid and epidermoid cyst, optic nerve glioma, orbital cellulitis.

Management workup should proceed on an emergency basis.

- CT scan shows bony destruction and a low-density tumor.
- Biopsy is via an anterior orbitotomy with minimal trauma to minimize dislodging cells as metastases.
- Metastatic workup includes physical examination, chest radiography, bone marrow biopsy, lumbar puncture (arrange with orbitotomy in the OR).

Treatment is initiated after urgent tissue diagnosis and metastatic workup to stage the disease. Treatment protocols consist of a combination of limited surgical removal of the tumor, radiation therapy, and combined adjuvant chemotherapy with variations depending on the location of the disease.

3.3.5 Cavernous Hemangioma—encapsulated lesions and the most common benign neoplasms of the orbit in adults.

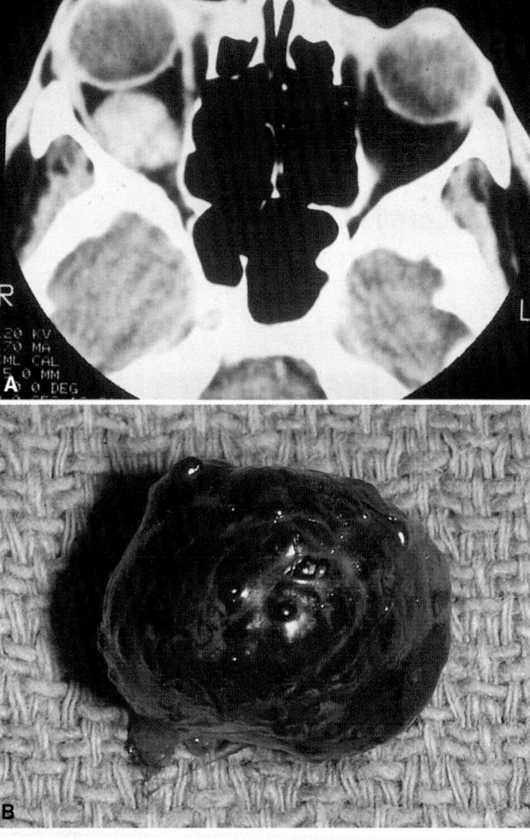

FIGURE 3.3.5a CT scan with well-circumscribed intraconal mass.
FIGURE 3.3.5b Surgical specimen: cavernous hemangioma.

Presentation predilection for middle-aged women in the intraconal area. Usually, there is a history of slowly progressive proptosis, although pregnancy may accelerate the growth. Large lesions can cause retinal striae, hyperopia and strabismus, and increased IOP and optic nerve compression.

Differential Diagnosis metastatic, mucocele, lymphoma, optic nerve meningioma, neurofibroma, schwannoma, fibrous histiocytoma, hemangiopericytoma, lymphangioma, dermoid cyst.

Management CT scan confirms the well-defined mass. The treatment of these lesions is surgical excision; at the time of surgery, the tumor appears as a plump, purplish, nodular mass with vascular channels on its surface.

3.3.6 Carotid Cavernous Fistula

—an abnormal communication between the previously normal carotid artery and cavernous sinus. These lesions can be either high flow or low flow and are caused by trauma, vascular disease, or tumors.

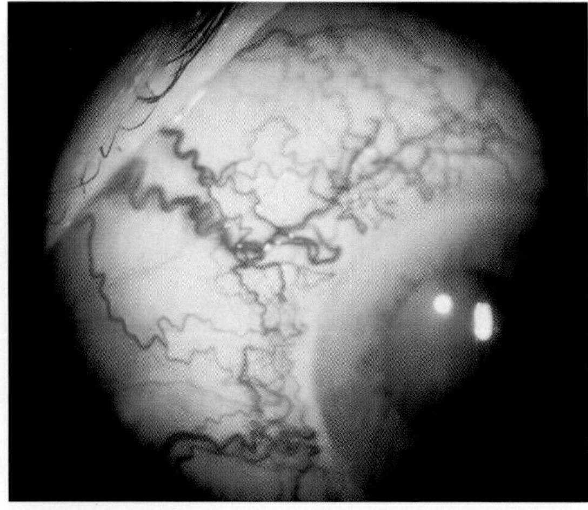

FIGURE 3.3.6 Episcleral venous congestion due to dural cavernous fistula.

Presentation

- High-flow lesions: usually caused by trauma, commonly due to a basal skull fracture that causes a tear within the cavernous portion of the internal carotid artery. Findings include an audible bruit, pulsatile proptosis associated with chemosis, orbital swelling, episcleral venous congestion, and IOP elevation. Limitation of extraocular motility secondary to cranial nerve palsies may occur. The ultimate rate of visual loss in untreated high-flow lesions may be as high as 50%.
- Low-flow lesions: small meningeal arteries that supply the dural wall of the cavernous sinus may rupture spontaneously as a degenerative process in patients with systemic hypertension and atherosclerosis, especially post-menopausal females. A dural–sinus fistula may ensue. The onset may be insidious with mild orbital congestion, proptosis, and low or no bruit. These lesions are prone to fluctuations, and spontaneous resolution may occur.

Differential Diagnosis

cavernous sinus thrombosis, orbital pseudotumor, metastatic disease, thyroid disease and other orbital lesions, Tolosa-Hunt syndrome, nasopharyngeal carcinoma.

Management

CT scan will demonstrate proptosis with enlargement of the superior ophthalmic vein and frequent enlargement of the extraocular muscles in proportion to the degree of shunting. However, angiography, which classically shows retrograde opacification of the cavernous sinus and the orbital venous system, is necessary to evaluate and plan treatment of arteriovenous fistulas of the orbit and cavernous sinus. Detachable balloon embolization is now the treatment of choice for post-traumatic, high-flow shunts. Intravascular embolization is the treatment of choice for high-flow lesions secondary to spontaneous arteriovenous shunts; however, the success rate is not as high as in the post-traumatic variety.

3.3.7 Orbital Varices—primary dilation of preexisting venous channels or secondary venous dilation due to arteriovenous fistulas.

Presentation usually near the end of the first decade or early in the second decade with hemorrhage or thrombosis, leading to sudden proptosis and pain with increased pressure on the orbital tissues: there may be swelling or disfigurement of the lids and conjunctiva, mechanical restriction of ocular movement, or visual deficit.

Differential Diagnosis orbital hemorrhages, including trauma and lymphangioma.

Management the diagnosis is usually confirmed with contrast enhanced CT or venography. The treatment is usually conservative and is reserved for cases in which the varix is threatening vision because of optic nerve damage. Surgical management consists of deep orbital exposure with evacuation of clotted blood and excision of the associated varix. Complete surgical excision is difficult because the varix often is intertwined with orbital structures. Bipolar cautery is useful to shrink and scar areas of the varix, and CO_2 and Nd:YAG lasers may facilitate removal of these lesions.

3.3.8 Mucocele—cystic, slowly expanding lesions originating from the sinuses and caused by obstruction of the sinus excretory ducts. The cysts are usually filled with mucous secretions; however, when filled with pus, they are called pyoceles.

Presentation frontal headache with a history of chronic sinusitis. The clinical features are due to an expansive cystic mass that slowly invades the orbit by eroding through the orbital bones. Most mucoceles arise from the frontal or ethmoid sinus and cause a slowly progressing, downward and outward displacement of the globe. They are often associated with a fullness in the superonasal and medial canthal region and a palpable mass.

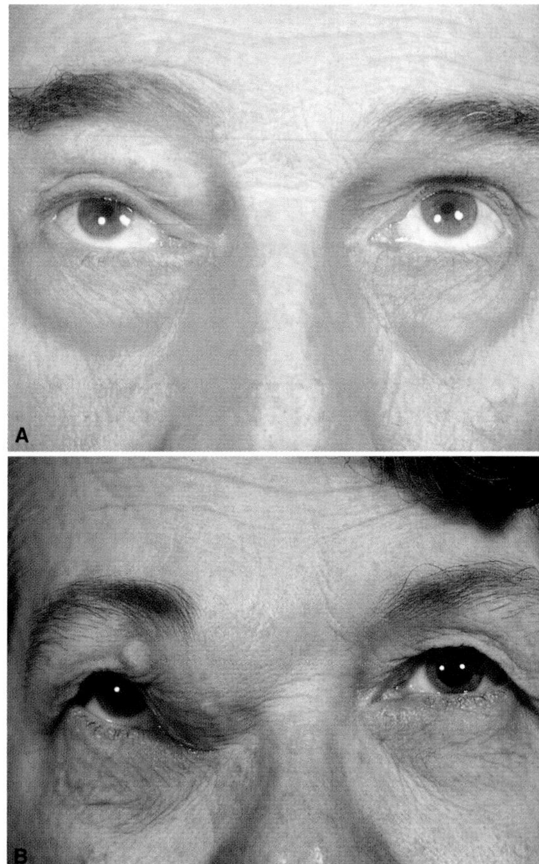

FIGURE 3.3.8a Fullness of the superonasal region with limited upgaze due to a mucocele.
FIGURE 3.3.8b Advanced mucocele.

Differential Diagnosis

in children: encephaloceles, lymphangioma, optic nerve glioma, leukemia, metastatic neuroblastoma, dermoid cysts. In adults: sinus polyposis, dermoid cysts, cavernous hemangioma, lymphomas, optic nerve sheath meningioma, neurofibroma, fibrous histiocytoma, hemangiopericytoma, metastatic disease.

Management ENT consultation. On CT scan, the sinus is homogeneously opacified by the material of soft tissue density. Findings on radiography are similar. Surgical treatment is directed toward complete removal of the cyst lining, reestablishment of normal drainage, or obliteration of the sinus.

3.3.9 Metastatic Orbital Lesions—metastasis of solid tumors to the orbit (compose between 2 and 10% of all orbital tumors). Metastatic carcinomas are more common than sarcomas.

Presentation frequently progress rapidly (generally months), leading to displacement of the globe and functional deficits, including motor abnormalities, diplopia, and ptosis. Sensory abnormalities include the occurrence of a dull, aching, pressure-like pain and paresthesia. Visual loss may be secondary to direct infiltration or increased IOP. Most solid cancers and metastases occur in the fifth, sixth, and seventh decades. Metastasis usually occur within 6 months to 1 year of the primary tumor. The most common orbital metastasis in women is breast carcinoma, which is also the most common orbital metastasis overall. Paradoxically, cicatrical enophthalmos occurs in metastatic breast carcinoma, as well as lung, gastrointestinal, and prostate cancers. The most common orbital metastasis in men is bronchogenic carcinoma. The most common metastatic carcinoma affecting the orbit in children, especially boys, is neuroblastoma and can be the presenting sign of the disease.

Differential Diagnosis orbital pseudotumor and lymphangioma in adults, and rhabdomyosarcoma, lymphangioma, and leukemia in children.

Management CT scan may show infiltrative or circumscribed masses that may be attached to specific structures, such as the lacrimal gland or the extraocular muscles. Bone destruction may be seen, but calcification is rare. Areas of necrosis may be identified. Contrast is helpful in detecting small lesions. B-scan is important in confirming the solid nature of the tumors. A systemic evaluation is mandatory and includes radiologic investigation of the chest and abdomen, bone scans, and, at times, bone marrow biopsy. Tumor-associated antigens may help detect primaries and assess tumor load. Specification of particular tumor types is important and may require a biopsy with immunohistochemical or tumor marking studies. Metastatic disease is usually incurable, and frequently only palliative therapy is possible.

3.3.10 Neurofibroma (of the Eyelid and Orbit)—peripheral nerve sheath hamartoma made up of mixtures of Schwann, perineural, and fibroblastoid cells, and often residual axons. Neurofibromas are plexiform, fusiform, or diffuse.

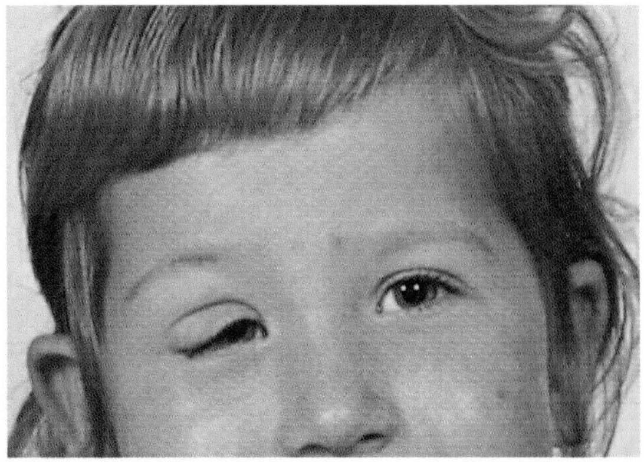

FIGURE 3.3.10 S-shaped ptosis due to a plexiform neurofibroma.

Presentation most common and most complex peripheral nerve tumors of the orbit. They are generally associated with neurofibromatosis and present in the first decade of life. The lesions are not encapsulated, grow along the nerves, and insinuate themselves throughout the orbital tissues. The overlying skin may be thickened (elephantine neuromatosa). The tortuous, ropy, tangled nerves produce a characteristically palpable "bag of worms." Plexiform neurofibromas frequently involve the lateral aspect of the lid and cause a pathognomonic S-shaped deformity. Localized neurofibromas infrequently present in the orbit. They are solid, isolated, circumscribed, slow-growing mass lesions. They tend to be seen in middle-aged persons.

Differential Diagnosis lymphangiomas, capillary hemangiomas, malignant neoplasms, nonspecific and specific inflammations of the orbit and amyloid.

Management check for signs of systemic neurofibromatosis. CT scan with contrast demonstrates irregular soft tissue infiltration of orbital and periorbital structures, frequently with extraocular muscle enlargement. Bony changes may consist of enlargement of the orbit and widening of the superior and inferior orbital fissures. Solitary neurofibromas appear as well-circumscribed, usually homogeneous masses. Plexiform neurofibromas and diffuse neurofibromas are difficult to excise owing to vascularity, close interdigitation with normal tissues, and a tendency for continued growth. Surgical management is usually cosmetic debulking of the tumor. Some clinicians recommend exenteration in the case of significant involvement. In contrast, solitary neurofibromas can be removed more easily because they are encapsulated.

3.4 Lacrimal Gland Enlargement

cases of lacrimal gland enlargement are 50% inflammatory and 50% neoplastic.

3.4.1 Lacrimal Gland Inflammation—the intrinsic inflammatory lesions of the lacrimal gland include: infectious (dacryoadenitis) and other causes. Infection includes bacterial and viral dacryoadenitis. The other causes include orbital pseudotumor, Sjögren's syndrome, and sarcoid.

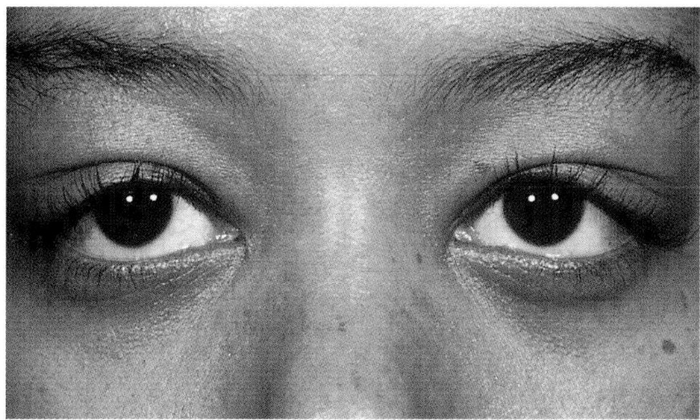

FIGURE 3.4.1 Superotemporal fullness due to sarcoid-induced lacrimal gland inflammation bilaterally.

Presentation acute or subacute inflammation with an associated palpable lacrimal gland and pain, tenderness, and injection of the temporal lid and conjunctival fornix.

- Infectious: suppuration, preauricular and cervical adenopathy, and systemic features of malaise, upper respiratory infection, fever, and leukocytosis. Dacryoadenitis may occur secondarily to infectious mononucleosis, herpes zoster, mumps, trachoma, syphilis, and tuberculosis. Acute dacryoadenitis may progress to chronic disease.
- Inflammatory: frequently have an S-shaped deformity of the lid. There is an overall tendency for lacrimation to be affected with the inflammatory lesions, unlike

lacrimal gland tumors. Patients with Sjögren's syndrome or sarcoid can present as having dacryoadenitis, along with symptoms of dry eye.

Differential Diagnosis

lacrimal gland neoplasms, lymphoma, lacrimal cysts, extrinsic lesions such as myeloma, Hodgkin's disease, granulomas, dermoid cysts, mucocele.

Management

- Infectious: CT scan reveals a diffuse lacrimal tumefaction with irregular margins, frequently demonstrating contrast enhancement and no bony defect. Bacterial dacryoadenitis may require aspiration from the local site or regional lymph node to identify the organism. Mild to moderate dacryoadenitis can be treated with oral antibiotics such as amoxicillin–clavulanate [Augmentin], 250 to 500 mg PO q8h (adults) or 20 to 40 mg/kg/day tid (children). If moderate to severe, patients should be hospitalized. One regimen is ticarcillin–clavulanate (Timentin) 3.2 g IV 4 to 6 h (adults) or 200 mg/kg/day IV in four divided doses (children). The antibiotic regimen should be adjusted according to the clinical response and culture and sensitivity results. IV antibiotics can be changed to comparable oral antibiotics, depending on the rate of improvement, but systemic antibiotics should be continued for a full 7- to 14-day course. If an abscess develops, incision and drainage are necessary.
- Inflammatory: CT scan reveals a compressed and molded enlargement of the lacrimal gland with obscuration of the lateral aspect of the globe and enhancement including at times the adjacent sclera. Motility is involved only minimally and generally reflects the mass effect alone. Systemic evaluation is necessary; consider biopsy. Sjögren's syndrome and sarcoid may be distinguished from orbital pseudotumor by their systemic manifestations. Treatment is with systemic steroids, starting with prednisone 0.5 to 1.0 mg/kg/day, depending on severity. Because of the potential association of autoimmune inflammatory disorders and lymphoma, patients with this syndrome should have lifelong follow-up.

3.4.2 Lacrimal Gland Tumors—neoplasms of epithelial origin are approximately: 50% benign mixed tumors (pleomorphic adenoma) and 50% carcinomas. Half of the carcinomas are adenoid cystic.

3.4.2.1 Benign Mixed Tumor (Pleomorphic Adenoma)—a benign epithelial neoplasm with mixed elements of mucinous, cartilaginous, and osseous origins.

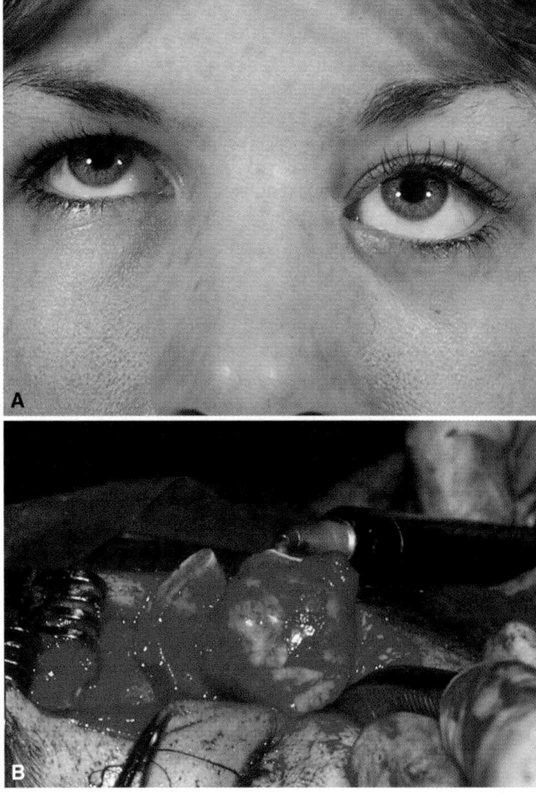

FIGURE 3.4.2.1a Limited upgaze due to benign mixed tumor.
FIGURE 3.4.2.1b Surgical specimen of benign mixed lacrimal gland tumor.

Presentation in the second to fifth decades, with the peak incidence in the fourth. There is a slight male:female preponderance. They commonly present as slow-growing (>1 year), non-inflammatory lesions with a progressive, painless downward and inward displacement of the globe and axial proptosis. Large tumors may be associated with blurring of vision, diplopia, retinal and choroidal striae, and, very occasionally, swelling of the optic nerve head.

Differential Diagnosis lymphoma, orbital pseudotumor, dacryoadenitis, orbital pseudotumor, sarcoid, Sjögren's syndrome, other lacrimal gland tumors.

Management CT scan may show evidence of enlargement or expansion of the lacrimal fossa due to pressure erosion. The lesion itself is well circumscribed and may have a slightly nodular configuration. Effective management involves extirpative biopsy by a modified lateral orbitotomy. The prognosis of pleomorphic adenoma is excellent, with approximately 99% survival after careful surgical excision without capsular rupture. There is a high rate of recurrence with possible malignant transformation when a margin of normal tissue is not removed along with the tumor. It is therefore important to establish the diagnosis before surgical intervention.

3.4.2.2 Adenoid Cystic Carcinoma—the most common epithelial carcinoma of the lacrimal gland (accounts for 50% of carcinomas).

Presentation in either sex, with a peak in the fourth decade. These tumors are dominated by mass effect with a rapid temporal sequence (<1 year) as opposed to benign mixed tumors (>1 year). Because of the propensity of this tumor to invade perineurally and into bone, pain and rarely paresthesis may be associated with it. Grossly, adenoid cystic carcinoma is grayish-white with a firm nodular surface. Five histologic patterns have been described: Swiss cheese (cribiform), sclerosing, basloid (solid), comedocarcinomatous, and tubular (ductal).

Differential Diagnosis lymphoma, orbital pseudotumor, dacryoadenitis, orbital pseudotumor, sarcoid, Sjögren's syndrome.

Management CT scan shows areas of pressure erosion, bony destruction, or calcification of the lacrimal fossa. Tumor may be diffuse and extend toward the orbital apex. The prognosis for adenoid cystic carcinoma is dismal, and the clinical course, despite treatment, is one of painful local and regional recurrences followed by systemization. The tumor should be completely excised, because radiation has not been shown to be efficacious. Because of its propensity to invade cranial nerves, the bounds of the excision may be breached. When the tumor is confined to the orbital tissues, the recommended therapy is en bloc excision of the orbit and its contents.

3.4.3 Lacrimal Cysts—ductal in origin.

Presentation characteristically blue-domed, cystic swellings visible through the conjunctiva that transilluminate. They can be bilateral.

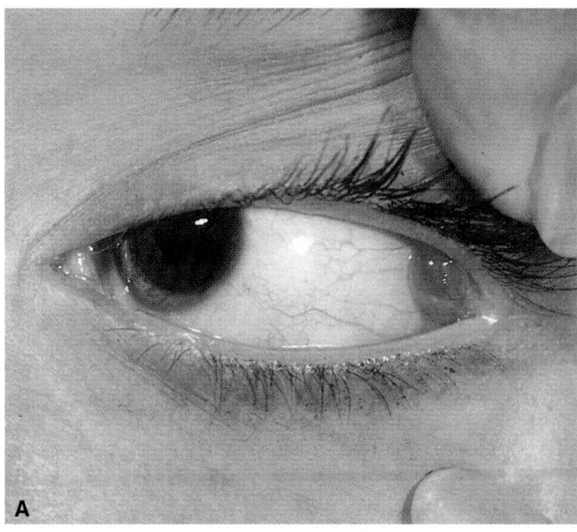

FIGURE 3.4.3a Lacrimal gland duct cyst.

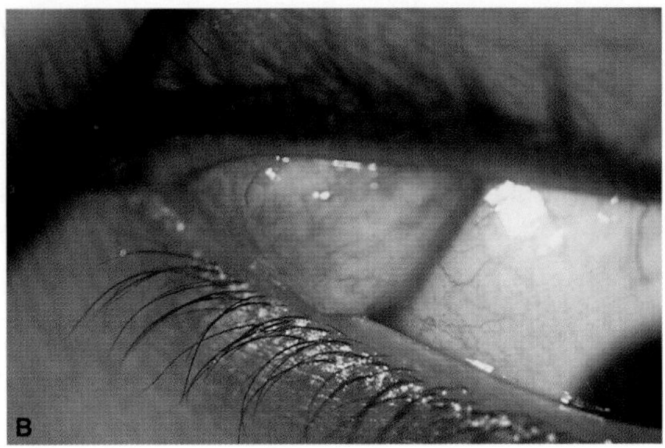

FIGURE 3.4.3b Lacrimal cyst with prolapse.

Differential Diagnosis

lymphoma, orbital pseudotumor, dacryoadenitis, orbital pseudotumor, sarcoid, Sjögren's syndrome.

Management

a limited, careful microscopic excision with caution to avoid other lacrimal ducts.

Chapter 4
EXTERNAL DISEASE

Kristin Pisacano, Michael B. Starr,
Eric E. Donnenfeld

4.1 Blepharitis and Ocular Rosacea

inflammation of eyelid margins caused by meibomian gland dysfunction related to ocular rosacea, seborrheic dermatitis, or chronic bacterial overgrowth (usually staphylococcal).

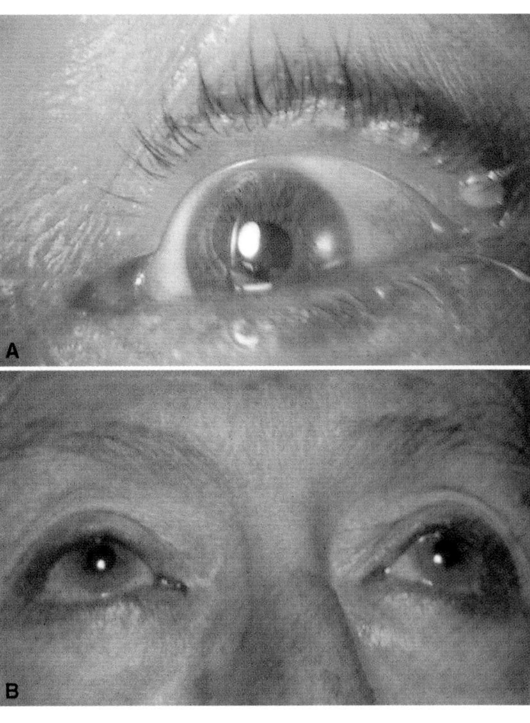

FIGURE 4.1a Collarettes with eyelid crusting.
FIGURE 4.1b Ocular rosacea with hyperemic eyelid margins.

Presentation lid crusting, redness, swelling, foreign-body sensation, burning, blurry vision, recurrent chalasia, itching.

- Infectious: collarettes, margin thickening and hyperemia, superficial punctate keratitis, conjunctival papillary hypertrophy, marginal corneal infiltrates, phlyctenules, corneal micropannus.
- Seborrheic: seborrheic dermatitis, greasy scales ("scurf"), tear-film instability.
- Meibomian dysfunction: inspissated glands, foam ("meibomian froth"), tear-film abnormalities, 60% with ocular rosacea.
- Ocular rosacea: telangectasia, pustules/papules and/or erythema of cheeks, forehead, and nose, eyelid margins; rhinophyma, superficial punctate keratitis, peripheral corneal "catarrhal" infiltrates of staphylococcal hypersensitivity, phlyctenules, rare iritis.

Differential Diagnosis infectious, allergic, or toxic conjunctivitis; dry eye.

Management warm compresses, lid hygiene (lid scrubs with diluted "tear-free" baby shampoo and cotton-tip applicator or wet washcloth), lubricants, antibiotic ointment (erythromycin or bacitracin, tapered according to symptoms).

- Tetracyclines: if not improved or if acne rosacea is present (i.e., doxycycline, 100 mg bid for 3 to 6 weeks; taper slowly once symptoms are relieved; not for children <8 years of age).
- Topical steroids: if severe inflammation, corneal infiltrates or phlyctenules (taper quickly, and only after appropriate treatment for any infectious component).

4.2 Conjunctivitis

any inflammation of the conjunctiva.

4.2.1 Viral—an acute infection of the conjunctiva. Causes include adenovirus (serotypes 8, 11, and 19—EKC; serotypes 3, 4, and 7—pharyngoconjunctival fever, usually in children); also influenza, rhinovirus, enterovirus, varicella, mumps, and others.

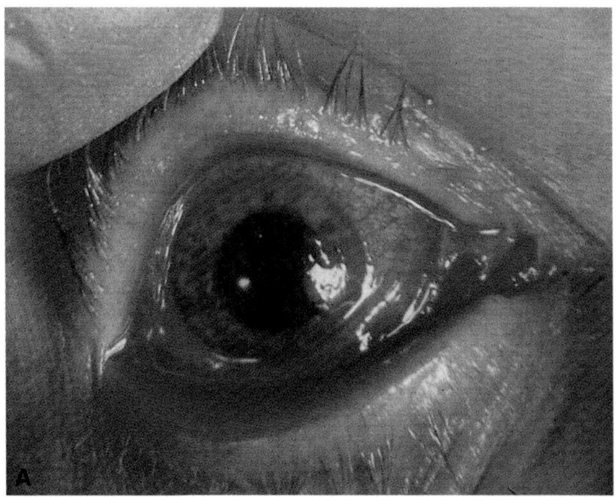

FIGURE 4.2.1a Watery discharge with redness and conjunctual chemosis.

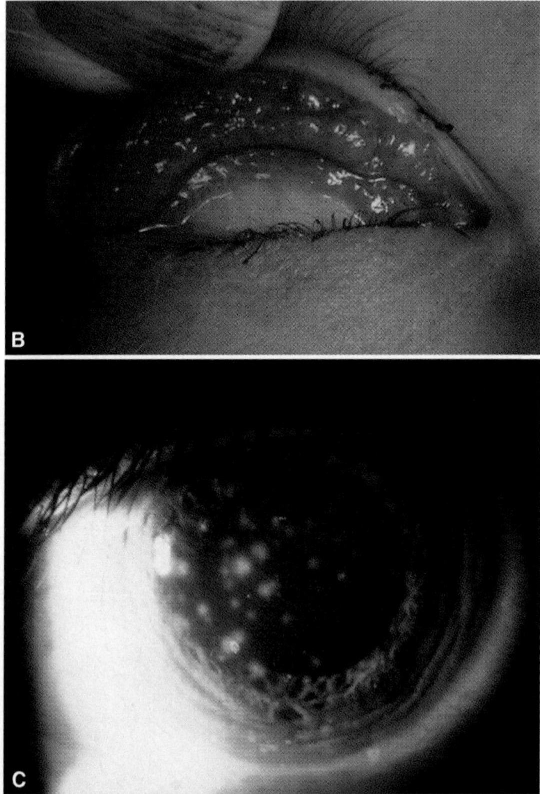

FIGURE 4.2.1b Superior tarsal papillofollicular reaction.
FIGURE 4.2.1c Subepithelial infiltrates.

Presentation watery discharge, photophobia, irritation, redness (peak at days 3 to 5). Signs include a papillofollicular conjunctival reaction, chemosis, preauricular lymph node, epithelial keratitis (indicates replicating virus), subepithelial infiltrates after 2 weeks (immune reaction classic for EKC), occasional membrane or pseudomembrane formation, pharyngitis, fever, subconjunctival hemorrhage, eyelid ecchymosis, edema.

Differential Diagnosis bacterial, herpes simplex, or allergic conjunctivitis. Of membranous conjunctivitis: severe viral (EKC) or bacterial (streptococcal, *Corynebacterium diphtheriae*) infection, Stevens-Johnson syndrome, ocular cicatricial pemphigoid, *Chlamydia*.

Management supportive therapy, cool compresses and artificial tears (preservative free, given q 1 to 2h, as needed) are helpful. Treat itching and irritation with topical vasoconstrictors/antihistamine/NSAIDs (e.g., Naphcon-A, Livostin, Acular). Encourage careful hygiene (the disease is contagious for 14 days or more after the onset of symptoms).

- If membrane or pseudomembrane, gently peel (using topical anesthetic and jeweller's forceps) and consider topical steroid for 1 week with slow taper.
- If subepithelial infiltrates affect vision, consider topical steroid (as above); note that infiltrates will likely recur with stopping of steroid and may be more prolonged.
- See Sections 5.1.1 and 5.1.2 for treatment of HSV and HZV keratitis.

4.2.2 Acute Bacterial—purulent, infectious conjunctivitis (only 5% of all conjunctivitis). Causative agents include *Staphylococcus aureus* (often with blepharitis, phlyctenules), *Streptococcus pneumoniae,* and *Haemophilus influenzae* (children).

Presentation moderate purulent discharge, chemosis, lid edema, subconjunctival hemorrhage for *H. influenzae* and *S. pneumoniae*), membrane formation (*Streptococcus*), peripheral corneal ulcers or stromal infiltrates (*H. influenzae*).

Differential Diagnosis other forms of conjunctivitis (viral, toxic).

Management for workup, laboratory studies are usually not indicated unless presentation is hyperacute or nonresolving. If gram

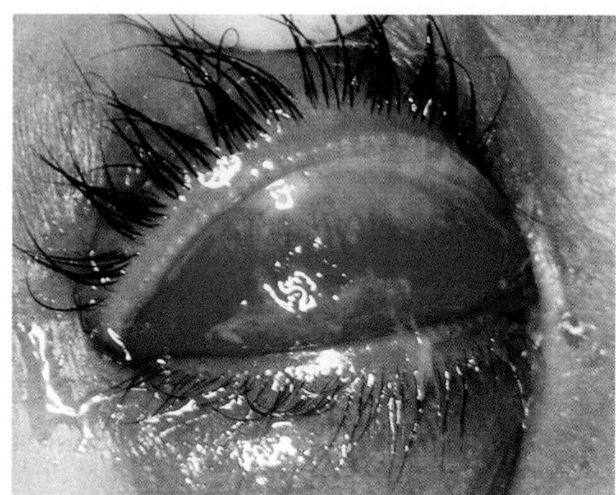

FIGURE 4.2.2 Purulent discharge with early pseudomembrane formation.

positive, treat with topical polymyxin–trimethoprim (Polytrim), erythromycin, or bacitracin qid for 5 to 7 days. If gram negative, treat with topical ciprofloxacin or aminoglycosides qid for 5 to 7 days. Oral amoxicillin–clavulanate (Augmentin) if pharyngitis or otitis is present concurrently.

4.2.3 Hyperacute (Gonococcal) Conjunctivitis—*Neisseria gonorrhoeae* infection from genital–ocular or genital–hand–ocular transmission.

Presentation sudden onset (<12 hours), severe purulent discharge, pain, redness. Signs include conjunctival papillae, chemosis, eyelid edema, adenopathy, keratitis (15 to 40%) including epithelial haze and defects, peripheral ulcers, possibly perforation.

Differential Diagnosis other forms of conjunctivitis (viral, toxic, other bacteria).

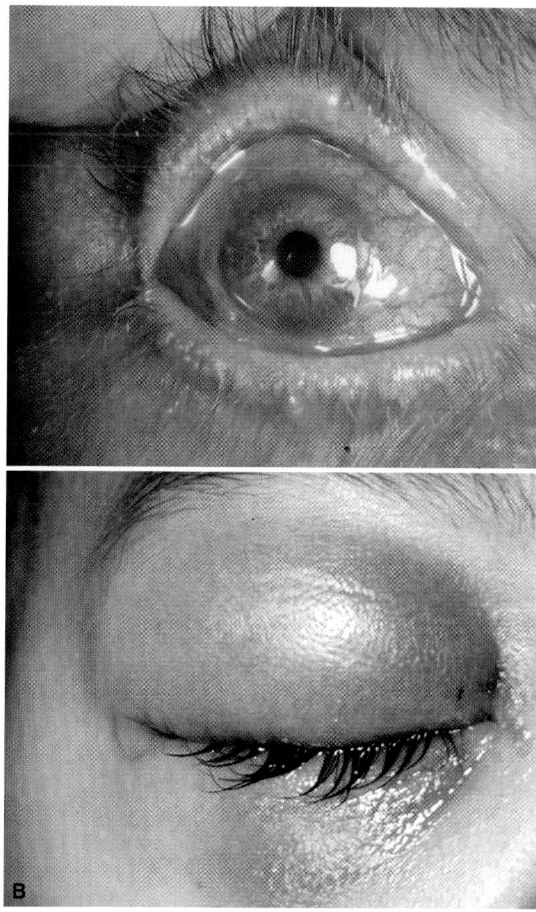

FIGURE 4.2.3a Purulent discharge in early gonococcal conjunctivitis.

FIGURE 4.2.3b Preseptal cellulitis secondary to gonococcal conjunctivitis.

Management

obtain conjunctival scrapings for culture and microscopy (blood agar, chocolate, Thayer-Martin). With Gram's stain, epithelial parasitism by gram-negative diplococci is seen.

Treat with ceftriaxone, 1 gm IM (single dose) or 1 gm IV q12h for 3 days if corneal ulceration exists; with penicillin allergy, ciprofloxacin, 500 mg PO bid for 5 days; topical ciprofloxacin q2h; doxycycline 100 mg bid for 1 week (for 33% chance of concurrent chlamydial venereal disease); cool water irrigation to flush out organisms and toxins; hospitalization for children or adults with corneal involvement.

4.2.4 Chronic Bacterial Conjunctivitis—prolonged infection with symptoms lasting longer than 1 month. Causes include *S. aureus, Moraxella lacunata, Proteus, Enterobacter,* and *Pseudomonas.*

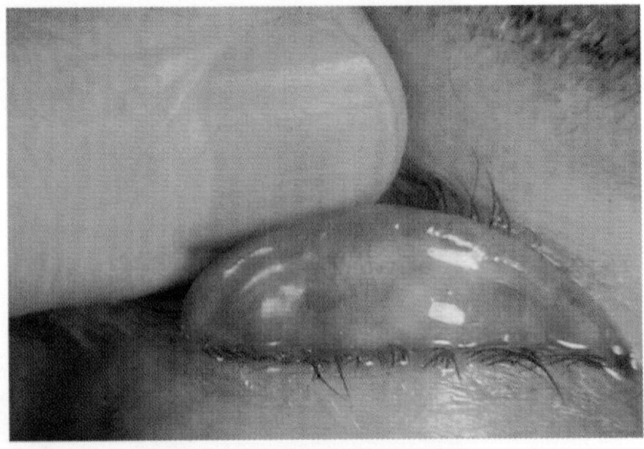

FIGURE 4.2.4 Chronic scarring of the superior tarsal conjunctiva.

Presentation mild injection, scant mucopurulent discharge, worse in morning. Crusting and ulceration of skin in lateral canthal angle is seen with *Moraxella* infection. Matted golden crusts with ulcerations on anterior eyelid margin, marginal corneal infiltrates, phlyctenule, or inferior superficial punctate keratitis indicate *S. aureus.* Often, associated risk factors are present, such as eyelid malposition, tear-film abnormalities, chronic dacryocystitis, chronic topical steroid use, systemic disease and/or immunosuppressive therapy, or ocular prosthesis.

Differential Diagnosis other forms of conjunctivitis.

Management obtain Gram's stain and culture (blood, chocolate agar) of palpebral conjunctiva. Avoid the use of preserved anesthetic, if possible. Begin treatment with topical bacitracin, erythromycin, polymyxin–trimethoprim (Polytrim) or aminoglycoside. Tailor according to culture and Gram's stain results.

4.2.5 *Chlamydia* Trachoma

—a leading cause of blindness due to a chronic, recurrent infection with *Chlamydia trachomatis* serotypes a to c. Endemic in arid areas with poor water supply and poor sanitation.

Presentation foreign-body sensation, redness, tearing, discharge. There are five clinical stages based on the extent of the following: tarsal follicular reaction (most prominent on superior tarsus, may become necrotic), limbal follicles (scarred limbal follicles are Herbert's pits), conjunctival scarring (Arlt's line), epithelial keratitis, subepithelial infiltrates, predominantly superior vascular pannus, corneal scarring.

Differential Diagnosis other forms of conjunctivitis, especially secondary to molluscum.

Management obtain Giemsa stain (macrophages with ingested debris, lymphocytes, and PMNs, basophilic intracytoplasmic inclusion bodies in epithelial cells), and chlamydial culture when diagnosis is not certain. Treat with topical tetracycline or erythromycin ointment bid for 1 to 2 months; or oral tetracycline or erythromycin (250 to 500 mg qid) or doxycycline (100 mg PO bid) for 3 to 4 weeks.

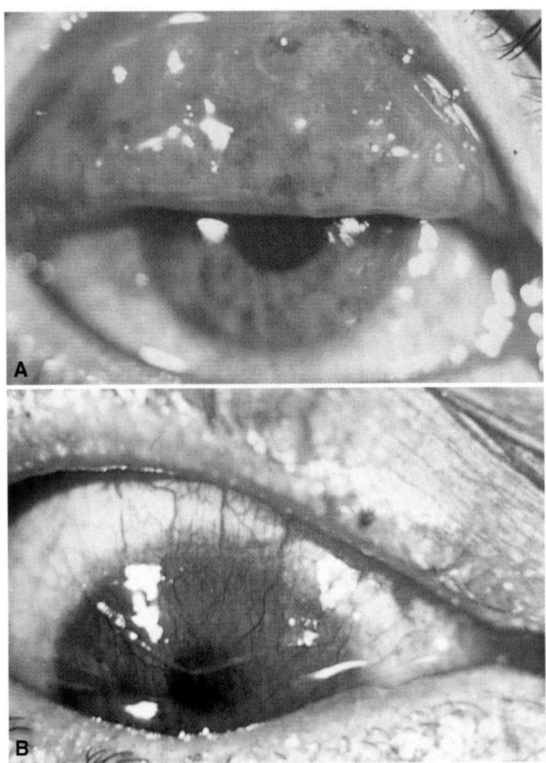

FIGURE 4.2.5a Superior tarsal follicular reaction in trachoma.
FIGURE 4.2.5b Corneal pannus formation in trachoma.

4.2.6 Chlamydia/Adult Inclusion Conjunctivitis—a chronic follicular conjunctivitis caused by *C. trachomatis* serotypes d to k; usually sexually transmitted.

Presentation chronic, bilateral, red, irritated eyes; follicular conjunctival reaction, preauricular lymph node, corneal pannus or micropannus ($<$2 mm), peripheral or central subepithelial corneal infiltrates, mucoid discharge.

Differential Diagnosis other forms of chronic conjunctivitis (bacterial, toxic, al-

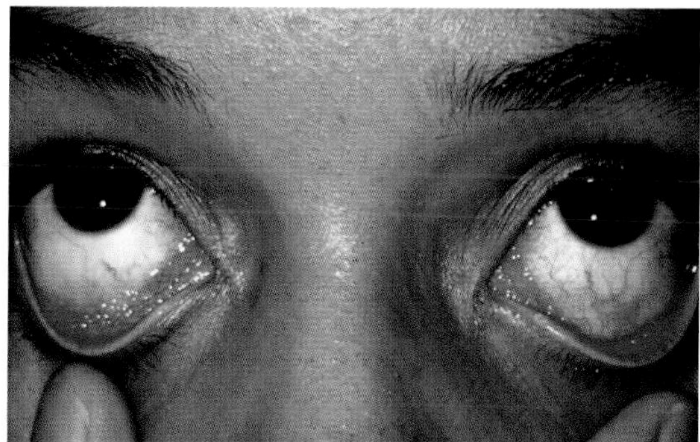

FIGURE 4.2.6 Prominent follicular reaction in adult inclusion conjunctivitis.

lergic). Of chronic follicular conjunctivitis: molluscum, drug induced, HSV (recurrent).

Management obtain history of vaginitis, cervicitis, urethritis, or possible exposure. Obtain conjunctival *Chlamydia* culture or DNA probe. Giemsa stain has macrophages with ingested debris, lymphocytes, and PMNs, basophilic intracytoplasmic inclusion bodies in epithelial cells. Treat both sexual partners concurrently with tetracycline or erythromycin (250 to 500 mg PO qid) or doxycycline (100 mg bid for 3 to 4 weeks). Consider topical erythromycin or tetracycline ointment bid–tid for 3 weeks.

4.2.7 Parinaud's Oculoglandular Syndrome—chronic granulomatous conjunctivitis with tender regional adenopathy, usually in children. The most common etiology is CSD (*Rickettsia, Rochalimaea henselae*). Others include tularemia and brucellosis.

Presentation painful adenopathy, usually a history of inoculation site and exposure to a cat; indolent and self-limited; granulomatous conjunctivitis.

Differential Diagnosis infectious mononucleosis, Kawasaki disease, infection with streptococci or staphylococci, mycobacterial infec-

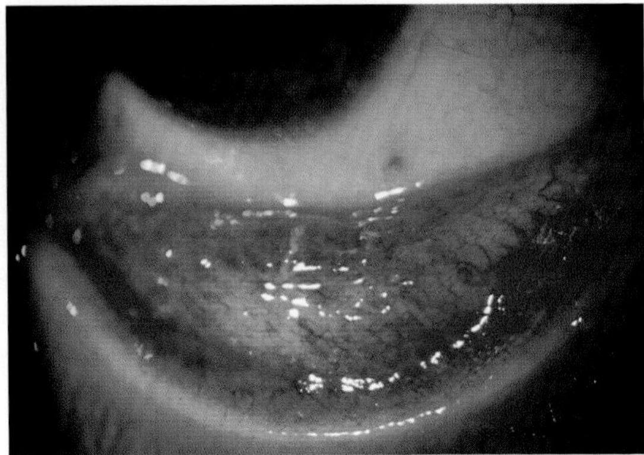

FIGURE 4.2.7 Conjuctival granuloma in tularemia.

tion. Of conjunctival granuloma: sarcoidosis, ocular rosacea, mycobacteria.

Management consider CSD skin test and/or workup for the aforementioned other causes of lymphadenopathy. Usually no treatment is necessary.

4.2.8 Molluscum Contagiosum Conjunctivitis—chronic conjunctivitis from toxic secretions of eyelid molluscum lesions due to a pox virus; spread by direct contact; increased incidence in AIDS.

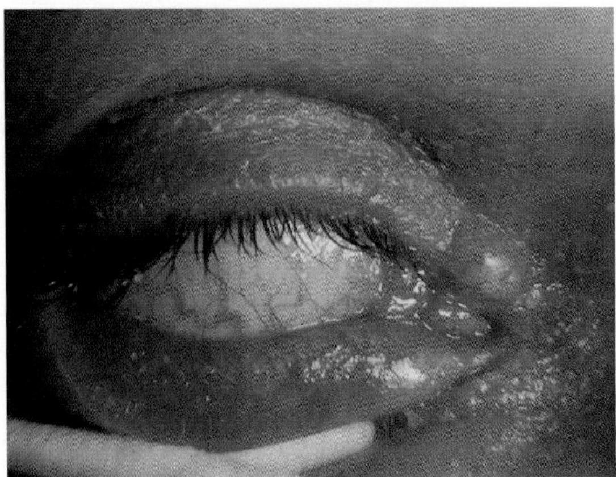

FIGURE 4.2.8 Molluscum conjunctivitis.

Presentation unilateral or bilateral chronically red, irritated eye; elevated, umbilicated, pearly nodules on eyelids, along with a follicular conjunctival reaction, superficial punctate keratitis, pannus.

Differential Diagnosis of chronic follicular conjunctivitis: molluscum, drug induced, HSV (recurrent).

Management excision, incision and curettage, or cryosurgery.

4.2.9 Allergic Conjunctivitis

4.2.9 Allergic Conjunctivitis—acute or chronic conjunctivitis due to IgE-mediated hypersensitivity reaction, usually to airborne or handborne allergens.

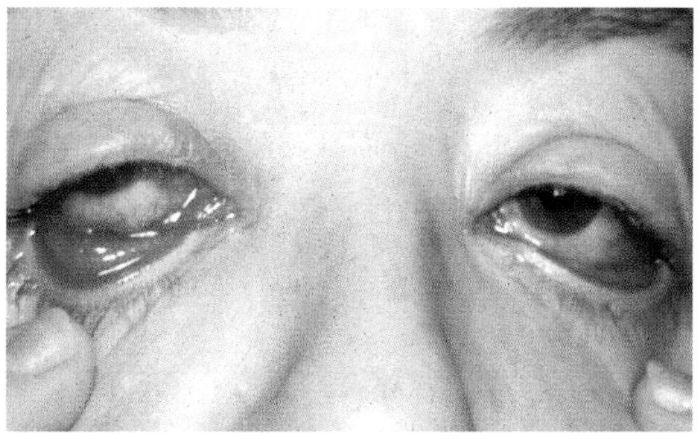

FIGURE 4.2.9 Acute allergic conjunctivitis.

Presentation itching, tearing, dry and sticky eyes. Findings are nonspecific and include lid swelling, conjunctival hyperemia, papillary reaction, chemosis, and ropy mucoid discharge. Other atopic conditions, such as rhinitis and asthma, are often present.

Differential Diagnosis bacterial, viral, or drug induced conjunctivitis; toxic, atopic.

Management usually a clinical diagnosis. A Wright's or Giemsa stain of conjunctival scraping confirms eosinophils. Treat with cold compresses; topical NSAIDs such as ketorolac (Acular qid) or mild steroids (fluoromethalone qid); topical vasoconstrictor–antihistamines (Naphcon or Vasocon A, or Livostin qid); oral antihistamines. Consider topical mast cell stabilizers (cromolyn or Alomide qid, Patanol bid), or hyposensitization injections if allergen is identified.

4.2.10 Vernal Conjunctivitis—moderate to severe seasonal inflammation in children and young adults.

Presentation typically a young male with itching, blepharospasm, photophobia, copious mucoid discharge, blurred vision, and red eyes. Slit-lamp examination shows a diffuse papillary hypertrophy on the palpebral conjunctiva (upper > lower), giant papillae, hyperemia, chemosis, thickened gelatinous limbal swelling (in black and Asian patients), superficial punctate keratitis, superior pannus, shield ulcer (epithelial ulcer with

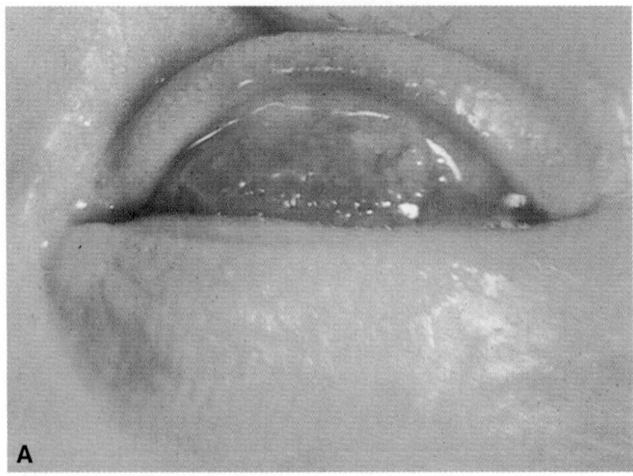

FIGURE 4.2.10a Diffuse papillary hypertrophy on the superior tarsus.

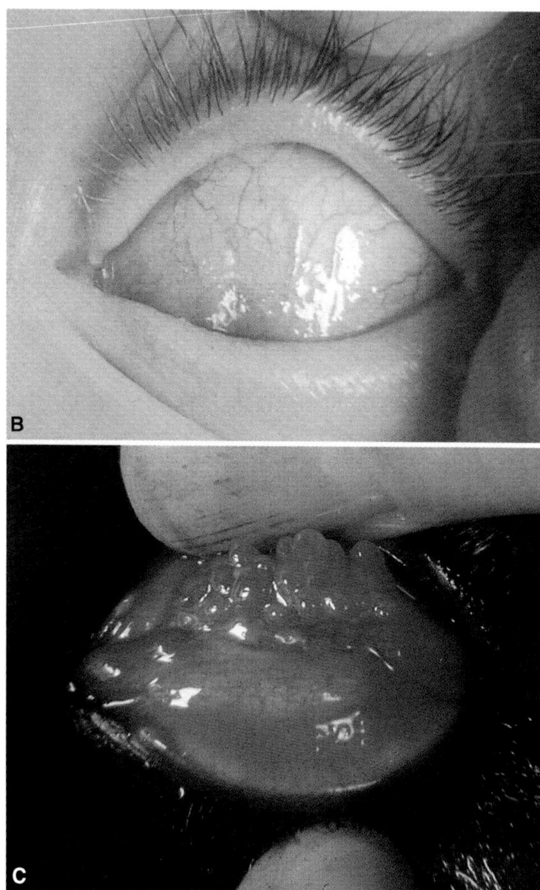

FIGURE 4.2.10b Horner-Trantas dots.
FIGURE 4.2.10c Giant papillary reaction of the superior tarsus.

underlying opacification), and Horner-Trantas dots (limbal or conjunctival eosinophil and epithelial cells).

Differential Diagnosis bacterial, viral, chlamydial, atopic conjunctivitis.

Management
- No shield ulcer: treat as described for allergic conjunctivitis; use of mast cell stabilizers and steroids is helpful.
- With shield ulcer: topical steroids 4 to 6 times a day with a prophylactic antibiotic and cycloplegic agent in addition to mast cell stabilizer and cool compresses.

4.2.11 Atopic Conjunctivitis—keratoconjunctivitis associated with atopic dermatitis.

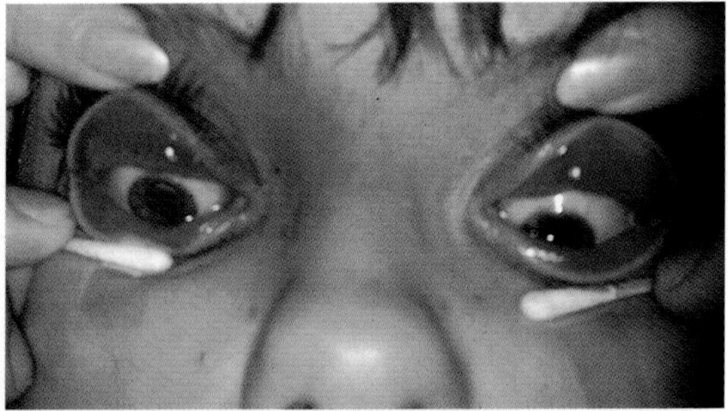

FIGURE 4.2.11 Smooth papillary reaction of the superior and inferior tarsal conjunctiva.

Presentation an atopic adult (multiple environmental allergies, asthma, allergic rhinitis, relapsing atopic dermatitis, family history of atopy) with chronic itchy, irritated eyes and acute flare-ups. Pruritus, photophobia, blurred vision, and tearing are common. Signs include relapsing dermatitis and extensor lichenification. Slit-lamp findings include a papillary reaction equally affecting upper and lower lid. Severe corneal vascularization, opacification, symblepharon, and a characteristic posterior or anterior subcapular cataract may develop.

Differential Diagnosis bacterial, viral, chlamydial, or vernal conjunctivitis; rosacea, trachoma, ocular cicatricial pemphigoid.

Management same as for vernal conjunctivitis but more need for and risk from topical steroids, because patients can be immunosuppressed and are susceptible to HSV infections, which are more commonly bilateral.

4.2.12 Giant Papillary Conjunctivitis—inflammation due to mechanical trauma or hypersensitivity due to contact lens wear (soft, 10%; rigid, 1%), prosthesis, exposed sutures.

Presentation contact lens intolerance, itching, mucoid discharge, blurred vision, lens decentration, ptosis. Slit-lamp examination shows hyperemia and large papillae (>0.3-mm diameter) on superior tarsal conjunctiva.

Management remove mechanical irritation (polish prosthesis and remove exposed sutures). Stop contact lens wear for at least 2 weeks or longer, depending on severity of disease. Consider refitting of contact lenses or daily wear lenses, disposable lenses, or RGP lenses if intolerant to soft disposable lenses. Also required is good lens hygiene with preservative-free solutions; perhaps topical steroids (for severe cases); Alomide qid, cromolyn sodium 4 to 6 times a day, or Patanol bid (for milder cases or for maintenance therapy).

4.2.13 Ligneous Conjunctivitis—rare, chronic membranous conjunctivitis of unknown etiology; possible association with β-hemolytic streptococci or a disorder of immune regulation (i.e., excessive T-helper cell response).

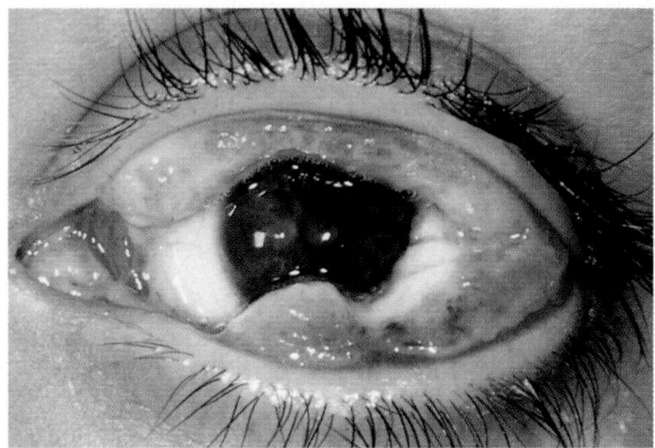

FIGURE 4.2.13 Cigneous conjunctivitis.

Presentation onset usually in children and young adults. A bilateral, abrupt development of fibrinous exudate accompanies other signs of conjunctivitis. Later, granulation tissue forms a thick, white, "woody" membrane, usually found on tarsal conjunctiva.

Differential Diagnosis other forms of conjunctivitis, especially streptococcal.

Management for workup, biopsy of membranes and any extraocular manifestations (buccal, nasopharynx, vaginal mucosal abnormalities) is usually diagnostic. No treatment is very effective. Surgical resection and frequent debridement increase comfort. Topical hyaluronidase, α-chymotrypsin, steroids, mucolytics, mitomycin C, and cyclosporine A have been used.

4.3 Cicatrizing Disorders

diseases causing conjunctival scarring.

4.3.1 Ocular Cicatricial Pemphigoid—a slowly progressive, chronic cicatrizing conjunctivitis. Etiology is idiopathic but possibly a type II hypersensitivity reaction.

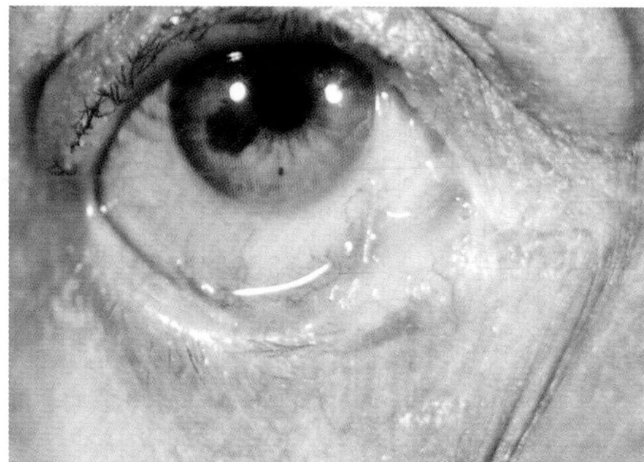

FIGURE 4.3.1 Stage 3 OCP with symblepharon.

Presentation usually in women over the age of 60 years; recurrent attacks of nonspecific conjunctival inflammation with mild redness, foreign-body sensation, tearing, photophobia; usually bilateral. There may be associated oral, pharyngeal, or vaginal or urethral mucosal lesions. Rarely, there is skin involvement. Palpebral conjunctival subepithelial fibrosis (stage 1), shortening of conjunctival fornices (stage 2), symblepharon, or palpebral–bulbar conjunctival adhesions (stage 3), and ankyloblepharon (stage 4). Other important findings are conjunctival bullae, entropion, trichiasis, tear-film abnormalities and corneal abrasions, vascularization, scarring, and ulceration.

Differential Diagnosis of cicatrizing disorders: Stevens-Johnson syndrome, chemical burn, post radiation, squamous cell carcinoma, postinfectious (trachoma, *C. diphtheriae,* streptococci, adenovirus); pseudopemphigoid (chronic topical medication use, such as pilocarpine, timolol, ecothiopate iodide, or epinephrine, reversible after discontinuation of drug).

Management for workup: conjunctival biopsy for direct immunofluorescence studies (C3, IgG, IgA, IgM on basement membrane). If negative and immunosuppressive therapy is necessary, consider rebiopsy for immunoperoxidase study. Treat with lubrication and aggressive blepharitis management. Treat trichiasis with lid rotation procedures, electrolysis, or cryodestruction.

- Dapsone: initial choice for mild cases; takes 5 weeks to have an effect; up to 80% response reported if the patient can tolerate 100 to 150 mg PO qid; side effect is hemolysis; avoid in sulfa allergies or G6PD deficiency.
- Cyclophosphamide: if dapsone is not effective or in conjunction with dapsone during initial 5 weeks while dapsone begins to take effect. (5 to 7 mg/kg, titrated for WBC count of about 3000 with careful monitoring).
- Steroids: prednisone (40 to 80 mg PO qd) to suppress acute exacerbations.
- Mucous membrane or limbal stem cell grafts: for forniceal or ocular surface rehabilitation.
- Keratoprosthesis: in end-stage eyes with good macular function.

4.3.2 Stevens-Johnson Syndrome—acute hypersensitivity reaction consisting of an inflammatory vesiculobullous reaction of the skin and mucous membranes. Immune complex deposition is incited by medications (sulfonamides, anticonvulsants, aspirin, penicillin, isoniazid, Diamox [acetazolamide], many more) and sometimes infectious organisms (HSV, streptococci, adenovirus, mycoplasma).

Presentation most common in children and young adults. An acute onset of fever, rash, and red eye with malaise, arthralgia, and respiratory symptoms is typical. Signs include "target" skin lesions, maculopapular or bullous skin lesions (commonly on hands and feet), severe mucosal lesions involving at least two sites (most commonly eyes and mouth), subsequent bulla with membrane or pseudomembrane formation and necrosis, mucopurulent conjunctivitis, symblepharon, trichiasis, tear-film abnormalities, corneal scarring, and/or ulceration. Mortality from the syndrome is about 20%.

Differential Diagnosis ocular cicatricial pemphigoid, Stevens-Johnson syndrome, chemical burn, after radiation, squamous cell carcinoma,

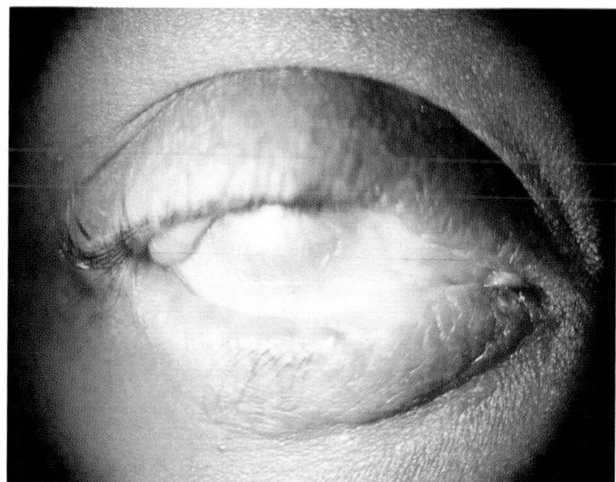

FIGURE 4.3.2 OSD in Stevens-Johnson Syndrome.

postinfectious (trachoma, *C. diphtheriae,* streptococci, adenovirus) pseudopemphigoid (chronic topical medication use such as pilocarpine, timolol, ecothiopate iodide, or epinephrine, reversible after discontinuation of drug).

Management supportive hospital therapy initially.

- Topical and systemic steroids, topical antibiotics, aggressive lubrication, cycloplegics.
- Surgical procedures for symblepharon, trichiasis; mucous membrane grafts and limbal stem cell transplant, and penetrating keratoplasty in stages after quiescence. Consider keratoprosthesis in end-stage eyes with visual potential.

4.4 Dry Eye Syndrome

an abnormality in the rate of production (<1.2 μl/min) or quality of the tear film. Etiology may be idiopathic, medications (antihistamines, β-blockers, anticholinergics, phenothiazines, psychotropics), lacrimal gland inflammation (sarcoid, mumps, HIV, Sjögren's syndrome), lacrimal gland dysfunction (congenital, traumatic, neuropathic), collagen

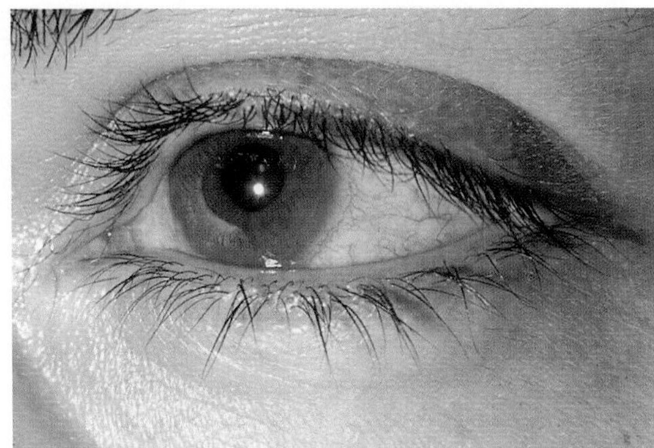

FIGURE 4.4 Conjunctival hyperemia.

vascular disease (rheumatoid arthritis, SLE), pemphigoid, chemical burns, vitamin-A deficiency, blepharitis.

Presentation symptoms include foreign-body sensation, tearing (increased reflex secretion), burning, blurry vision; often worse after prolonged use of eyes, at the end of the day, and in cold weather. Signs include decreased tear meniscus height, PEK, filaments, bulbar conjunctival staining in exposure palpebral fissure zone, conjunctival hyperemia, papillary hypertrophy, fluorescein tear-film breakup time less than 10 seconds.

Differential Diagnosis conjunctivitis, blepharitis, exposure keratopathy.

Management

- Schirmer's test: Anesthetize the eye and absorb excess tears and anesthetic with a cotton swab. Place filter paper strips in the outer lower fornix and wait 5 minutes. Wetting of < 5 mm is highly suggestive of Sjögren's syndrome. Less than 10 mm indicates dry eye but is neither highly sensitive nor specific.
- Stain ocular surface with fluorescein, rose begal, or lissamine green dyes.
- Treat stepwise with preservative-free artificial tears and lubricants, punctal occlusion (temporary or permanent

plugs, argon laser, thermal cautery), moist chamber spectacles and humidification of ambient environment, tarsorraphy (temporary or permanent suturing of the eyelids).

4.5 Vitamin A Deficiency

xerosis (dryness of conjunctiva) related to malnutrition, decreased intake, or decreased absorption (cystic fibrosis, pancreatitis, after gastrectomy, after intestinal bypass surgery, chronic liver disease).

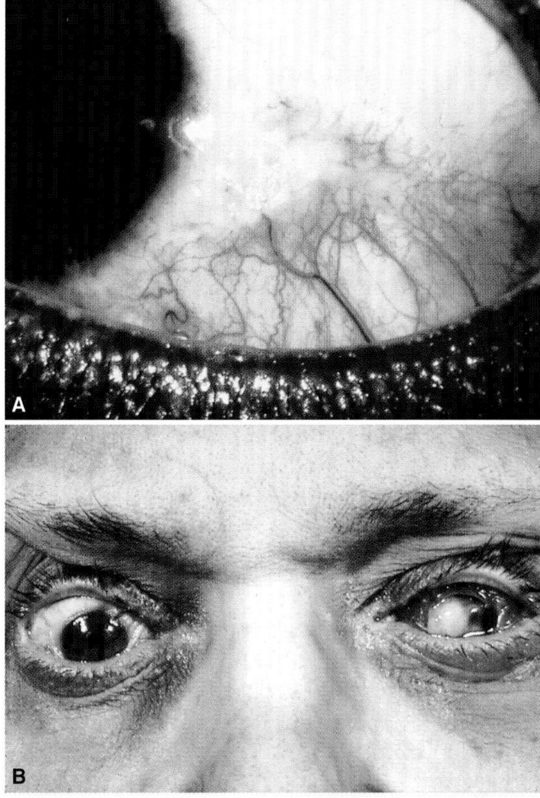

FIGURE 4.5a Bitot's spot.
FIGURE 4.5b Xerophthalmia secondary to vitamin A deficiency.

Presentation foreign-body sensation, ocular pain, night blindness. Bitot's spots (superficial, foamy, gray area on bulbar conjunctiva consisting of keratinized epithelial and inflammatory cells), tear-film abnormalities, corneal ulcers, scars, and eventually necrosis are seen.

Differential Diagnosis other causes of dry eye syndrome; pingueculum.

Management for workup, determine the serum vitamin-A level, dark adapted ERG. Treat with vitamin-A replacement (PO or IM and topical), lubrication.

4.6 Pingueculum or Pterygium

a pingueculum is an elastoic degenerative lesion of bulbar conjunctiva. A pterygium is a wing-shaped fold of conjunctiva and fibrovascular tissue invading the superficial cornea, sometimes produced by pinguecula. The cause may be actinic exposure; exposure to wind, dust, and other irritants; chronic dryness; inflammation.

Presentation patients are usually asymptomatic but may complain of redness and irritation or interference with contact lens wear.

- Pingueculum: yellow-white, amorphous subepithelial deposits at the limbus in the interpalpebral zone, usually nasal. May slowly enlarge with time.
- Pterygium: fibrovascular growth into the anterior cornea; pigmented iron line (Stocker's line) or dellen at advancing edge. Pterygium may induce astigmatism (classically against the rule).

Differential Diagnosis conjunctival intruepithelial neoplasia, dermoid, pannus

Management for workup, measure corneal involvement to document advancing pterygium, careful refraction and keratometry or computerized corneal topography. Treat with UV sun-

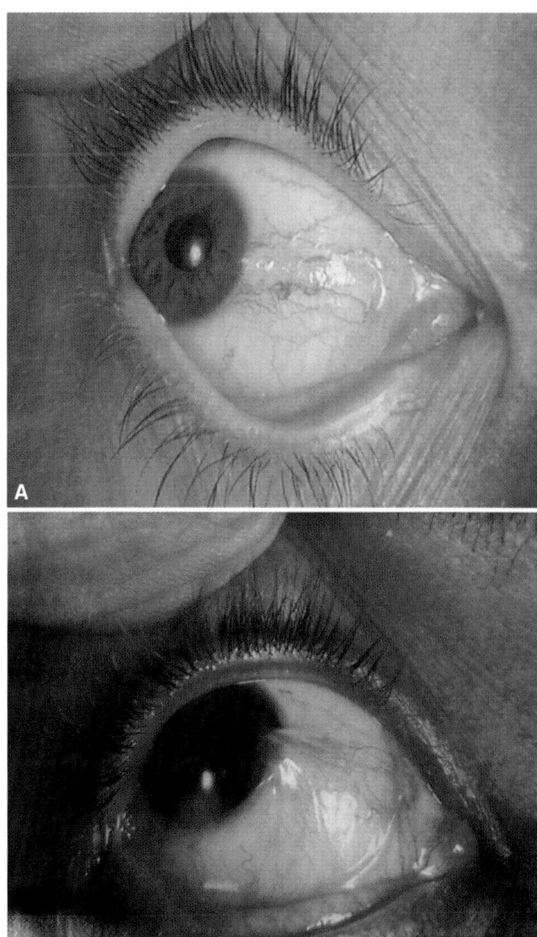

FIGURE 4.6a Nasal pingueculum.
FIGURE 4.6b Nasal pterygium.

glasses to protect eyes from wind and sun; lubrication, vasoconstrictors, topical NSAIDs or mild steroids (taper according to symptoms). Surgical removal is indicated if the lesion is interfering with contact lens wear, severe inflammation is not responding to medical therapy, or pterygium is threatening the visual axis. Adjunctive conjunctival autograft or mitomycin C reduces the recurrence rate from 40% to approximately 5%.

4.7 Phlyctenule

a lymphocytic inflammatory nodule located on the limbus, cornea, or bulbar conjunctiva caused by a type IV hypersensitivity reaction usually to staphylococcal antigen. Other associations are TB, HSV, ocular rosacea, extraocular candida infections, and lymphogranulum venereum.

Presentation pronounced photophobia, tearing, and irritation. Signs include the following:

- Conjunctival: focal, round or triangular, elevated small white nodule in center of hyperemic area.
- Corneal: white nodule at the limbus; may grow toward central cornea, producing wedge-shaped corneal pannus and leading edge ulceration and scarring. All lesions initially have intact overlying epithelium that ulcerates after 2 to 3 days.

Differential Diagnosis inflamed pingueculum, corneal ulcer, interstitial keratitis.

Management work up for signs of blepharitis, rosacea, and HSV. Obtain history for TB. Consider PPD and/or chest radiography. Treatment is indicated only if symptomatic. Topical steroids are usually very effective (taper according to symptoms); lid hygiene, lubrication, antibiotic ointment; doxycycline (100 mg bid) if severe blepharitis is present. Refer to internist if PPD or chest radiography is positive. Treat central corneal scarring with PK, manual keratectomy, excimer laser keratectomy.

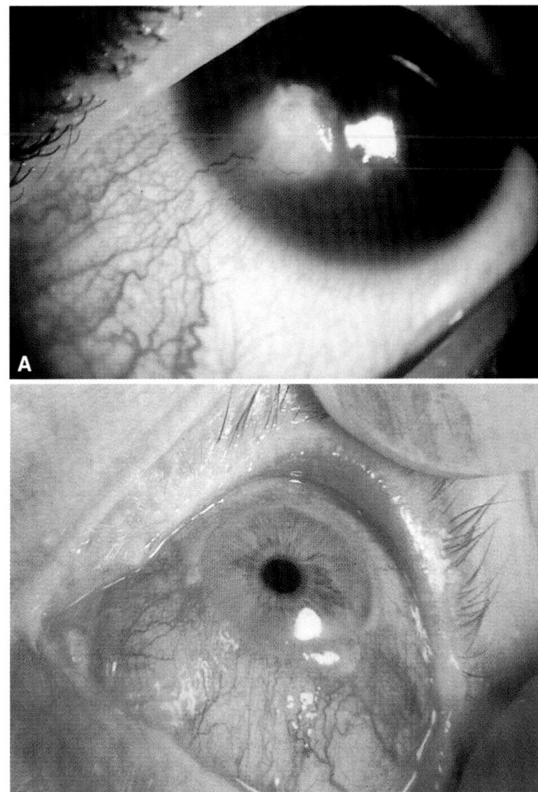

FIGURE 4.7a Cornea phylctenule in HSV.
FIGURE 4.7b Conjunctival and limbal phlyctenule secondary to staphylococcus.

4.8 Superior Limbic Keratoconjunctivitis (SLK)

chronic, recurrent irritation more common in adult women; idiopathic, but associated with thyroid dysfunction in approximately 50% of cases.

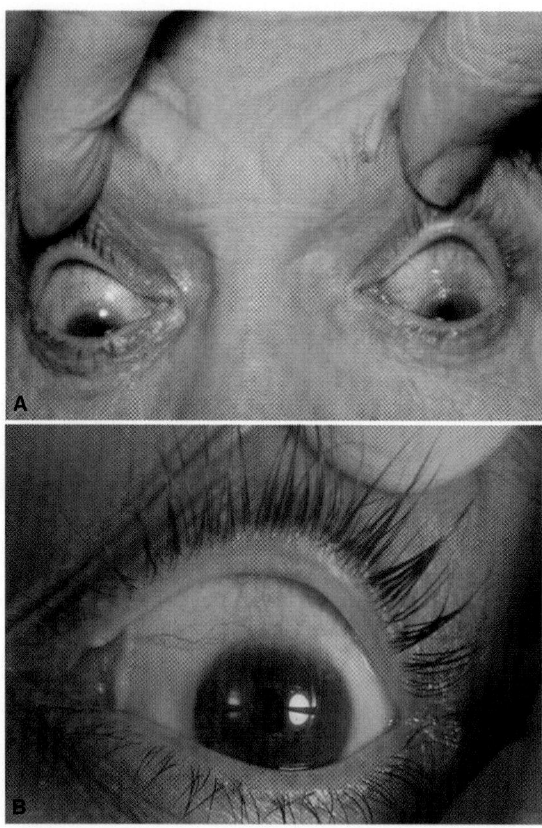

FIGURE 4.8a Superior conjunctival injection in SLK.
FIGURE 4.8b Superior conjunctival thickening in SLK.

Presentation

recurrent irritation, redness. There is a papillary conjunctivitis of superior tarsal conjunctiva. Injection, thickening, redundancy, and fine punctate staining of superior bulbar conjunctiva are present. PEK of superior cornea is seen with fluorescein and rose bengal. Filamentary keratitis and tear-film abnormalities are common.

Differential Diagnosis dry eye syndrome, atopic, other forms of conjunctivitis.

Management perform thyroid function tests (50% of patients have associated thyroid disease). Treat with lubrication (artificial tears 4 to 8 times a day, lubricating ointment qhs); silver nitrate 0.5 to 1% solution (from wax ampules) on a cotton swab applied to the superior tarsal and bulbar conjunctiva, either irrigated out after 60 seconds or not if stronger effect desired. Consider mechanical scraping, cryotherapy, cautery, or surgical resection of superior bulbar conjunctiva. Consider acetylcysteine (Mucomyst 10%) 3 to 5 times a day (for significant filaments) and a large-diameter therapeutic contact lens.

4.9 Episcleritis

self-limited inflammation of the episclera generally not associated with systemic disease; usually idiopathic, but may rarely be associated with gout, previous HZV, or collagen vascular disease.

Presentation red eye with minimal or no irritation; may be recurrent; inflamed episcleral vessels (straight, radiate posteriorly from the limbus, can be moved with a cotton-tip applicator over sclera and will blanch with phenylephrine 2.5 to 10%). Inflammation is localized to one sector (70%) or diffuse (30%). A mobile nodule may develop (nodular episcleritis). No aqueous cells or flare are present.

Differential Diagnosis scleritis, conjunctivitis, foreign body.

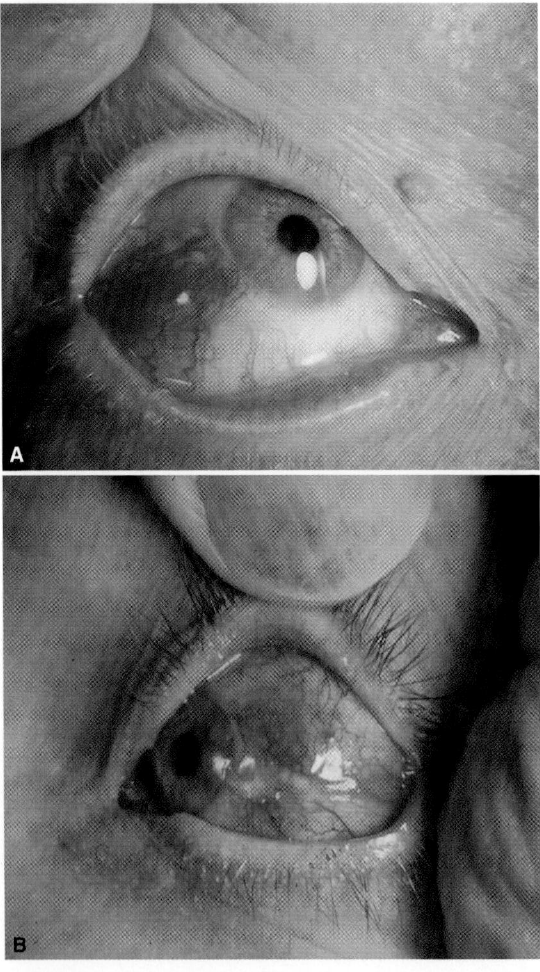

FIGURE 4.9a Nodular episcleritis.
FIGURE 4.9b Diffuse episcleritis.

Management

will spontaneously resolve. If symptomatic, treat with lubrication, topical NSAIDs (Acular qid), or oral NSAID (ibuprofen, 200 to 600 mg tid; Indocin [indomethacin], 25 mg tid) or mild topical steroids (fluoromethalone) for discomfort. Vasoconstrictors for short-term cosmesis.

4.10 Scleritis

inflammation of the sclera associated with underlying systemic autoimmune disease more than 50% of the time; more common in women.

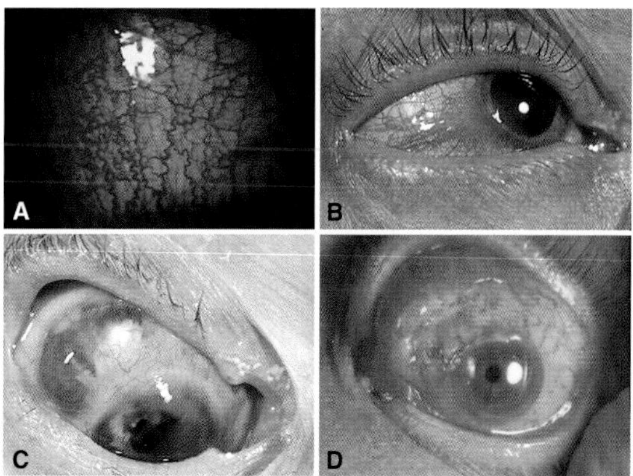

FIGURE 4.10a Diffuse anterior scleritis.
FIGURE 4.10b Nodular anterior scleritis.
FIGURE 4.10c Scleromalacial perforans.
FIGURE 4.10d Necrotizing inflammatory scleritis.

Presentation

ocular pain (worse at night), photophobia, pain on eye movements. Signs include a violaceous hue to sclera, inflamed scleral vessels (crisscrossing, nonmobile vessels), do not blanch with phenylepherine 2.5 to 10%; scleral edema by slit lamp, scleral ischemia. Concurrent keratitis and iritis with complications (cataract, synechiae, glaucoma) may be present.

- Nodular anterior (44%): deep red or purple immobile nodule; may be multiple
- Diffuse anterior (40%): most benign course; 30% of patients have underlying systemic disease.
- Necrotizing inflammatory (10%): most destructive; high association with systemic disease and increased mortal-

ity if untreated. Thin, transparent sclera may be seen (choroid visible). Perforation may occur.
- Necrotizing noninflammatory (scleromalacia perforans) (4%): usually associated with RA (55%), usually few to no symptoms, transparent sclera, rarely perforates.
- Posterior (2%): mild proptosis, visual loss, choroidal thickening, folds, retinal detachment, papilledema, restricted extraocular movements, usually unrelated to systemic disease.

For workup, check for underlying infection (syphilis, tuberculosis, HZV).

- Underlying collagen vascular disease: rheumatoid arthritis, lupus, ankylosing spondylitis, Wegener's granulomatosis, polyarteritis nodosa.
- Underlying metabolic disease: gout.
- Recommended tests: CBC, ESR, ANA, ANCA, RF, urinalysis, uric acid, FTA/VDRL, PPD, CXR, B-scan to check for posterior extension.

Differential Diagnosis

episcleritis, choroiditis, uveal effusion syndrome, endophthalmitis, orbital cellulitus, trauma, orbital pseudotumor, uveitis conjunctivitis.

Management

treatment includes the following:

- Mild or moderate scleritis: oral NSAIDs (ibuprofen, 400 to 600 mg tid–qid) or oral steroids (prednisone, 60 to 80 mg qd). Taper according to symptoms or inflammation. Topical steroids may help, especially if iritis is present.
- Severe or necrotizing keratitis or sclerokeratitis: PO or IV steroids. May require systemic immunosuppressives (i.e., methotrexate, cyclophosphamide, cyclosporin A).
- Scleromalacia perforans: no ocular treatment is available. Refer to a rheumatologist for control of systemic disease. Consider eye shield with significant risk of perforation with minor trauma. Subconjunctival steroid in-

jections and topical steroids are contraindicated due to risk of perforation if thinning is present or suspected.

4.11 Dilated Episcleral Vessels

See Section 3.3.6, Carotid Cavernous Fistula.

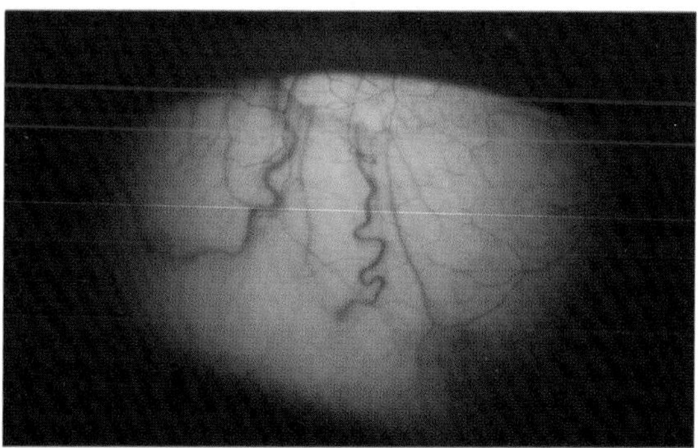

FIGURE 4.11 Dilated episcleral vessels.

4.12 Pigmented Conjunctival Lesions

4.12.1 Ocular or Oculodermal Melanocytosis (Congenital Melanosisi Oculi)—congenital blue nevus of episcleral and sclera.

Presentation multiple slate-gray patches on sclera, episclera, and deep conjunctiva. May be associated with periocular cutaneous melanosis, called nevus of Ota or oculodermal melanocytosis. Darker ipsilateral iris and choroid are present; rare malignant transformation in white patients; glaucoma (10%).

Differential Diagnosis racial pigmentation, primary acquired melanosis, nevus, malignant melanoma.

Management biopsy if the diagnosis is uncertain. Follow the size of the nevus. Perform a fundus examination for malignant transformation. Monitor for glaucoma.

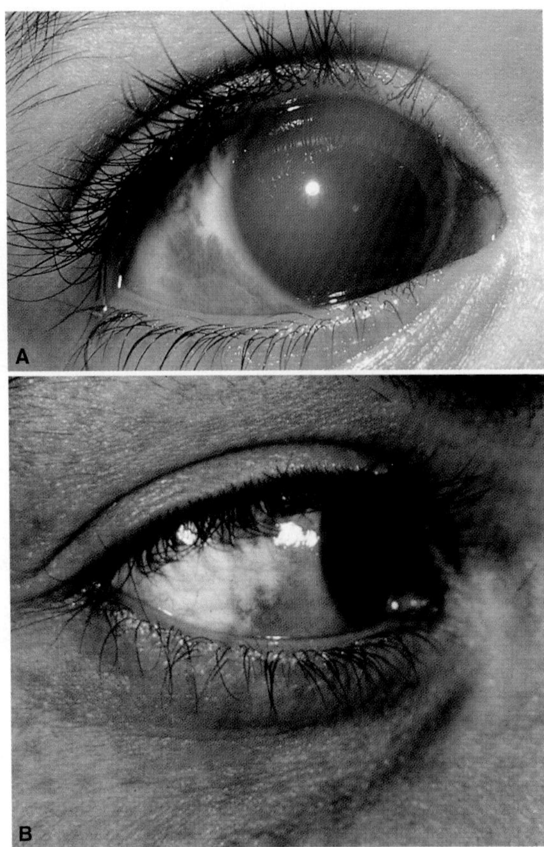

FIGURE 4.12.1a Ocular melanocytosis.
FIGURE 4.12.1b Oculordermal melanocytosis.

4.12.2 Primary Acquired Melanosis—proliferation of intraepithelial melanocytes in conjunctiva of middle-aged white patients.

Presentation multiple flat, brown intermittently changing patches of unilateral pigmentation within the superficial conjunctiva; 20 to 30% of patients develop malignant melanoma (40% mortality rate).

Differential Diagnosis racial melanosis, secondary acquired melanosis (caused by Addison's disease, radiation, pregnancy), malignant melanoma.

Management careful observation, photographic comparison; careful map biopsy, repeated when changes occur; surgical excision of any pathologically atypical lesions.

4.12.3 Racial Pigmentation—perilimbal benign pigmentation developing after birth in dark-skinned individuals.

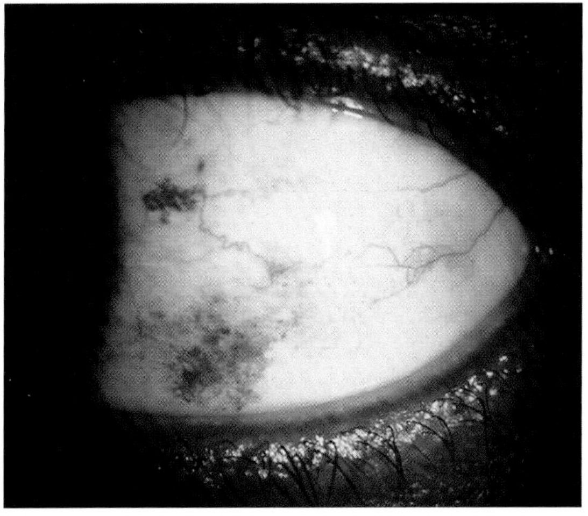

FIGURE 4.12.3 Perilimbal benign pigmentation.

Differential Diagnosis primary acquired melanosis, conjunctival melanoma or nevus.

Management there is no treatment.

4.12.4 Conjunctival Nevus—congenital overgrowth of epithelial pigment that commonly develops during puberty.

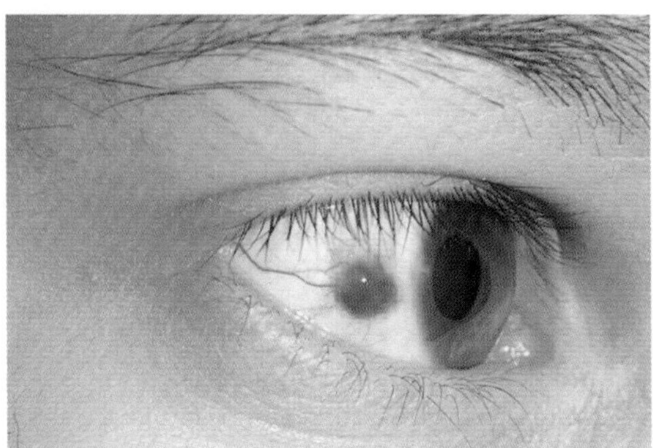

FIGURE 4.12.4 Suspicious conjunctival nevus.

Presentation well-demarcated, pigmented conjunctival lesion (usually bulbar, palpebral), which may contain small cysts; rare malignant potential, but when they do progress there is about a 20% mortality rate.

Differential Diagnosis primary acquired melanosis, malignant melanoma, racial pigmentation.

Management careful observation, photographic comparison; biopsy if growing or atypical appearance. Treatment includes a baseline photograph, follow-up of 4 to 6 months, and elective excision.

4.12.5 Adenochrome Deposits—pigmentation secondary to chronic epinephrine compound use.

Presentation dark brown to black deposits, usually in the inferior conjunctiva; usually in glaucoma patients using epinephrine or dipivefrin.

Differential Diagnosis primary acquired melanosis, malignant melanoma, racial pigmentation, cosmetic pigments.

Management may discontinue medication is cosmesis is affected.

4.12.6 Malignant Melanoma of Conjunctiva—malignant tumor of the conjunctiva. About one-third arise from nevi, one-third arise from primary acquired melanosis, and one-third arise de novo (mortality rate, about 40%).

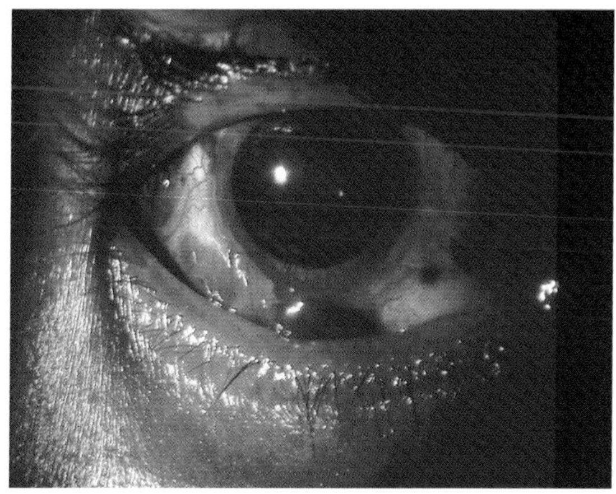

FIGURE 4.12.6 Conjunctival melanoma.

Presentation usually a bulbar or inferior palpebral conjunctival, variably pigmented lesion, which is usually elevated or nodular. Sentinel blood vessels are common. Extension may occur into the globe.

Differential Diagnosis primary acquired melanosis, conjunctival nevus, racial pigmentation, iris or ciliary body melanoma with extension outside of the globe.

Management any suspicious lesions should be biopsied. Treat with complete excision with adjunctive cryotherapy or β-irradiation. With local invasion, enucleation or evisceration may be necessary.

Chapter 5
CORNEA

Gavin Bahadur, Suresh Mandava,
Eric E. Donnenfeld, Richard P. Gibralter

5.1 Cornea Infections

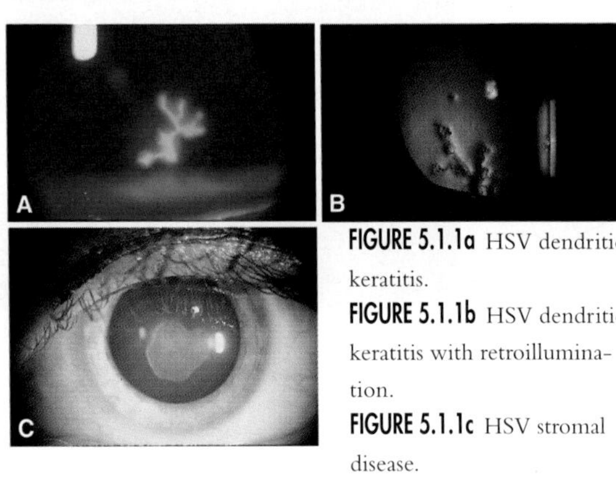

FIGURE 5.1.1a HSV dendritic keratitis.
FIGURE 5.1.1b HSV dendritic keratitis with retroillumination.
FIGURE 5.1.1c HSV stromal disease.

5.1.1 Herpes Simplex Virus

5.1.1 Herpes Simplex Virus—a virus that may cause primary systemic infection with ocular involvement or recurrent ocular involvement due to latent infection. HSV infection may manifest a variety of corneal findings.

Presentation

- *Primary disease:* viral prodrome with fever, URI, and possible follicular conjunctivitis, preauricular node, and cutaneous vesicles on eyelids, rarely with corneal epithelial punctate lesions or dendrites.
- *Recurrent disease:* many manifestations; recurrences may vary in presentation.
  Iridocyclitis: see Section 6.2.2.

Blepharitis: vesicular lesions with erythema and ulceration on eyelid margins (see Section 4.1).

Conjunctivitis: recurrent, unilateral follicular conjunctivitis, frequently with corneal involvement (see Section 4.2).

Epithelial infectious keratitis: dendritic or geographic ulcers presenting with pain, photophobia, tearing, redness, and blurry vision. Dendrites are true ulcers that are thin and branching with terminal bulbs and swollen borders. Fluorescein stains centrally, and rose bengal stains at the edges. Geographic ulcers are similar to dendrites but are larger, widened lesions.

Marginal ulcer: perilimbal epithelial lesion and infiltrate with pannus and thinning. More severe pain and chronic symptoms are typical.

Neurotrophic ulcer: a persistent epithelial defect caused by impaired corneal innervation. Smooth, rolled borders distinguish neurotrophic from geographic ulcers.

Necrotizing stromal keratitis: direct viral stromal infection causing necrosis, an epithelial defect, and a dense infiltrate.

Immune stromal (or interstitial) keratitis: blurry vision due to hazy stromal infiltrate, scarring, and thinning, with later neovascularization and lipid deposits. Epithelium is usually intact.

Endotheliitis: focal or "disciform" stromal edema with underlying endothelial KP and anterior chamber cells.

Differential Diagnosis

- Epithelial disease: HZV, healing recurrent erosions or other corneal abrasions including post-PRK, pseudodendrites secondary to contact lens wear, preservatives in ophthalmic preparations, or *Acanthamoeba* infection.
- Marginal ulcer: staphylococcal marginal disease, peripheral melt associated with collagen vascular disease, Mooren's ulcer.

- Neurotrophic ulcer: see Section 5.5 on neurotrophic ulcer.
- Stromal disease: acute bacterial or other corneal ulcers.

Management diagnosis is usually clinical. Consider scrapings of corneal or skin lesions for Giemsa stain and Papanicolaou smear. Consider viral cultures or fluorescent antigen studies when the diagnosis is uncertain.

- Epithelial disease: debridement of involved epithelium. Trifluridine 1% (Viroptic) drops 9 times daily. May substitute oral antiviral (valcyclovir, 500 bid). Consider long-term prophylactic (e.g., valcyclovir, 500 qd). Cycloplegic agent. Avoid topical steroids.
- Neurotrophic keratopathy: nonpreserved lubricant drops and ointments. Consider erythromycin ointment qhs and possibly pressure patching. Tarsorrhaphy frequently heals persistent epithelial defects. Severe corneal thinning may require hospitalization and ultimately patch grafting, or lamellar or penetrating keratoplasty. If chances of visual rehabilitation are poor, consider conjunctival flap.
- Immune stromal disease: for moderate to severe inflammation with symptoms and decreased visual acuity, corticosteroids are indicated. Prednisolone acetate 1% dosage is tailored to the patient and tapered slowly with close follow-up until a minimum "flare" dosage is achieved. Oral steroids are indicated for severe cases. Prophylactic trifluridine 1% is sometimes matched drop for drop with steroid above qd dosage. A suppression dosage of oral antiviral (i.e., valcyclovir, 500 qd) avoids corneal toxicity and is useful for long-term prophylaxis.

5.1.2 Herpes Zoster Virus

5.1.2 Herpes Zoster Virus—varicella-zoster viral infection of the cornea generally occurs as a reactivation of latent virus but does not recur like HSV. Primary infection is chicken-pox and may have a nonspecific follicular conjunctivitis and rare corneal vesicles.

Presentation vesicular skin lesions in a cranial nerve V ophthalmic dermatomal distribution generally preceding complaints of

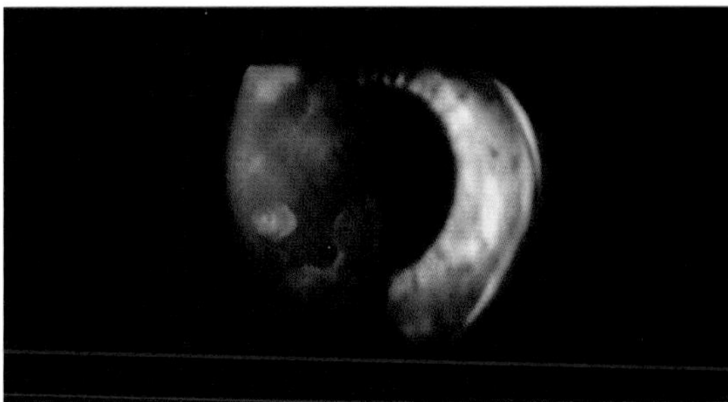

FIGURE 5.1.2 HZV keratitis.

blurry vision, eye pain, and redness. Corneal lesions may consist of punctate epithelial keratitis, or ulcers, generally associated with severe neurotrophic disease. Involvement of the tip of the nose is often associated with corneal involvement and is termed Hutchinson's sign. Other corneal signs include corneal mucous plaques and pseudodendrites, anterior stromal infiltrates, and an immune stromal keratitis.

Differential Diagnosis

HSV (pseudodendrites are broader than dendrites, "stuck-on" appearance, no ulceration, less fluorescein uptake, and no terminal end-bulbs), bacterial or fungal keratitis, immunologic or inflammatory ulcers.

Management

diagnosis is usually clinical, but a Tzanck type smear may be performed. For greatest effect, treatment should be initiated within 3 days of onset: valcyclovir 1000 mg tid (adjust for renal insufficiency) or acyclovir, 800 mg, PO 5 times daily for 7 to 10 days; broad-spectrum topical antibiotics to skin lesions. Severely immunocompromised individuals are at risk for disseminated or severe ocular complications and should receive acyclovir, 15 to 30 mg/kg/day IV. Topical steroids are used for uveitis or immune stromal keratitis.

5.1.3 Epstein Barr Virus—herpesvirus infection generally transmitted via saliva, which may cause epithelial keratitis or multifocal stromal keratitis.

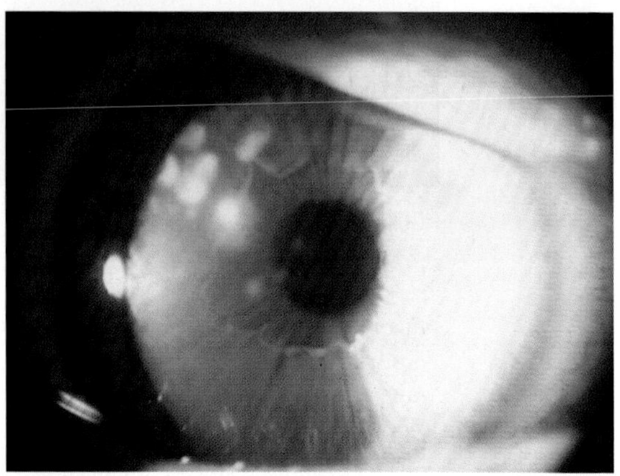

FIGURE 5.1.3 EBV keratitis.

Presentation pain, redness, decreased vision. Findings may include epithelial keratitis or multifocal nummular stromal opacities (larger and more coarse than those seen in EKC).

Differential Diagnosis EKC, HSV, HZV, sarcoidosis, contact lens hypersensitivity, *Acanthamoeba*.

Management consider IgG and IgM antibodies to viral capsid and nuclear antigens for diagnosis. Supportive treatment consists of lubrication and topical erythromycin ointment for epithelial keratitis. Chronic subepithelial infiltrates may respond to corticosteroids.

5.1.4 Bacterial Corneal Ulcer—an infectious infiltrate of the corneal stroma. Common bacterial causes include *Staphylococcus aureus, Staphylococcus epidermidis, Streptococcus pneumoniae,* other streptococci, *Pseudomonas aeruginosa* (most common etiology in soft contact-lens wearers), *Proteus, Enterobacter, Serratia,* and others. Less commonly, *Neisseria,*

Moraxella, Mycobacterium, Nocardia, non–spore-forming anaerobes, and *Corynebacterium* are involved.

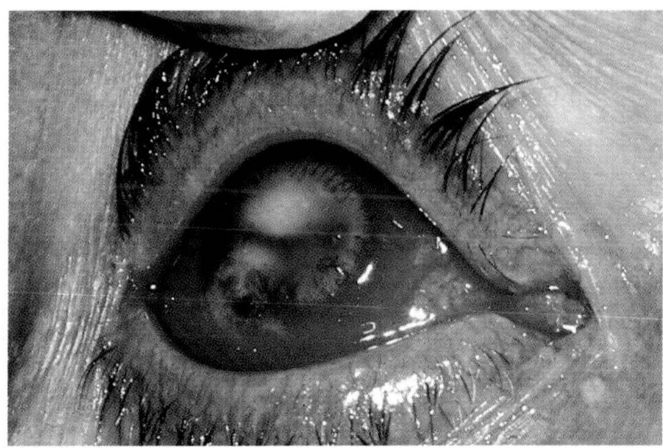

FIGURE 5.1.4 Bacterial ulcer with perforation.

Presentation

pain, redness, photophobia, decreased vision, discharge, tearing. Focal white opacity (infiltrate) of the corneal stroma with varying degrees of thinning and/or edema, overlying epithelial defect that stains with fluorescein, surrounding superficial punctate keratitis, Descemet's folds, conjunctival injection, mucopurulent discharge, anterior chamber reaction with hypopyon in severe cases, posterior synechiae, increased intraocular pressure, upper eyelid edema, and less commonly hyphema and corneal perforation.

Differential Diagnosis

fungal keratitis (usually after post-traumatic injury with tree branch or other vegetable matter, or in chronic corneal disease), *Acanthamoeba* keratitis, viral infection (HSV), atypical mycobacteria infection (penetrating injuries or in corneal grafts), staphylococcal marginal disease, sterile ulcer, (collagen vascular disease, Mooren's ulcer, neutrophic ulcer vernal conjunctivitis, vitamin-A deficiency), immune infiltrates (EKC, Wesseley ring).

Management

- Investigate history of contact lens wear (poor lens hygiene, overnight wear), corneal injury or foreign body, exposure keratitis, previous corneal disease, or systemic illness. Document location and size of infiltrate(s) and overlying epithelial defect, degree of anterior chamber reaction, and intraocular pressure. Corneal scrapings for culture on a variety of media and Gram's stain (see Section 18.11 for procedure). Also consider culturing current contact lenses, lens cases, solutions, or eyedrops.

- Corneal ulcers should be treated as bacterial initially unless a high index of suspicion of another cause exists. Monotherapy with a fluoroquinolone (ciprofloxacin, ofloxacin 0.3% every 5 minutes for 2 doses, and then every half-hour with at least two doses overnight) is becoming more accepted, especially in small, peripheral ulcers and with mild anterior chamber reaction. Fortified antibiotics are the mainstay of therapy and are indicated for larger ulcers, central location, exuberant anterior chamber reaction, or severe purulent discharge: fortified cefazolin (50 mg/ml) (may substitute vancomycin [33 mg/ml] in penicillin allergy) and tobramycin (15 mg/ml) or a fluoroquinolone. Load with one drop of each every 15 minutes for the first 2 hours and then alternate every half-hour (including overnight) until clinical or symptomatic improvement is seen on daily follow-up, and then taper.
- Cycloplegic (homatropine 2% bid to tid) for pain, photophobia, and prevention of posterior synechiae.
- Discontinue contact lenses until resolution. Hospitalize patients unable to comply, with impending or true perforations, or with suspected gonococcal infection.

5.1.5 Acanthamoeba

5.1.5 Acanthamoeba—corneal infection by an ubiquitous amoebic parasite associated with poor contact lens hygiene, the use of homemade saline solutions, or exposure to stagnant water (e.g., lakes, pools, hot tubs).

Presentation marked pain (although cornea may be anesthetic), redness, tearing, photophobia, blurry vision, often over the course of weeks. Findings include epithelial keratitis, subepithelial infiltrates, radial corneal perineuritis, pseudodendrites; ring infiltrate in stroma late in disease course.

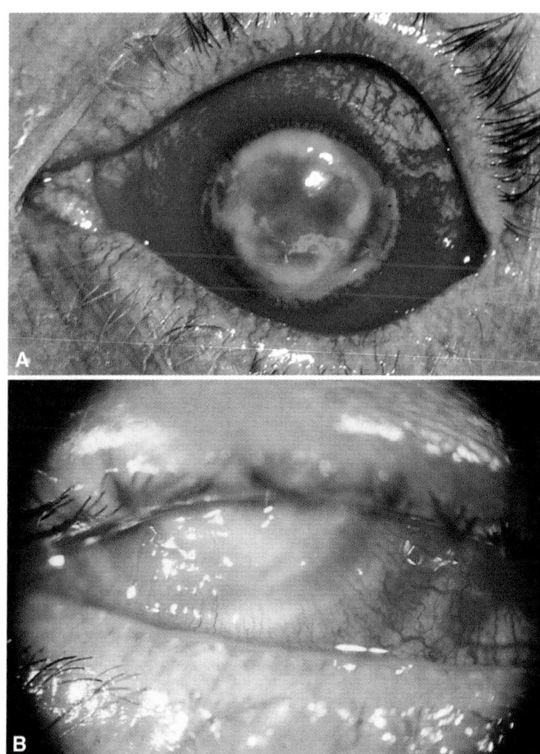

FIGURE 5.1.5a *Acanthamoeba* ulcer.
FIGURE 5.1.5b Advanced keratitis with neovascularization.

Differential Diagnosis

HSV, bacterial keratitis, fungal keratitis, immune ulcer.

Management

- Corneal scraping (or biopsy) for Calcofluor white, Giemsa, and Gram's stains; culture on nonnutrient agar with overlay of *Escherichia coli*.
- Discontinue contact lens use.
- Treatment options are many and are used in combination: PHMB 0.02%, propamidine isothionate 0.1% (Brolene solution, also ointment) and neomycin–polymyxin B–gramicidin (Neosporin), one drop every 30 minutes to 2 hours over the first week. Clotrimazole 1%, micona-

zole or ketoconazole drops, and oral fluconazole (200 to 400 mg PO qd) have also been used with some success. Some patients may need pain management and therapeutic penetrating keratoplasty.

5.1.6 Fungal Keratitis

5.1.6 Fungal Keratitis—fungal infection affecting corneal epithelium and stroma, usually from plant or soil source, or in chronic corneal disease with corticosteroid use.

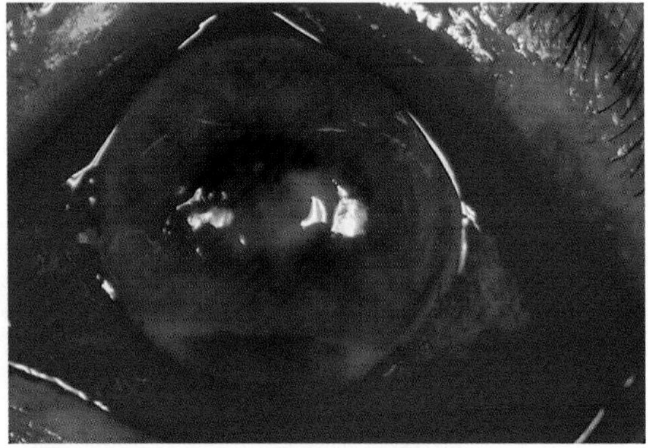

FIGURE 5.1.6 *Fusarium* ulcer with hypopyon and hyphema.

Presentation eye pain, redness, tearing, photophobia, blurred vision, discharge. Light gray-white stromal opacity with feathered margins and epithelial defect may be present. Satellite lesions are often seen along with anterior uveitis, endothelial plaque, and hypopyon.

Differential Diagnosis see Section 5.1.4 on bacterial, viral (HSV), or *Acanthamoeba* corneal ulcer.

Management

- Giemsa, PAS, or GMS stains of corneal scraping at base of infiltrate. Consider corneal biopsy.
- Mechanical debridement daily.
- Infectious corneal ulcers should be treated as bacterial until proved otherwise. Treat with natamycin 5% drops

q 1 to 2h and/or consider amphotericin B 0.1 to 0.15% qh. Fluconazole or itraconazole (200 mg qd) is useful. Add a cycloplegic agent. Avoid steroids and patching. Patients may require admission for close follow-up and medications.

5.2 Corneal Inflammation and Surface Disorders

5.2.1 Interstitial Keratitis—a group of inflammatory disorders of the corneal stroma, may be acute or may show signs of scarring from old disease, classically caused by congenital syphilis.

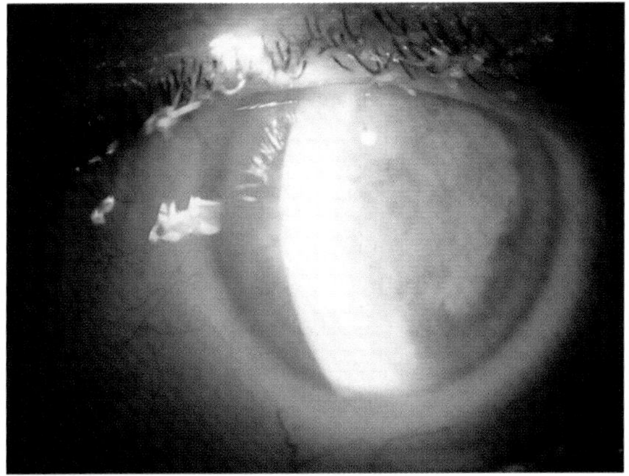

FIGURE 5.2.1 Interstitial keratitis.

Presentation acute disease may demonstrate red painful eye, tearing, and photophobia. Findings include stromal blood vessels and thickening or haze from edema. There may be fine KP and anterior uveitis. In congenital syphilis, the disease is bilateral and begins in the first decade of life.

Differential Diagnosis syphilis (usually congenital and bilateral; in acquired disease, usually unilateral), TB, leprosy, Cogan's syndrome (autoimmune disease, bilateral IK, vestibuloauditory symptoms, negative [FTA-ABS]test), mumps, rubeola, EBV, sarcoidosis, Lyme disease, HSV, HZV, and others.

Management check for history of venereal disease and hearing loss. Test for FTA-ABS, VDRL, PPD, viral antibody titers. Treat underlying systemic disease. Topical steroids shortens the usually self-limited active inflammation. (See sections on HSV or HZV for specific treatment.)

5.2.2 Thygeson's Superficial Punctate Keratitis—idiopathic chronic condition demonstrating multiple, punctate snowflake-shaped epithelial opacities.

Presentation foreign-body sensation, tearing, photophobia. Conjunctiva may appear only minimally injected. SPK stain with fluorescein. Relapsing episodes, tends to be self-limited, usually bilateral.

Differential Diagnosis subepithelial infiltrates of EKC, EBV, staphylococcal hypersensitivity.

Management exquisitely responsive to topical steroids (e.g., fluorometholone qid). Other options are lubricating drops and bandage contact lenses.

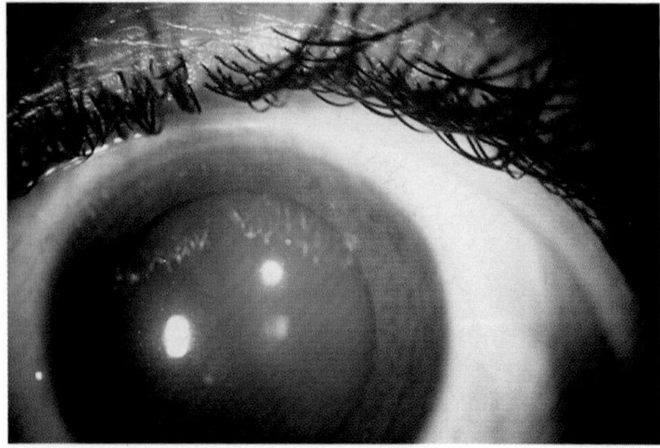

FIGURE 5.2.2 Thygeson's SPK.

5.2.3 Shield Ulcer—oval opacification in superior portion of cornea, which occasionally occurs in the setting of vernal keratoconjunctivitis and GPC.

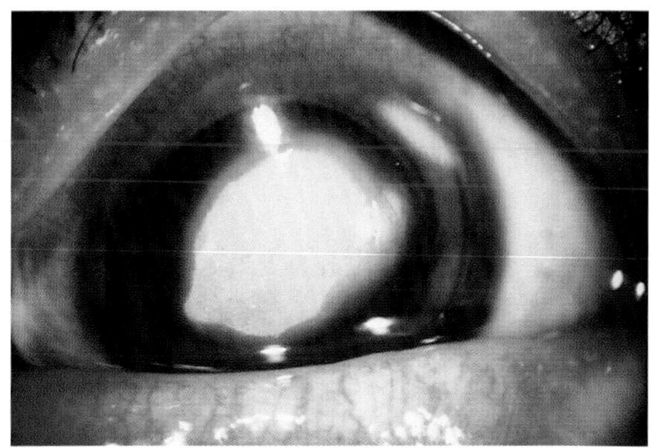

FIGURE 5.2.3 Shield ulcer in vernal keratoconjunctivitis.

Presentation itching, photophobia, mucus discharge. Usually seen in children and young adults. Seasonal, recurring symptoms, possible with a history of GPC. There may or may not be an epithelial defect.

Differential Diagnosis infectious ulcer.

Management cold compresses, lubricant drops. Consider topical antihistamines (Livostin), mast cell stabilizers (Alomide, cromolyn sodium, Patanol), or corticosteroids.

5.3 Exposure Keratopathy

corneal dehydration and epithelial disruption resulting from poor blink or eyelid closure from thyroid-related immune orbitopathy, seventh nerve palsy, ectropion, nocturnal lagophthalmos, floppy eyelid syndrome, proptosis, or postsurgical causes.

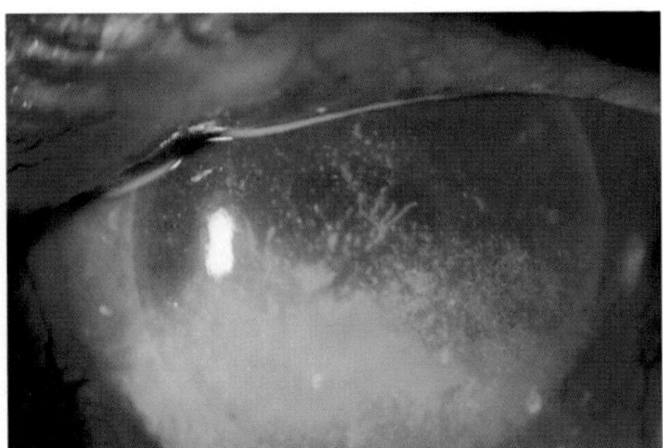

FIGURE 5.3 Exposure keratopathy due to trichiasis.

Presentation irritation, burning, redness, foreign-body sensation. Punctate fluorescein or rose bengal staining of corneal and conjunctival epithelium generally in interpalpebral zone. There may be a frank epithelial defect.

Differential Diagnosis dry eye syndrome (see Section 4.4).

Management identify and treat etiology. Treat aggressively with lubricating drops q 1 to 2h and lubricant ointment hs. Consider punctal occlusion, punctal cauterization, and tarsorrhaphy.

5.4 Filamentary Keratitis

inflammatory condition in which mucus strands and epithelial debris accumulate on the corneal surface. Associated with inadequate blinking, lagophthalmos, dry eye, postsurgical trauma, contact lens overwear, atopic dermatitis, superior limbic keratoconjunctivitis, and prolonged patching.

Presentation pain, foreign-body sensation, redness, photophobia. Filaments stain with fluorescein. There is often an inadequate tear film.

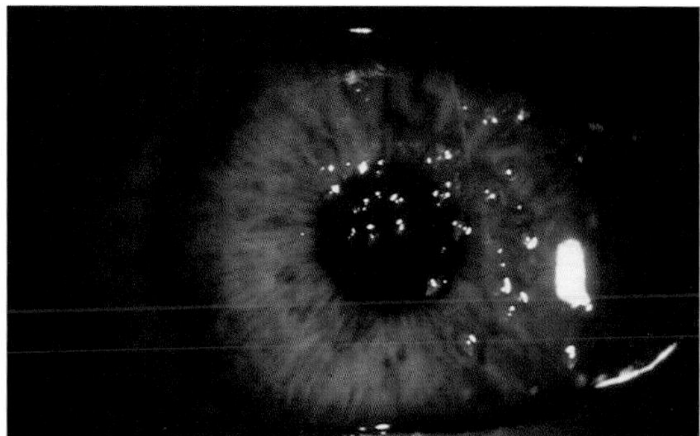

FIGURE 5.4 Filamentary keratitis.

Management scraping or debridement of mucus and filaments. Lubricating drops at least qid or ointment. Consider sodium chloride 5% drops qid or acetylcysteine (Mucomyst) 10 to 20% drops qid. Patients may benefit from use of bandage contact lens.

5.5 Neurotrophic Keratopathy

epithelial defects or stromal ulceration occurring in a cornea with reduced sensation. May be secondary to HSV or HZV infection, leprosy, lesion affecting trigeminal nerve (acoustic neuroma, trauma), topical anesthetic abuse, diabetes, ciliary nerve trauma from retinal photocoagulation, chemical burns, or postorbital radiation therapy.

Presentation blurry vision, redness, possible eye irritation. Findings include PEK and neurotrophic ulcers with varying degrees of corneal thinning and scarring.

Differential Diagnosis corneal abrasion, recurrent erosions, infectious ulcer, collagen vascular diseases, dry eye syndrome.

Management identify and treat underlying lesion responsible for decreased corneal sensation. Treat with lubricating drops and

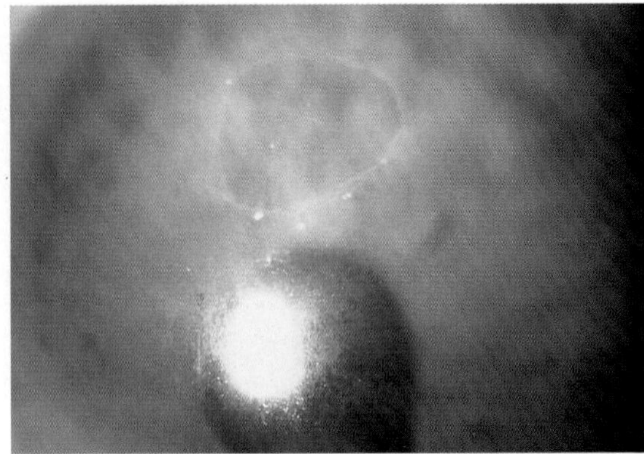

FIGURE 5.5 Neurotrophic keratitis.

erythromycin ointment qid. Consider pressure patch, bandage contact lens, tarsorrhaphy, or conjunctival flap. Lamellar or penetrating keratoplasty may be performed for vision but is a high-risk procedure.

5.6 Recurrent Erosion

relapsing epithelial defects secondary to abnormal attachments between epithelial and basement membrane, often due to previous trauma or epithelial basement membrane dystrophy.

Presentation episodes of recurring pain, tearing, photophobia. Onset is usually on awakening. Findings of epithelial basement membrane or other cornea dystrophy may be present. Epithelial defect may have healed prior to presentation.

Differential Diagnosis corneal abrasion, neurotrophic ulcer.

Management initial treatment is similar to that for corneal abrasion. Add sodium chloride 5% ointment qhs. Consider bandage contact lens, anterior stromal puncture, epithelial scraping, or excimer PTK for refractory cases.

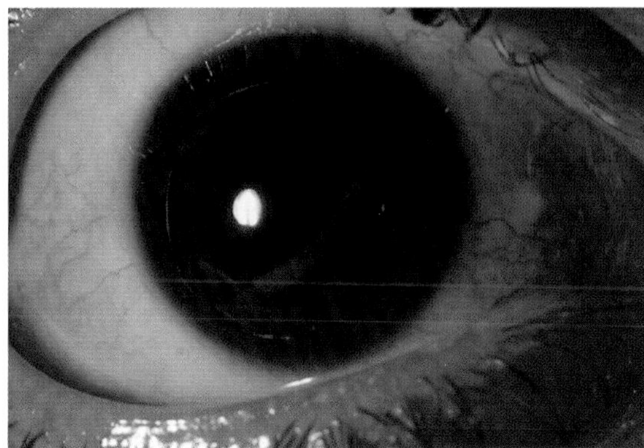

FIGURE 5.6 Traumatic corneal abrasion.

5.7 Congenital Anomalies

see Chapter 12.

5.8 Dystrophies

5.8.1 Anterior Corneal Dystrophies

5.8.1.1 Epithelial Basement Membrane Dystrophy—

common (2% incidence) autosomal dominant dystrophy or degeneration of the corneal epithelial basement membrane characterized by various patterns in the epithelium (also map-dot-fingerprint or Cogan's microcystic dystrophy).

Presentation patients may be asymptomatic or may present with decreased visual acuity, foreign-body sensation, photophobia, and tearing. Examine both eyes for fine cysts (dots), refractile lines (fingerprints), or patches of gray (maps), best seen on retroillumination. Erosions may recur.

Differential Diagnosis recurrent erosion syndrome, Meesmann's dystrophy, Thygeson's SPK, Fuchs' dystrophy.

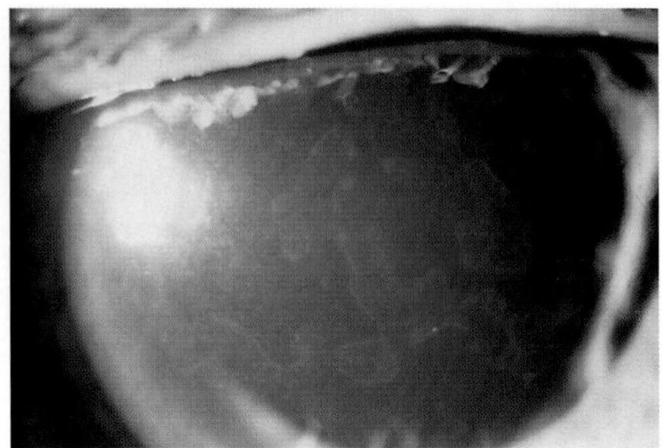

FIGURE 5.8.1.1 Epithelial basement membrane dystrophy.

Management if symptomatic, consider bandage contact lens or lubricants. For decreased vision or recurrent erosions, consider epithelial scraping or PTK.

5.8.1.2 Meesmann's Dystrophy—rare autosomal dominant dystrophy affecting corneal epithelium.

Presentation patients may have decreased vision, usually in middle age. Fine cysts at the level of the corneal epithelium are best seen on retroillumination. Patients may present with recurrent erosion symptomatology.

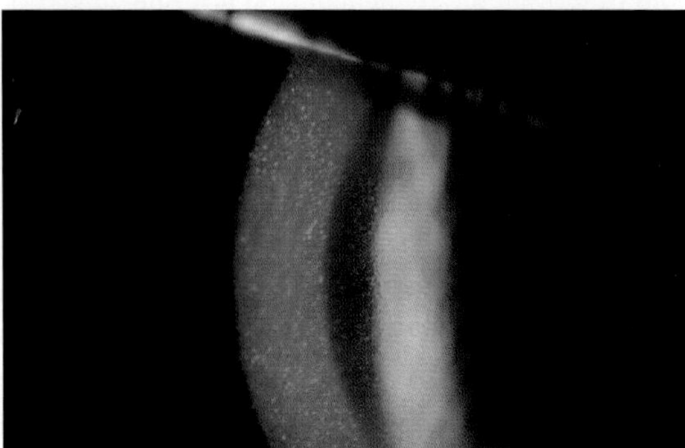

FIGURE 5.8.1.2 Meesmann's dystrophy.

Differential Diagnosis punctate epithelial keratitis, microcystic edema.

Management usually no treatment is necessary. Treat with lubrication. Consider corneal scraping if vision is affected. Recurrence is common.

5.8.1.3 Reis-Bücklers Dystrophy—bilateral, progressive, autosomal dominant corneal dystrophy causing fibrosis of Bowman's layer.

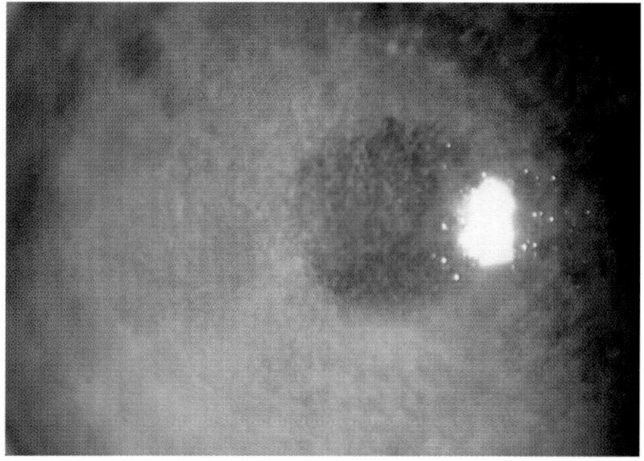

FIGURE 5.8.1.3 Reis-Bückler dystrophy.

Presentation patients may be asymptomatic, complain of blurry vision, or may experience the symptoms of recurrent erosions. Superficial gray-white, reticular opacities largely affect the central cornea.

Differential Diagnosis recurrent erosion syndrome and scarring from other causes, anterior basement membrane dystrophy.

Management standard treatment for recurrent erosions if necessary. If decreased vision is significant, consider excimer PTK or lamellar keratoplasty. Recurrence is common, and retreatment with PTK is possible.

5.8.2 Stromal Corneal Dystrophies

5.8.2.1 Granular Dystrophy—bilateral, autosomal dominant corneal stromal dystrophy characterized by hyaline degeneration.

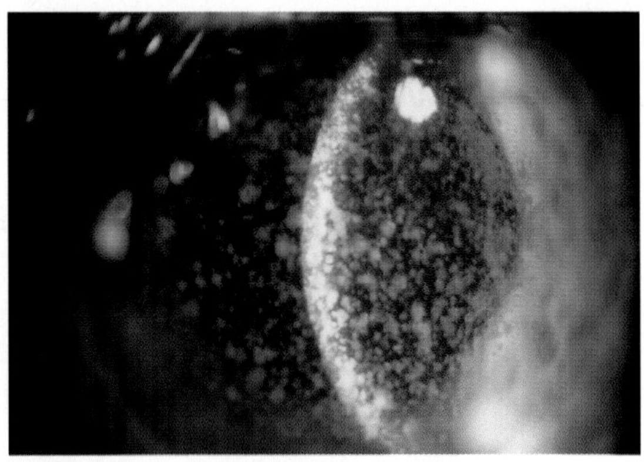

FIGURE 5.8.2.1 Granular dystrophy.

Presentation becomes clinically apparent in childhood but is generally asymptomatic until late adulthood. Decreased vision or asymptomatic incidental finding. Discrete, well-defined, white anterior stromal opacities mainly in the central cornea with intervening clear zones. May present with recurrent erosion symptomatology.

Differential Diagnosis macular dystrophy, Avellino dystrophy.

Management deposits stain with Masson trichrome stain in corneal biopsy. Patients may require penetrating keratoplasty for significant visual loss. Consider excimer PTK.

5.8.2.2 Lattice Dystrophy—bilateral autosomal dominant corneal stromal dystrophy involving amyloid deposition.

Presentation decreased vision or signs and symptoms of recurrent corneal erosions. Fine refractile lines, seen best with

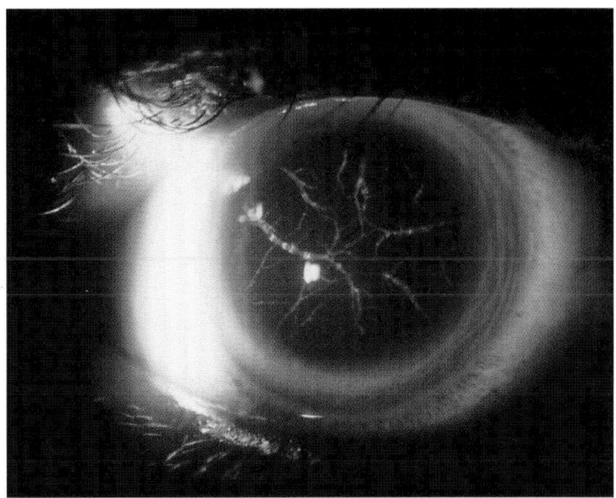

FIGURE 5.8.2.2 Lattice dystrophy.

retroillumination; scarring of the central cornea, usually with peripheral sparing.

Differential Diagnosis systemic or primary localized amyloidosis, enlarged corneal nerves.

Management amyloid stains with Congo red. Treat corneal erosions (see section 5.6 on recurrent erosions). Consider excimer PTK or PK in refractory cases.

5.8.2.3 Macular Dystrophy—rare, bilateral, autosomal recessive stromal dystrophy with abnormal stromal mucopolysaccarides.

Presentation decreased vision early in course. White or gray stromal opacities with poorly defined margins separated by hazy or cloudy areas. Lesions may be at any stromal level, tend to coalesce with time, and often involve the entire cornea to the limbus.

Differential Diagnosis granular or lattice dystrophy.

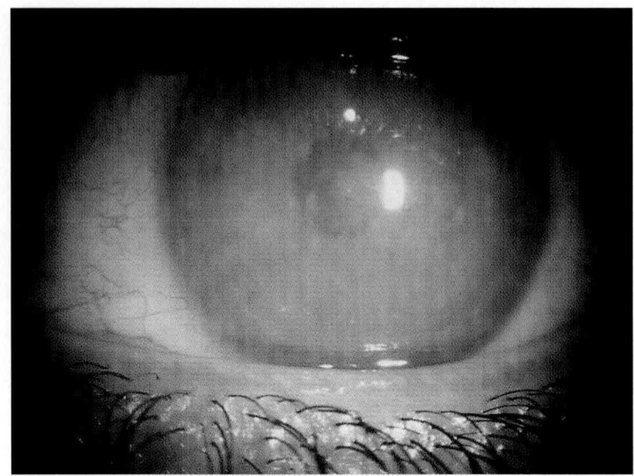

FIGURE 5.8.2.3 Macular dystrophy.

Management mucopolysaccharides stain with alcian blue. Treatment of recurrent erosions, if indicated. Penetrating keratoplasty may frequently be required for significantly decreased vision. Larger donor buttons may decrease likelihood of recurrence.

5.8.2.4 Central Crystalline Dystrophy of Schnyder—

gradually progressive, bilateral, autosomal dominant stromal dystrophy usually detectable by the age of 1 year.

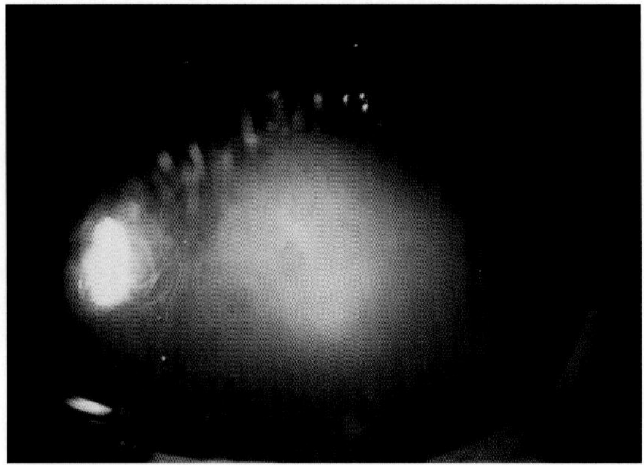

FIGURE 5.8.2.4 Central crystalline dystrophy of Schnyder.

Presentation normal or blurred vision. Signs include small, yellow-white stromal crystals that form a round or oval central opacity. Diffuse haze, significant arcus, and limbal girdle are common. Opacities appear posterior to Bowman's layer in a ring-like pattern. Corneal lesions are accumulations of cholesterol and neutral fats and there can be an association with elevated lipid profile.

Differential Diagnosis arcus senilis, limbal girdle of Vogt, other stromal dystrophies.

Management vision is rarely significantly affected, but penetrating keratoplasty may be indicated in some patients.

5.8.2.5 Fleck Dystrophy—nonprogressive, usually autosomal dominant stromal dystrophy, which may be asymmetric or unilateral and is sometimes evident at birth.

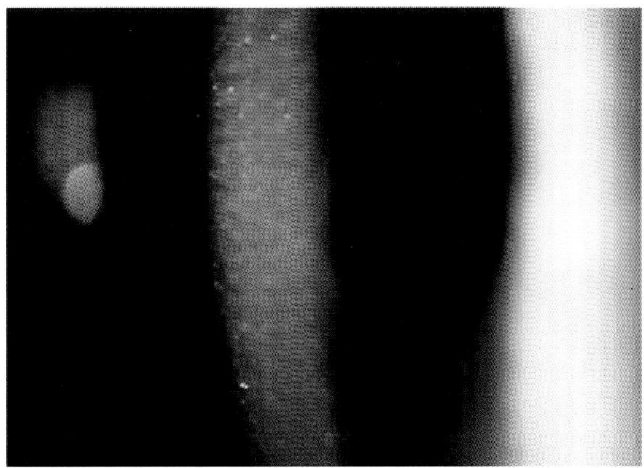

FIGURE 5.8.2.5 Fleck dystrophy.

Presentation vision is generally unaffected. Slit-lamp examination reveals well-defined, gray-white specks, sometimes ring shaped, which appear diffusely in the corneal stroma. It may have any of several associations: reduced corneal sensation, limbal dermoids, keratoconus, central cloudy corneal dystrophy of Schnyder, cortical cataracts, pseudoxanthoma elasticum, or atopy.

Differential Diagnosis posterior polymorphous dystrophy, pre-Descemet's dystrophy, ichthyosis.

Management there is no effect on vision and no association with recurrent erosions. No treatment is necessary.

5.8.2.6 Central Cloudy Dystrophy of François—bilateral, nonprogressive, stromal opacity of unknown histopathology. Although only sometimes a true dystrophy with autosomally dominant inheritance, this condition is a variant of crocodile shagreen.

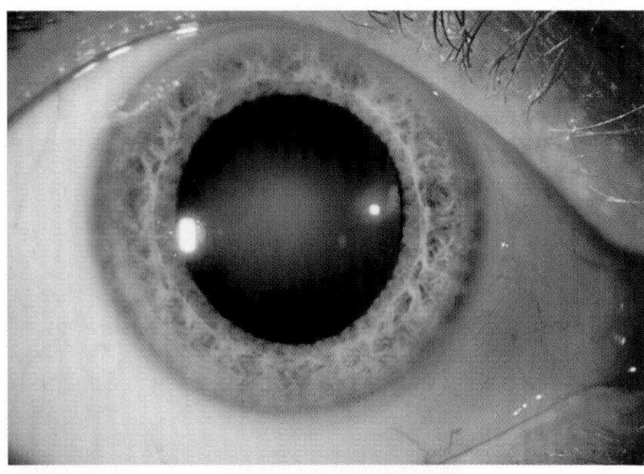

FIGURE 5.8.2.6 Central cloudy dystrophy of François.

Presentation multiple, ill-defined, gray polygonal opacifications. Opacities are most prominent centrally and posteriorly, separated by clear zones.

Differential Diagnosis Fuchs' dystrophy with corneal edema, posterior crocodile shagreen.

Management vision is rarely affected; however, PK may be considered in severe cases.

5.8.2.7 Pre-Descemet's Dystrophy—posterior stromal dystrophy, which may be acquired rather than hereditary.

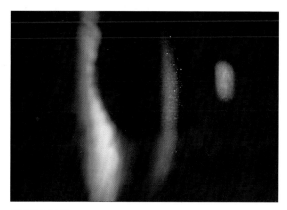

FIGURE 5.8.2.7 Pre-Descemet's dystrophy.

Presentation generally asymptomatic but can affect visual acuity. Findings include small linear or punctate gray-white flecks in the deep stroma, anterior to Descemet's membrane. Associated findings include keratoconus, posterior polymorphous dystrophy, central cloudy dystrophy, and anterior basement membrane dystrophy.

Differential Diagnosis fleck dystrophy, posterior polymorphous dystrophy, ichthyosis.

Management look for other associations: posterior polymorphous, anterior basement membrane, central cloudy corneal dystrophy of Schnyder, keratoconus, or ichthyosis. Usually no treatment is necessary.

5.8.2.8 Posterior Amorphous Stromal Dystrophy—rare bilateral, autosomal dominant stromal dystrophy, which may be slowly progressive, is evident in childhood, and can be congenital.

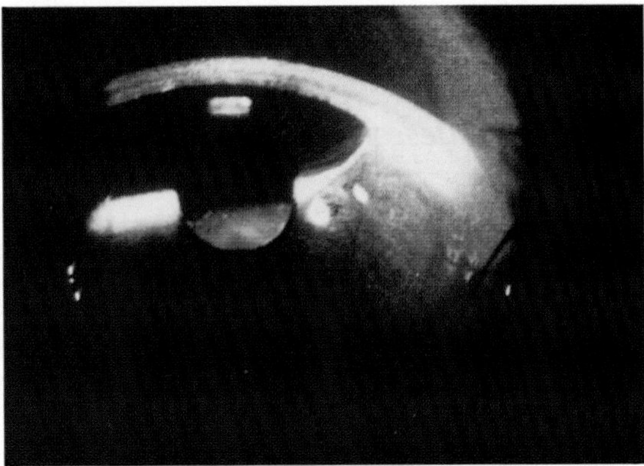

FIGURE 5.8.2.8 Posterior amorphous stromal dystrophy.

Presentation diffuse, gray-white lesions in the posterior corneal stroma, mostly involving the central cornea, but involvement occurs to the limbus (although there may be areas of endothelial involvement). Other signs may include corneal thinning with flat topography and resulting hyperopia, central stromal thinning, and peripheral iris processes.

Management RGP contact lenses for any significant irregular astigmatism. Best-corrected visual acuity is rarely impaired.

5.8.2.9 Congenital Hereditary Stromal Dystrophy—autosomal dominant, bilaterally symmetric stationary stromal dystrophy characterized by abnormal collagen lamellae evident in the newborn.

Presentation infant with central corneal clouding. Nebulous flakelike opacities affect the anterior stroma. The peripheral stroma is spared. Infants may demonstrate nystagmus and strabismus.

Differential Diagnosis congenital hereditary endothelial dystrophy, congenital glaucoma, mucopolysaccharidosis, birth trauma, PPMD.

Management consider early penetrating keratoplasty.

5.8.3 Posterior Corneal Dystrophies

5.8.3.1 Cornea Guttata—thickening or reduplication of Descemet's membrane, associated with endothelial dysfunction, corneal clouding, and resulting visual loss.

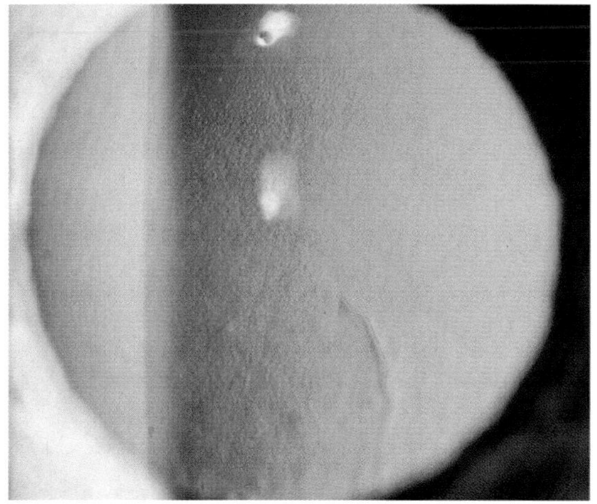

FIGURE 5.8.3.1 Cornea guttata.

Presentation rounded excrescences or dark areas in Descemet's membrane and the endothelium. Fine pigment deposits are common. May present as a hazy thickened cornea.

Differential Diagnosis Fuchs' endothelial dystrophy, Hassall-Henle bodies (peripheral guttata, a normal finding in the elderly.

Management consider specular microscopy. Use caution when performing intraocular surgery, because this may hasten endothelial compromise.

5.8.3.2 Fuchs' Endothelial Dystrophy—sporadic or autosomal dominant bilateral dystrophy affecting the corneal endothelium.

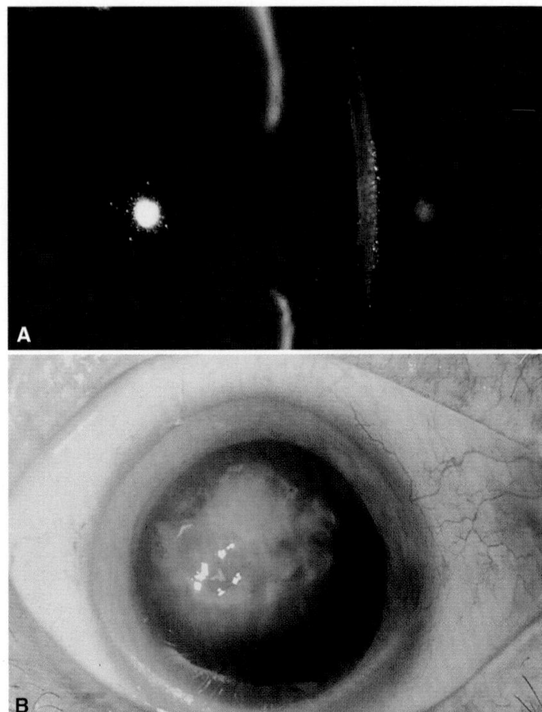

FIGURE 5.8.3.2a Early Fuch's endothelial dystrophy.
FIGURE 5.8.3.2b Advanced Fuch's endothelial dystrophy with bullae.

Presentation

blurry vision, sometimes halos, most common on awakening or early in the day. Patients are generally symptomatic in their sixth decade. Slit-lamp examination reveals central guttata, usually best noted on retroillumination, and stromal thickening or edema. Subepithelial scarring and fibrosis may occur.

Differential Diagnosis

ABK or PBK, posterior polymorphous dystrophy, endothelial pigmentation, other causes of cornea decompensation (chronic inflammation, glaucoma, intraocular surgery).

Management sodium chloride 5% drops (Muro-128) qid and ointment hs. A hair dryer to gingerly circulate warm air across the corneal surface to promote evaporation may be tried. Consider PK, depending on visual acuity and degree of corneal thickening. Exercise caution with intraocular surgery, because corneal decompensation may occur.

5.8.3.3 Posterior Polymorphous Dystrophy—gradually progressive autosomal dominant dystrophy affecting the corneal endothelium and Descemet's membrane.

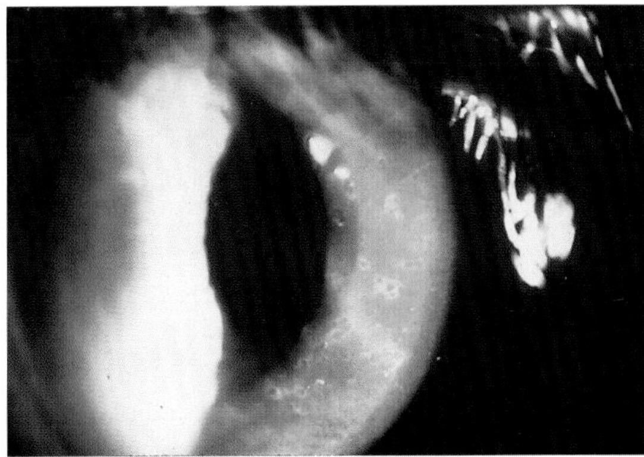

FIGURE 5.8.3.3 Posterior polymorphous dystrophy with posterior corneal vesicles.

Presentation usually bilateral, although findings may be asymmetric. Examination reveals deep clusters of vesicular lesions, map-shaped gray opacities, scalloped borders, stromal thickening and haze, and pupil displacement. The cornea may have appearance of beaten metal on retroillumination. PPMD may present as cloudy corneas in an infant.

Differential Diagnosis ABK, PBK, Fuchs' endothelial dystrophy, cornea vesicles (isolated, monocular incidental finding).

Management PK in patients with significant visual impairment.

5.8.3.4 Congenital Hereditary Endothelial Dystrophy—

in utero abnormalities in corneal endothelium and Descemet's membrane.

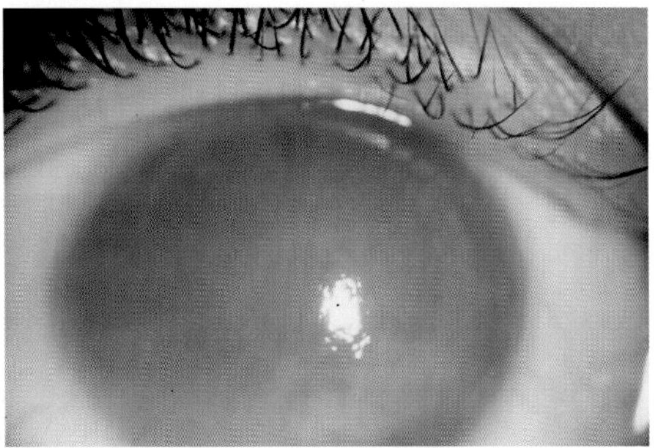

FIGURE 5.8.3.4 Congenital hereditary endothelial dystrophy.

Presentation

- Diffuse epithelial and stromal edema and haze, with bluish tint. Descemet's membrane may have peau d'orange appearance.
- Autosomal recessive form: bilateral corneal edema at birth with nystagmus. Dystrophy does not progress. No tearing or photophobia.
- Autosomal dominant form: usually evident by age 2. Marked by gradual progression. Pain and tearing present without photophobia and normal IOP.

Differential Diagnosis congenital glaucoma, mucopolysaccharidosis, congenital hereditary stromal dystrophy, PPMD, birth trauma.

Management topical 5% NaCl drops or ointment. Consider penetrating keratoplasty. There is a guarded visual prognosis secondary to amblyopia.

5.9 Ectatic Disorders

5.9.1 Keratoconus—a slowly progressive paracentral thinning and steepening of the cornea.

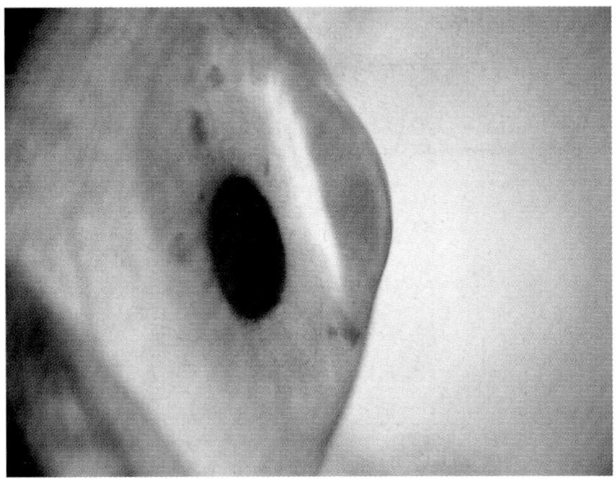

FIGURE 5.9.1 Keratoconus/Vogt's striae.

Presentation generally begins in adolescence and progresses slowly. Decreased vision. Acute hydrops may cause pain, tearing, and photophobia. Slit-lamp examination reveals thinning and bulging of central cornea, causing cone and astigmatism. Other signs include Vogt's striae (stromal stress lines), Fleischer ring (iron deposit line), Rizzuti's sign (conical reflection on nasal cornea), and Munson's sign (lower lid bulge on downgaze). Acute hydrops is caused by rupture of Decemet's membrane and influx of fluid into the stroma. It appears as a bluish, white area in the stroma.

Differential Diagnosis pellucid marginal degeneration, keratoglobus of acute hydrops: corneal ulcer, scarring secondary to contact lens.

Management retinoscopy, keratoscopy, or corneal topography may be of help in early diagnosis. RGP contact lenses until not tolerated and then therapeutic PK. For acute hydrops, observation only, because it usually resolves.

5.9.2 Keratoglobus

—congenital deformation of the cornea, similar to keratoconus except that the area of corneal thinning occurs in the mid-periphery.

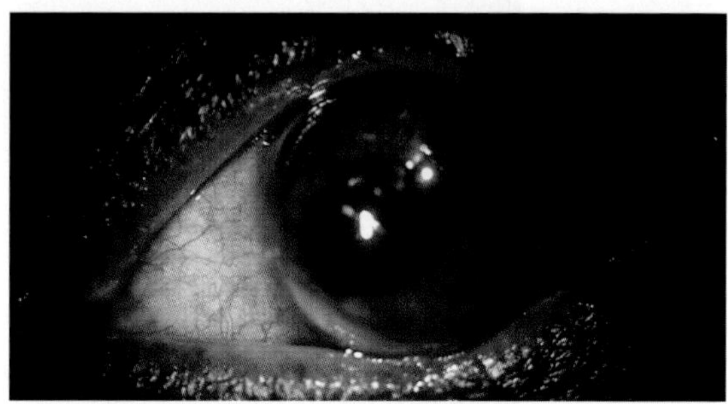

FIGURE 5.9.2 Keratoglobus with diffuse thinning.

Presentation corneal diameter may be larger than normal. Spherical protrusion or bulging on the central cornea. Usually not associated with a Fleischer ring. Folds may be observed in Descemet's membrane.

Differential Diagnosis keratoconus.

Management generally requires penetrating keratoplasty (possibly with preceding lamellar keratoplasty) for visual rehabilitation, but prognosis is guarded.

5.9.3 Pellucid Marginal Degeneration

—slowly progressive bilateral thinning of the inferior peripheral cornea.

Presentation age 20 to 40 years, blurry vision, corneal protrusion superior to thinned zone, which is inferior. Corneal topography may demonstrate inferior steepening with central flattening at axis 90° (against-the-rule astigmatism).

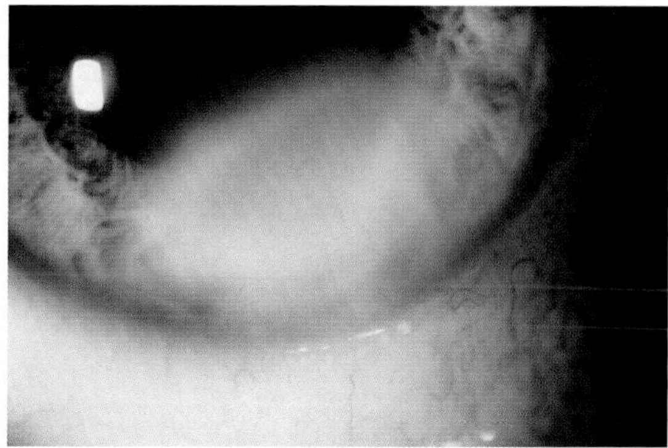

FIGURE 5.9.3 Pellucid marginal degeneration after acute hydrops.

Differential Diagnosis collagen vascular disease, keratoconus, furrow degeneration, Terrien's marginal degeneration.

Management RGP contact lenses. Consider crescentic lamellar or penetrating keratoplasty.

5.10 Corneal Degenerations and Deposits

5.10.1 Arcus Senilis or Corneal Arcus—accumulation of extracellular lipids in peripheral stroma.

Presentation asymptomatic, ringlike hazy opacity that begins in inferior and superior periphery with a clear zone between a self-defined peripheral border and the limbus. Asymmetric arcus may signify carotid disease.

Differential Diagnosis hyperlipoproteinemia, arcus juvenilis (present at birth and usually appears as a localized arc).

Management usually a normal involutional change. Obtain a lipid profile in patients younger than age 40 years. No treatment is necessary unless the patient has an elevated lipid profile.

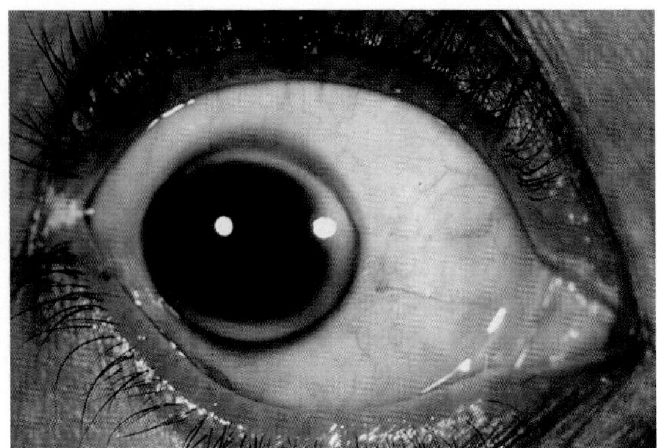

FIGURE 5.10.1 Arcus senilis.

5.10.2 Limbal Girdle of Vogt—elastotic degeneration of collagen in the anterior stroma, thought to be related to actinic exposure.

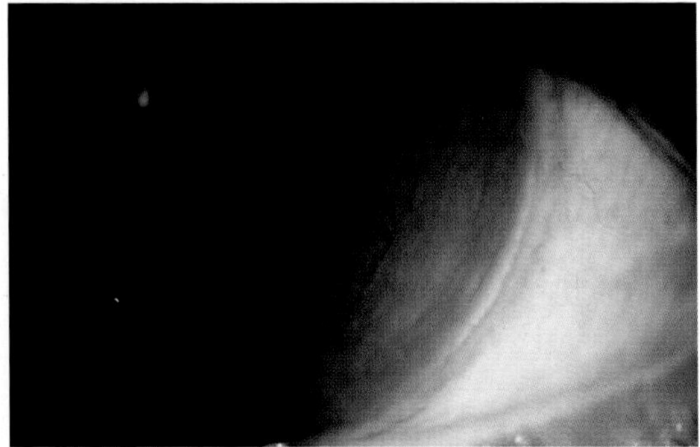

FIGURE 5.10.2 Limbal girdle of Vogt.

Presentation asymptomatic. Slit-lamp examination reveals needlelike opacities parallel to the limbus in the peripheral stroma usually nasally and temporally.

Management visual function is not affected. No treatment is required.

5.10.3 Hassall-Henle Bodies—minute elevations of Descemet's membrane found in the peripheral cornea due to focal exuberant production of Descemet's membrane.

Presentation asymptomatic, rare before the third decade. Seen best on retroillumination.

Differential Diagnosis cornea guttata (found centrally), Fuchs' endothelial dystrophy, PBK, ABK.

Management no treatment required.

5.10.4 Crocodile Shagreen—an alteration in the arrangement of stromal collagen fibers resulting in central polygonal opacifications of the cornea (usually anteriorly) with intervening clear zones.

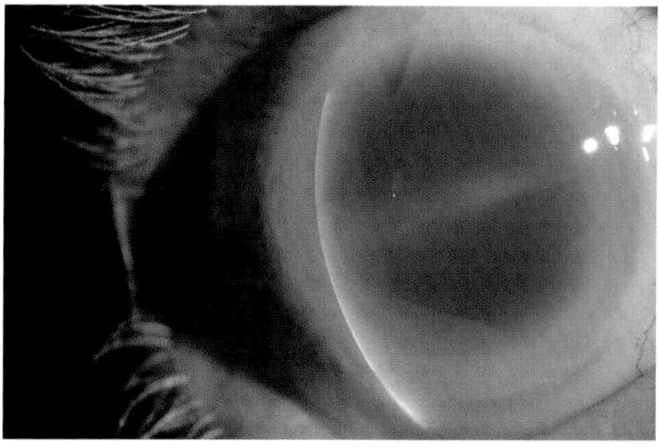

FIGURE 5.10.4 Crocodile shagreen.

Presentation rarely reduces visual acuity. Lesions may be anterior or posterior and appear as a mosaic pattern of hazy gray-white, multisided opacities in the central cornea.

Differential Diagnosis central cloudy dystrophy of François, PPMD.

Management no treatment required.

5.10.5 Calcific Band Keratopathy—degeneration affecting Bowman's layer with calcium hydroxyapatite deposition.

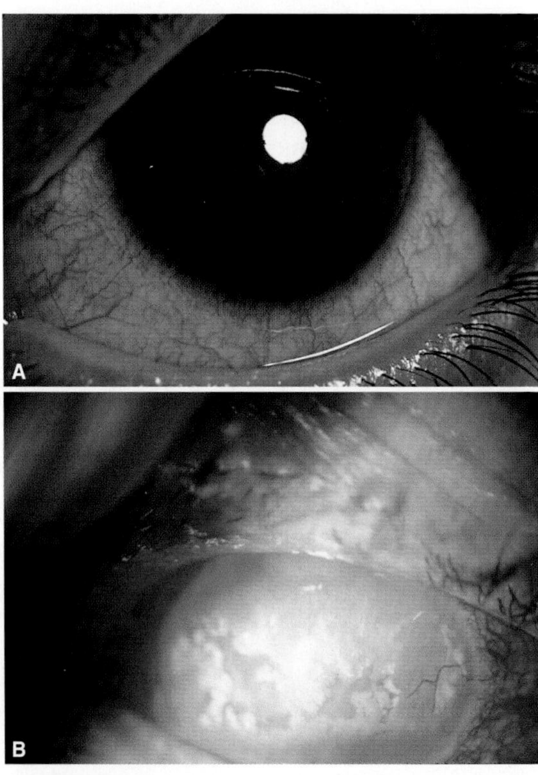

FIGURE 5.10.5a Mild calcific band keratopathy.
FIGURE 5.10.5b Severe calcific band keratopathy.

Presentation fine punctate opacities in the periphery within Bowman's layer, which later coalesce to form a band in the interpalpebral zone. A clear zone exists between the lesions and the limbus. Clear holes may be seen where corneal nerves perforate Bowman's layer.

Management

- Determine underlying cause: chronic inflammation, systemic hypercalcemia, primary hereditary band keratopathy, elevated phophorus levels, chronic mercury exposure, gout, sarcoidosis.
- For reduced vision or severe pain, 1.5% EDTA may be used for chelation and subsequent debriding of the lesions. Lidocaine 4% is often useful for removal of the epithelium.

5.10.6 Salzmann's Nodular Degeneration

—resolved inflammatory condition in which nodules occur following chronic keratitis of various etiologies, including blepharitis, interstitial keratitis, and idiopathic; usually acquired, but may be inherited as autosomal dominant.

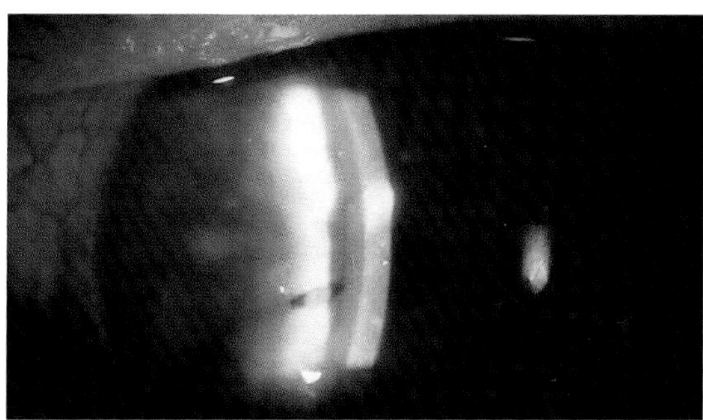

FIGURE 5.10.6 Salzmann's nodular degeneration with raised nodules.

Presentation usually found in middle-aged and elderly women. Bilateral, elevated lesions appear light blue or gray.

Differential Diagnosis spheroidal degeneration, phlyctenulosis.

Management treat any underlying conditions. If visual acuity is reduced, consider superficial keratectomy. Infrequently, lamellar or penetrating keratoplasty is required for visual rehabilitation (nodules can recur in grafted tissue). Also consider excimer PTK.

5.10.7 Spheroidal Degeneration—idiopathic golden brown spherical deposits in the anterior stroma; also referred to as Labrador keratopathy, Bietti's nodular dystrophy, and climatic droplet keratopathy.

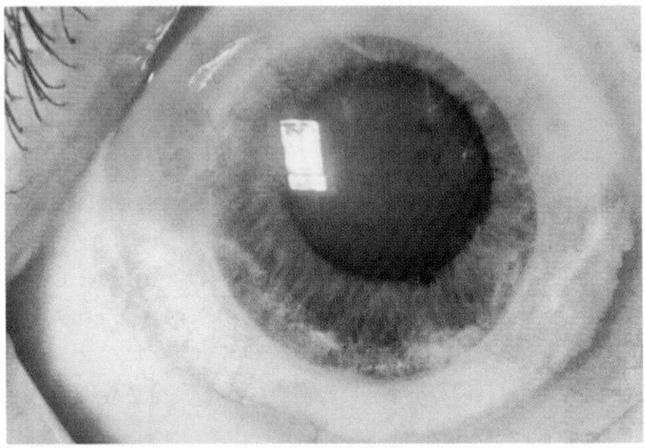

FIGURE 5.10.7 Spheroidal degeneration.

Presentation pain, photophobia, tearing. Semispherical protuberances are seen on corneal surface and conjunciva. More common in males, who may demonstrate a hereditary predisposition. Various factors are thought to play a role in pathogenesis, including sun exposure, aging, and microtrauma. Neovascularization may occur late in disease.

Management if vision is significantly reduced, consider PK (may recur in graft).

5.10.8 Coats' White Ring—circle, 1-mm diameter or smaller, of well-defined punctate lesions representing iron deposits appearing in the anterior stroma or in Bowman's layer, following injury with an iron-containing foreign body.

Presentation asymptomatic unless affecting visual axis.

Differential Diagnosis infectious cornea ulcer, retained foreign body.

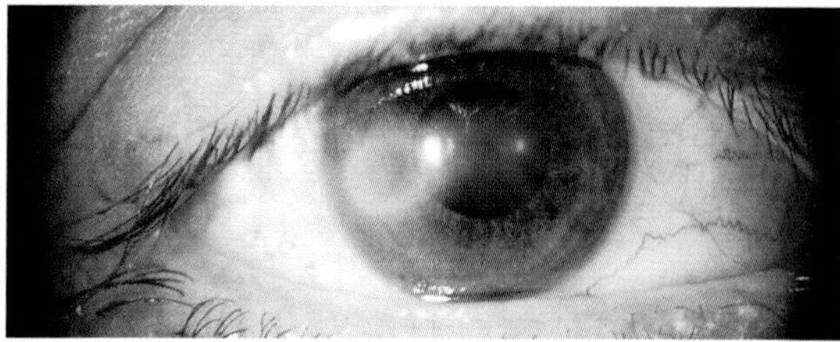

FIGURE 5.10.8 Coats' white ring.

Management vision is rarely affected. Consider debridement with corneal burr.

5.10.9 Iron Lines—iron deposition related to tear film abnormalities or deposition from perilimbal vessels.

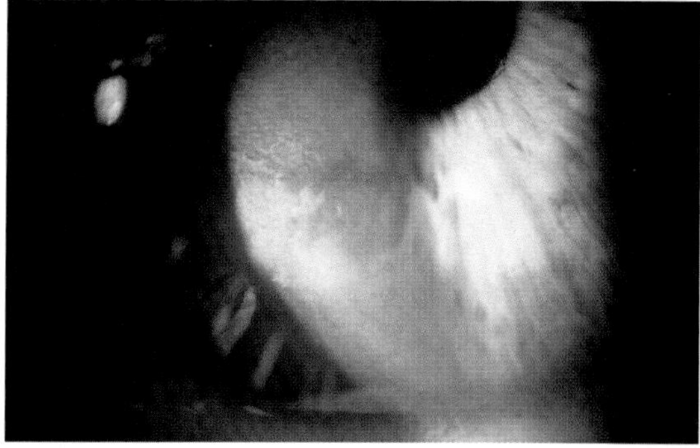

FIGURE 5.10.9 Hudson-Stähli iron line.

Presentation

- Ferry line: filtering bleb.
- Fleischer ring: surrounds the cone in keratoconus.
- Hudson-Stähli line: epithelial breakdown; often appears as a horizontal line in inferior one-third of the cornea in elderly patients.
- Stocker-Busacca line: central to the head of the pterygium.
- Iron lines may occur with other disruptions of the ocular surface such as radial keratotomy.

Management no treatment is necessary.

5.10.10 Cornea Farinata—probably dominantly inherited predisposition to developing stromal deposits, usually bilaterally.

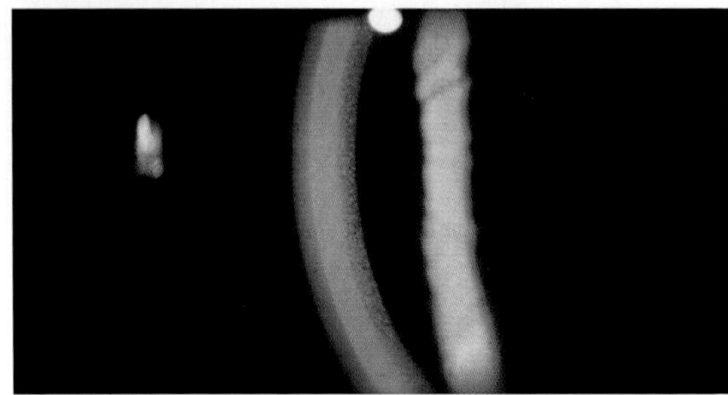

FIGURE 5.10.10 Cornea farinata.

Presentation asymptomatic. Findings include very fine, elusive punctate or comma-shaped lesions in the central corneal stroma.

Differential Diagnosis pre-Descemet's dystrophy, fleck dystrophy, ichythyosis.

Management vision is not affected. No treatment is necessary.

5.10.11 Kayser-Fleischer Ring—green or brown discoloration of peripheral cornea at the level of Descemet's membrane, which may extend all the way to the limbus, seen in the setting of systemic diseases.

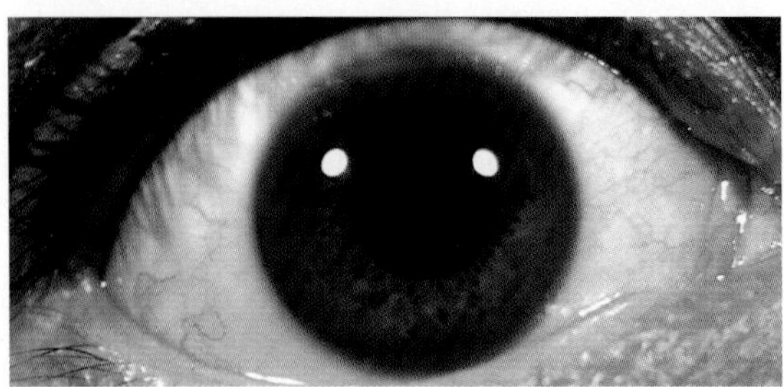

FIGURE 5.10.11 Kayser-Fleischer ring in Wilson's disease.

Presentation usually no ophthalmic symptoms. Found in Wilson's disease (elevated urine and serum copper levels), primary biliary cirrhosis, hepatitis, and multiple myeloma.

Management vision is not affected. No ocular treatment is required. Treat systemic disease.

5.10.12 Corneal Verticillata—a pattern of melanin deposition characterized by precipitates in a swirling pattern.

Presentation usually asymptomatic, although it can cause decreased visual acuity. Patients often report a history of family member with similar findings or a history of medication use.

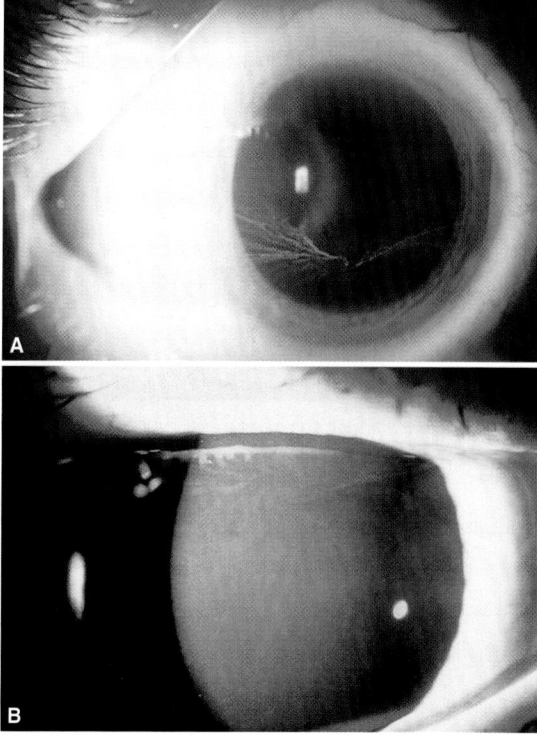

FIGURE 5.10.12a Cornea verticilatta related to amiodarone therapy.
FIGURE 5.10.12b Cornea verticilatta in Fabry's disease.

Differential Diagnosis use of amiodarone, chloroquine, or phenothiazines; Fabry's disease.

Management if visual acuity is not affected, follow clinically. If visual impairment occurs, consider epithelial debridement. In severe cases, consider discontinuing the offending medication unless absolutely essential for systemic condition.

5.11 PERIPHERAL THINNING

5.11.1 Mooren's Ulcer—chronic progressive ulceration involving peripheral epithelium and stroma.

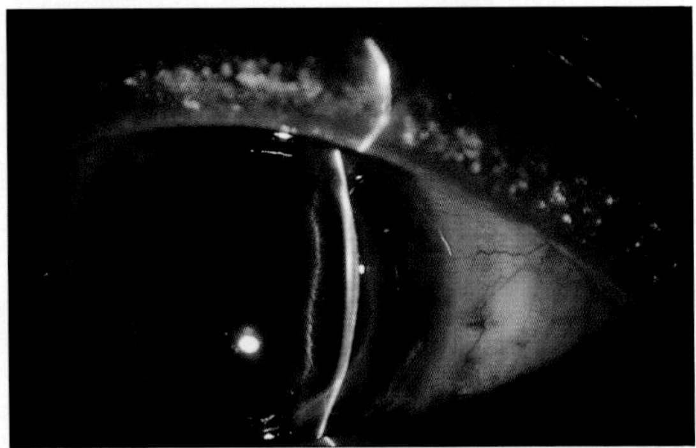

FIGURE 5.11.1 Chronic Mooren's ulcer.

Presentation

- Red painful eye. Ulceration proceeds in a circular fashion along the peripheral cornea and gradually extends centrally over 3 to 12 months with a leading edge of necrotic tissue.
- In young black males, there is usually bilateral, aggressive disease, and treatment is largely ineffective.
- Older patients experience a less severe form of the disease, which is usually unilateral and more responsive to therapy.

Differential Diagnosis infectious keratitis, Terrien's marginal degeneration, marginal keratolysis, furrow degeneration.

Management therapeutic contact lens, conjunctival or corneal debridement or resection, topical steroids. Consider immunosuppressives.

5.11.2 Peripheral Ulcerative Keratitis—peripheral corneal ulceration in the setting of autoimmune diseases, most commonly rheumatoid arthritis.

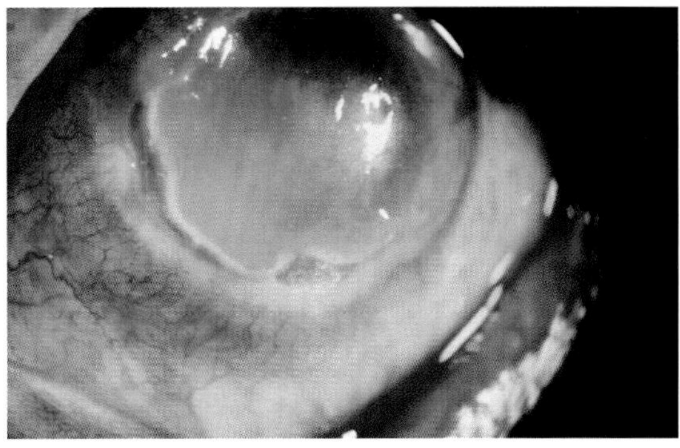

FIGURE 5.11.2 Marginal keratolysis/peripheral corneal melt.

Presentation pain, redness, decreased vision. Lesions are usually sectorial and unilateral but may be bilateral and can involve extensive areas of the cornea. Epithelial defects with stromal thinning with or without infiltrates are seen. Perforation may occur.

Differential Diagnosis Mooren's ulcer, infectious keratitis, Terrien's marginal degeneration, furrow degeneration.

Management aggressive lubricating drops q 1 to 2h, lubricant ointments, topical steroids, collagenase inhibitors (such as oral doxycycline), patching, tarsorrhaphy, or bandage contact lens may be indicated, depending on severity. For severe thinning or perforation, lamellar or penetrating keratoplasty may be necessary along with immunosuppressive therapy.

5.11.3 Terrien's Marginal Degeneration—usually bilateral idiopathic peripheral corneal thinning, which is characterized by minimal signs of inflammation.

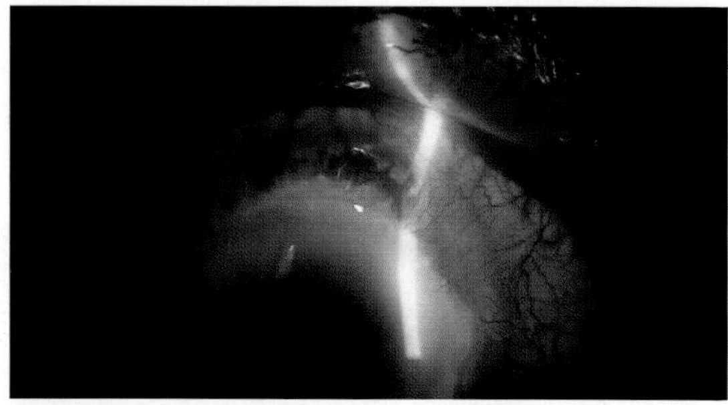

FIGURE 5.11.3 Terrien's marginal degeneration with impending perforation.

Presentation usually occurs in older children and young adults, more commonly in males. Initially begins as fine peripheral lipid opacities, which coalesce and become areas of thinning, usually in the superior stroma (with intact overlying epithelium). The thinning proceeds gradually in an annular pattern, usually accompanied by a vascular pannus. The cornea is often flatter in the 90° meridian and exhibits against-the-rule and irregular astigmatism.

Differential Diagnosis furrow degeneration, pellucid marginal degeneration.

Management watch for associated episcleritis, atypical pterygia, necrosis or neovascularization of corneal periphery. Lamellar or penetrating corneoscleral grafting may be necessary in advanced cases.

5.11.4 Furrow Degeneration—a thinned appearance of the peripheral cornea in the clear zone peripheral to corneal arcus.

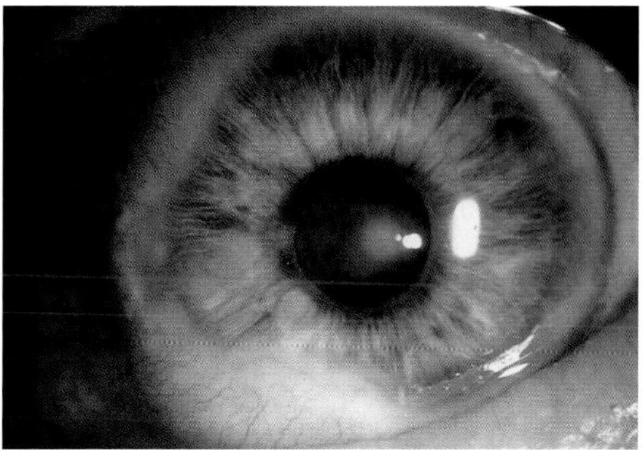

FIGURE 5.11.4 Furrow degeneration from 2- to 6-o'clock position.

Presentation asymptomatic. Usually seen in older patients with corneal arcus. May be an optical illusion of relative thinning, although a mild degree of true thinning may occur.

Differential Diagnosis Terrien's marginal degeneration.

Management no treatment is required.

5.12 Aphakic and Pseudophakic Bullous Keratopathy

cornea edema as a complication after cataract surgery (see Section 7.8.1).

5.13 Corneal Surgery

5.13.1 Penetrating Keratoplasty—full-thickness procedure in which the majority of the affected cornea is trephined and removed and then replaced with a corneal "button" created from a corneoscleral donor. Indications for penetrating keratoplasty are numerous and include corneal edema, corneal dystrophies, keratoconus, scarring, ulcerative conditions, previously failed transplants, and other conditions. Techniques demonstrate considerable variation but generally involve a series of equally spaced interrupted sutures (10–0 or 11–0 monofilament nylon or polypropylene), continuous running sutures, or a combination of the two.

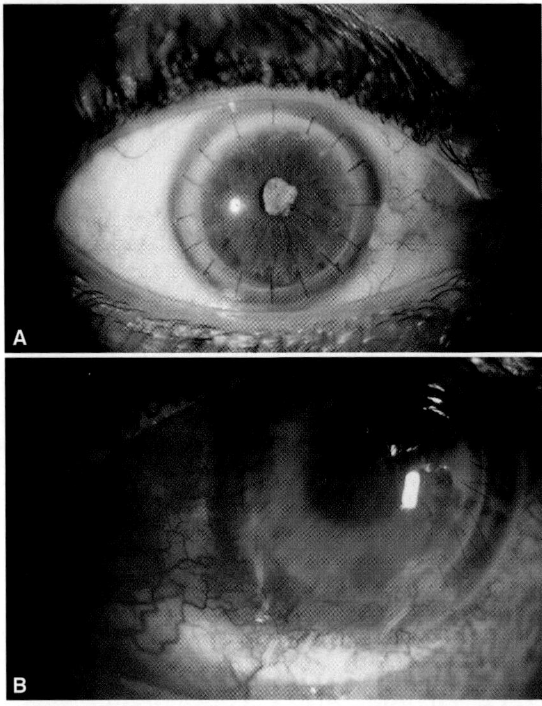

FIGURE 5.13.1a PK with cataract, interrupted sutures.
FIGURE 5.13.1b PK with broken running suture complicated by previous suture abscess.

5.13.2 Graft Failure—nonspecific edema and resulting loss of clarity of the donor tissue generally resulting from endothelial dysfunction due to mechanical trauma or host characteristics.

Presentation pain, tearing, photophobia, redness. Findings include stromal thickening and opacification. Guttata may be observed on the donor endothelium.

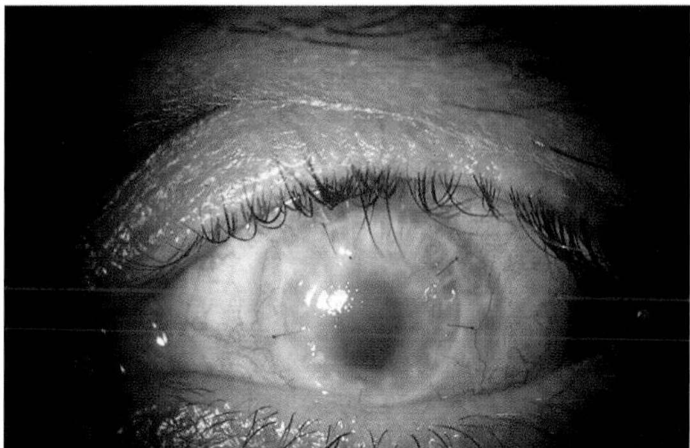

FIGURE 5.13.2 Graft failure with generalized edema.

Management careful observation and steroids are sufficient in some cases where the edema resolves with time. Persistent loss of clarity may require repeat transplantation.

5.13.3 Graft Rejection—the most common cause of graft failure; a type IV or delayed hypersensitivity reaction in which host lymphocytes attack donor epithelial, stromal, or endothelial cells.

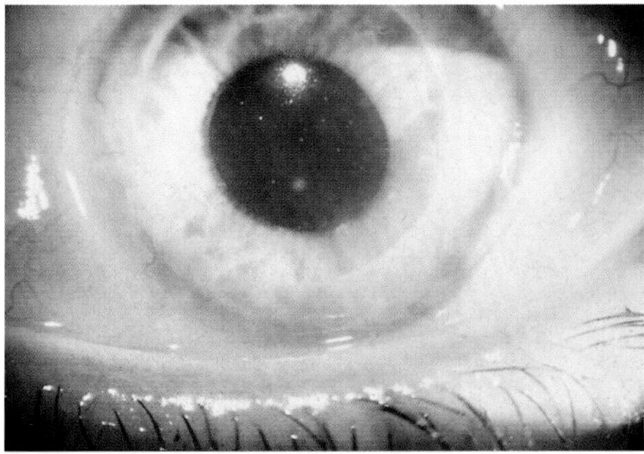

FIGURE 5.13.3 Graft rejection with subepithelial infiltrates and Koudadoust line (inferior pupillary margin).

Presentation tearing, photophobia, redness, decreased vision. Graft rejection generally does not take place within the first 10 days postoperatively. Findings include perilimbal injection, anterior chamber cell and flare, keratic precipitates, and corneal thickening and loss of clarity. Subepithelial infiltrates may also be seen. In endothelial rejection, keratic precipitates oriented linearly (Khodadoust line) may be noted along with localized edema and KP. Epithelial rejection may be seen as an advancing line of staining or late-staining epithelium.

Management rejection can usually be reversed with careful titration of steroid regimen, possibly with addition of cyclosporin A or other immunomodulators.

5.13.4 Suture Abscess—a sterile or infectious infiltrate at a usually exposed suture.

Presentation pain, tearing, decreased vision, redness. Intraocular inflammation and other signs of rejection may be present.

Differential Diagnosis sterile immune infiltrate.

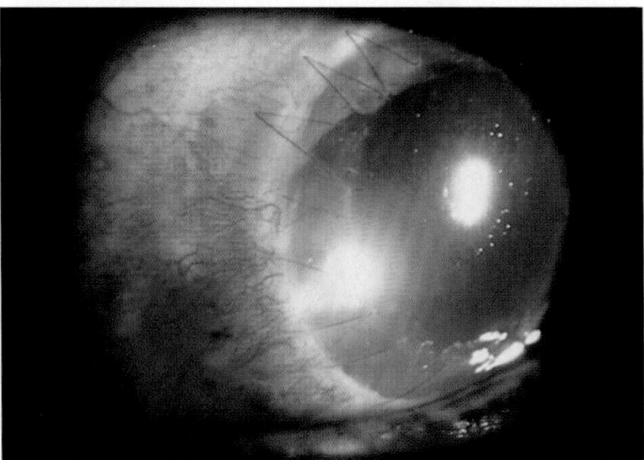

FIGURE 5.13.4 Suture-related abscess.

Management remove suture with fine forceps, and culture the suture on a variety of media. Follow management for bacterial corneal ulcer. Increase steroid regimen by 1 drop per day immediately or after 1 day. Consider more rare etiologies such as fungus or HSV recurrence if no improvement.

5.13.5 Gundersen Flap

5.13.5 Gundersen Flap—a conjunctival transposition procedure used in the management of multiple epithelial nonhealing disorders. The corneal epithelium is scraped and debrided. The area of the conjunctival flap is carefully dissected from Tenon's fascia. A 360° limbal peritomy is performed, and the conjunctival flap is mobilized across the entire cornea and sutured into place.

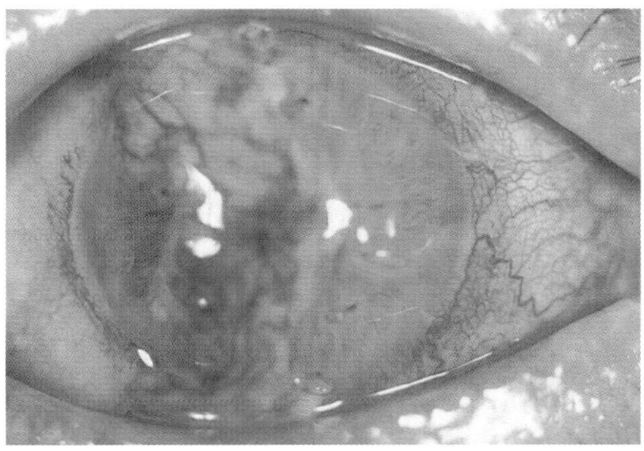

FIGURE 5.13.5 Well-vascularized vertical conjunctival flap.

5.14 Enlarged Corneal Nerves

prominent corneal nerves seen as fine white opacities radiating centrally in the corneal periphery.

Differential Diagnosis multiple endocrine neoplasia type IIb, ichthyosis, Refsum's disease, leprosy, keratoconus, Fuchs' endothelial dystrophy, osteogenesis imperfecta.

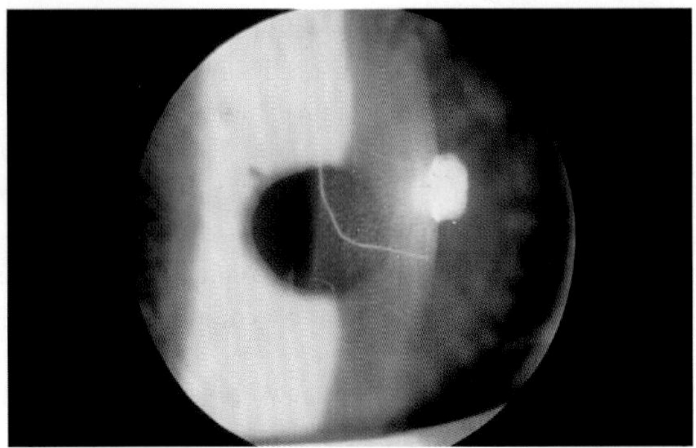

FIGURE 5.14 Enlarged corneal nerves.

5.15 Pannus

vascular invasion into cornea from limbal vessels.

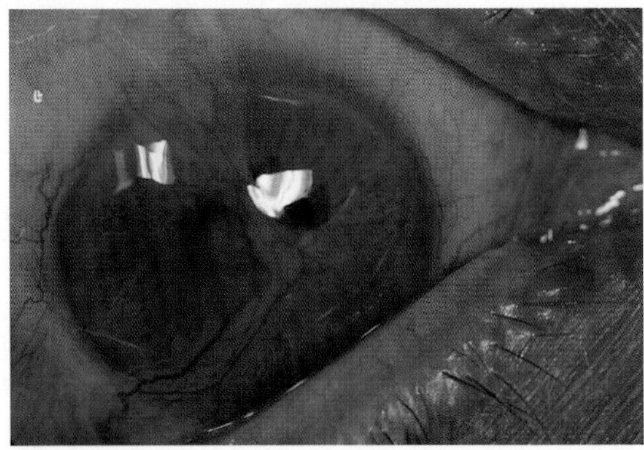

FIGURE 5.15 Pannus.

Differential Diagnosis

keratitis sicca, blepharitis, HSV or HZV keratitis, trachoma, Paget's disease, contact lens overwear, vernal and atopic keratoconjunctivitis, SLK, rosacea, chemical burns, toxic injuries, and others.

5.16 Leukocornea

an opacification of the cornea, which may be evident on clinical examination even without using a slit lamp. Leukocornea is a general and nonspecific finding, which may result from a wide variety of etiologies.

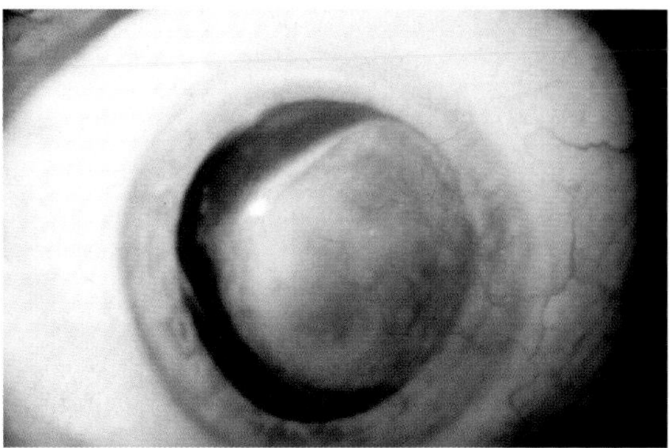

FIGURE 5.16 Leukocornea.

Differential Diagnosis

- Infections: bacterial, fungal, herpetic ulcers or stromal scarring, trachoma, *Acanthamoeba*.
- Inflammatory: ABK, PBK, graft rejection, Stevens, Johnson, ocular cicatricial pemphigoid.
- Hereditary: Fabry's disease, corneal dystrophies, congenital hereditary endothelial dystrophy, PPMD, mucopolysaccharidosis.
- Congenital: glaucoma, Peter's anomaly.
- Trauma: chemical burns, thermal injury.

5.17 Chemical Burn

see Section 1.1.4.

Chapter 6

INTRAOCULAR INFLAMMATION

Stephen Brown, Thomas Flynn,
Alfred E. Mamelok

6.1 Acute Anterior Nongranulomatous Uveitis

cell and flare confined to the anterior chamber without mutton-fat keratic precipitates for less than 6 weeks.

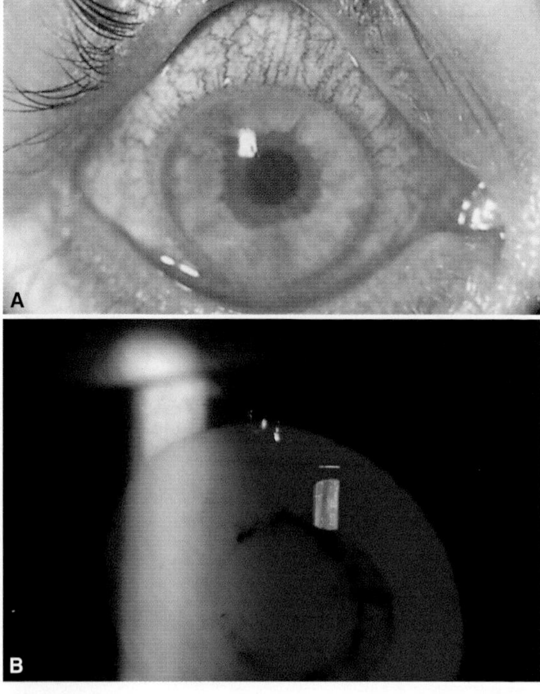

FIGURE 6.1a Acute iritis.
FIGURE 6.1b Posterior synechiae.

Presentation pain, photophobia, ciliary flush. May have decreased vision. Keratic precipitates may be present and the IOP may be abnormally low or elevated.

Differential Diagnosis idiopathic, infectious (syphilis, HSV, HZV, EBV, Lyme disease, early endophthalmitis, mumps, measles, adenovirus) HLA-B27-associated diseases (ankylosing spondylitis, Reiter's syndrome, IBD, psoriatic arthritis), traumatic iritis, SLE, Behçet's disease, renal disease (interstitial nephritis, IgA nephropathy), Posner-Schlossman syndrome, Kawasaki disease, medication hypersensitivity (streptokinase, rifabutin, sulfonamides), granulomatous disease that initially presents as nongranulomatous, masquerade syndromes.

Management careful medical history and review of systems for the aforementioned etiologies. Treat systemic diseases aggressively.

- First episode of unilateral disease: no workup. Treat with topical steroids and cycloplegics to control inflammation and prevent synechiae formation.
- Bilateral disease or recurrent unilateral disease: medical and/or rheumatologic evaluation and workup (CBC with differential, ESR, ANA, RF, VDRL, FTA, ACE, lysozyme, CXR, and PPD). Consider Lyme titer and HLA-B27.
- Prolonged inflammation: sub-Tenon's steroids, oral steroids, and/or oral nonsteroidals; immunosuppressive therapy may be required to prevent long-term sequelae of IOP abnormalities, posterior synechiae, cataract formation, and CME.

6.1.1 HLA-B27-Associated Uveitis—anterior chamber reaction in the presence of one of the HLA-B27 syndromes (ankylosing spondylitis, Reiter's syndrome, IBD, or psoriatic arthritis). HLA-B27 is present in 1 to 6% of the population. The pathogenesis of the inflammation in these diseases is unknown, but there is a molecular similarity between gram-negative bacteria and the HLA-B27 antigen.

6.1.1.1 *Ankylosing Spondylitis*—sacroiliac disease that may occur with ocular inflammation; the most common of the four HLA-B27-associated syndromes.

Presentation

- Ocular inflammation may precede all other symptoms and can be severe with pain, heavy cell and flare, and hypopyon.
- Men commonly present with lower back pain and stiffness that improves with activity.
- Women usually have minimal back pain.

Management treat uveitis with topical steroids and cycloplegics. Sacroiliac radiographs reveal sclerosis and narrowing of the sacroiliac joint space and ossification of the spinal ligaments; 90% of patients are HLA-B27 positive and should be comanaged with a rheumatologist.

6.1.1.2 *Reiter's Syndrome*—ocular inflammation in conjunction with urethritis and polyarthritis.

Presentation arthritis is typically asymmetric and oligoarticular, usually involving the knees, feet, wrists, and sacroiliac joints. Keratoderma blenorrhagicum (a scaly, erythematous disorder of the palms and soles) and circinate balanitis (a scaly, erythematous, circumferential rash of the penis) may be found. Less common findings are plantar fasciitis, Achilles tendonitis, sacroiliitis, nail-bed pitting, and palate or tongue ulcers. Ocular involvement ranges from conjunctivitis and keratitis to anterior, nongranulomatous inflammation.

Management history for exposure to *Yersinia, Salmonella, Shigella,* or other gram-negative organisms. Treat uveitis with topical steroids and cycloplegics. HLA-B27 is present in 75% of patients, and patients should be comanaged with a rheumatologist.

6.1.1.3 *Inflammatory Bowel Disease*—ulcerative colitis (diffuse inflammation of the colonic mucosa) or Crohn's disease (focal granulomatous disease of the entire GI tract).

Presentation ten percent of ulcerative colitis and 2% of Crohn's disease patients suffer from anterior uveitis. Sacroiliitis occurs in 20% of IBD.

- Ocular involvement may precede other symptoms and is generally not related to GI disease activity. Ocular involvement may include anterior uveitis, conjunctivitis, keratitis, episcleritis, scleritis, extraocular muscle palsies, optic neuropathy, retinal vasculitis, neuroretinitis, and orbital inflammation.
- Systemic symptoms include bloody diarrhea, crampy abdominal pain, skin rash, and arthralgias. GI complications such as toxic megacolon and colon cancer may occur; 25 to 40% of patients manifest extraintestinal disease, including erythema nodosum and pyoderma gangrenosum, sacroiliitis, renal stones, and hepatobiliary abnormalities.

Management treat uveitis with topical steroids and cycloplegics. Comanage with a GI specialist and/or rheumatologist.

6.1.1.4 *Psoriatic Arthritis*—psoriasis and arthritis.

Presentation an erythematous, hyperkeratotic rash, nail pitting, and distal phalangeal joint arthritis. Ocular involvement may include nongranulomatous, anterior inflammation, nodular episcleritis, keratitis, and keratoconjunctivitis sicca. Uveitis is not associated with psoriasis without arthritis. This is the least common of the HLA-B27-related disorders.

Management seventy percent of patients are HLA-B27 positive. Treat uveitis with topical steroids and cycloplegics. Comanage with a rheumatologist and/or dermatologist.

6.1.2 Glaucoma-Related Uveitis—anterior chamber inflammation in the presence of glaucoma.

6.1.2.1 *Posner-Schlossman Syndrome*—glaucomatocyclitic crisis.

Presentation unilateral mild pain and blurred vision with halos around lights are often the initial symptoms. There may be a history of previous episodes. Mild iritis and possible trabeculitis with a markedly elevated IOP and corneal edema are present. Minimal conjunctival injection and iris heterochromia may be present. Gonioscopy reveals a normal angle.

Differential Diagnosis infectious uveitis, acute angle-closure glaucoma, pigment dispersion syndrome, Fuchs' heterochromic glaucoma, neovascular glaucoma.

Management topical steroids and pressure-lowering agents. Pilocarpine may cause increased inflammation. No treatment is required between acute attacks. Good prognosis.

6.1.2.2 Uveitis–Glaucoma–Hyphema Syndrome—IOL irritation of the iris or ciliary body causes the UGH triad.

Presentation elevated IOP, anterior chamber inflammation, and hyphema formation in the presence of an IOL. Rarely caused by modern IOLs.

Management treat with topical steroids, cycloplegics, and pressure-lowering agents. Consider IOL removal or exchange.

6.1.2.3 Phacolytic Uveitis/Glaucoma—clogging of the trabecular meshwork by lens protein and foamy macrophages, which leak through an intact lens capsule of a hypermature cataract.

Presentation low-grade anterior chamber inflammation, increased IOP, refractile bodies in the anterior chamber, without the formation of keratic precipitates or synechiae.

Management treat with topical and systemic agents to control IOP. Perform emergent cataract extraction.

6.2 Chronic Nongranulomatous Uveitis

anterior chamber reaction that persists beyond 6 weeks despite proper treatment.

6.2.1 Juvenile Rheumatoid Arthritis-Associated Uveitis

Uveitis—a heterogeneous group of diseases with onset before 16 years of age.

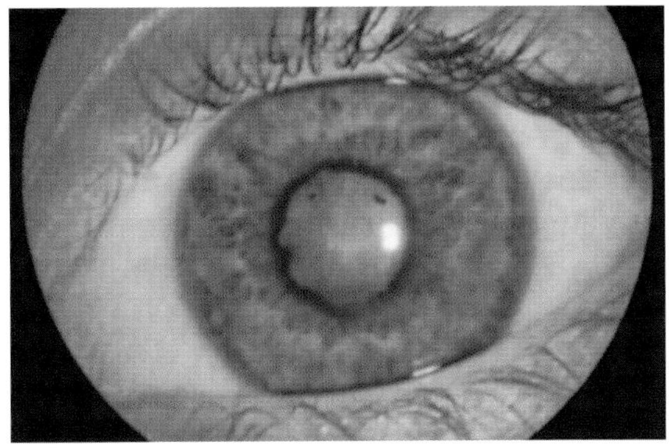

FIGURE 6.2.1 JRA: "quiet" eye with active inflammation and cataract formation.

Presentation the major subtypes are determined by symptoms present within the first 6 weeks:

- Systemic onset (Still's disease): < 2% with uveitis; rash, fever, lymphadenopathy, hepatosplenomegaly, pericarditis, anemia, psoriasis.
- Polyarticular: 7 to 37% incidence of iridocyclitis; fewer than 5 joints involved, inflammation of flexor tendon sheath of hands.
- Pauciarticular: the majority of ocular cases, especially girls 2 to 5 years of age; < 5 joints involved, usually large joints; late pauciarticular disease is more common in boys.
- Children are often asymptomatic, with insidious disease onset. There may be mild ocular pain, headaches, pho-

tophobia, and decreased vision. A white eye with active anterior chamber inflammation, keratic precipitates, posterior synechiae, cataract formation, glaucoma, and band keratopathy may even be found on the first examination.

- Ocular involvement usually occurs within 5 to 7 years of onset of arthritis, but the risk remains into adulthood. Ocular inflammation occurs in 2 to 12% of all cases and is usually bilateral. Unilateral cases often progress to bilateral within 12 months. The uveitis precedes arthritis in roughly 10% of cases with ocular involvement. The ocular and joint disease activity are not associated. A chronic iridocyclitis of children with similar symptoms and course exists without arthritis.

Management laboratory testing:

- ANA (+) in 65 to 88% of cases, usually with a low titer
- RF (−) except in older, polyarticular disease resembling adult disease
- HLA-B27 (−)
- HLA-DR5 (+) associated with eye disease
- HLA-DR1 (+) associated with the absence of eye disease

Rheumatology consultation is mandatory. Treat with topical steroids and cycloplegics; systemic or periocular steroids are sometimes needed. Perform EDTA chelation for band keratopathy. Cataract remains the most difficult management issue, because there is a high rate of surgical complications. Overall prognosis is better if disease is diagnosed and treated early; 25% have a good prognosis, 25% respond poorly, and 50% have moderate to severe disease that requires prolonged treatment; 12 to 40% of involved eyes are ultimately functionally blind.

6.2.2 Fuchs' Heterochromic Iridocyclitis—unilateral, chronic iridocyclitis that presents in the third or fourth decade.

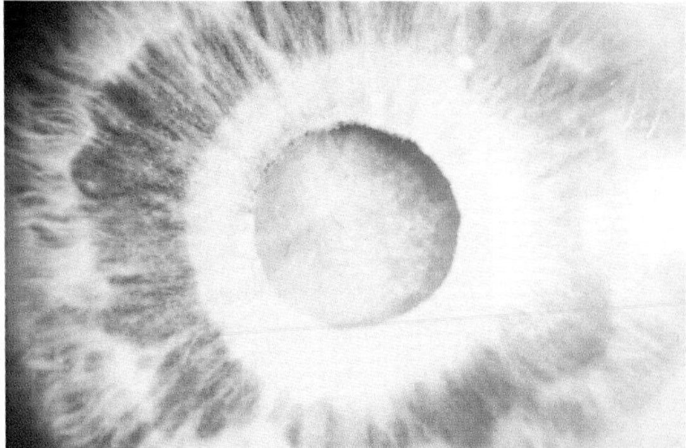

FIGURE 6.2.2 Fuchs' heterochromic iridocyclitis: note the cataract formation and absence of posterior synechiae.

Presentation may be asymptomatic or have mild decreased vision with minimal discomfort. Diffuse iris atrophy results in heterochromia with the involved iris usually being lighter. Small, white, diffuse, stellate, keratic precipitates with minimal aqueous cell and flare are present. Anterior vitreous cells and opacities may also be found. Glaucoma and cataract often occur secondary to the inflammation, but synechiae almost never occur.

Management do not treat aqueous flare; only treat the cells with topical steroids. Inflammation may persist for years. Although these patients often respond well to cataract surgery, the associated glaucoma may be difficult to control. Perform gonioscopy for angle neovascularization, which is present in chronic disease. Anterior vitrectomy may be indicated for severe vitreous opacities.

6.3 Granulomatous Uveitis

anterior chamber inflammation with the presence of mutton-fat keratic precipitates. May have Koeppe (granulomas at the pupillary border) and Busacca nodules (granulomas on the iris surface).

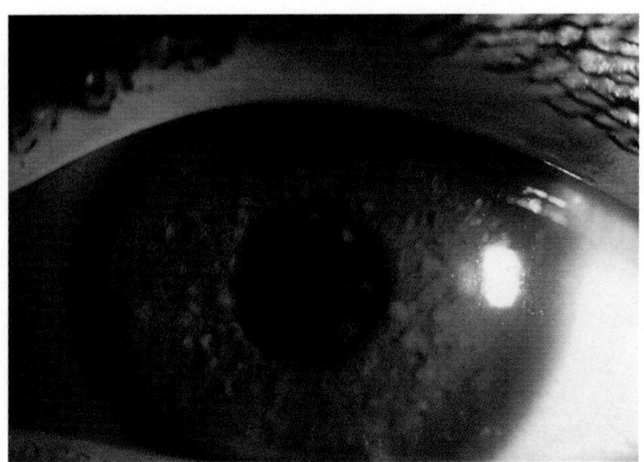

FIGURE 6.3 Granulomatous uveitis: note the iris nodules.

Differential Diagnosis sarcoidosis, syphilis, TB, Lyme disease, leprosy, multiple sclerosis, VKH syndrome, lens-induced or medication (metipranolol, quinidine)-induced inflammation.

Management treat underlying systemic disorder. May require more aggressive steroid or immunosuppressive therapy.

6.3.1 Syphilis—infection caused by *Treponema pallidum*.

Presentation may be congenital or acquired.

- Congenital: intense pain and photophobia with impaired visual acuity. Bilateral interstitial keratitis, keratouveitis, or iridocyclitis usually present at 5 to 25 years of age. Secondary glaucoma, chorioretinitis ("salt and pepper fundus" that may mimic congenital rubella), chorioretinal scars, vitritis, and choroidal neovascularization may occur. Hutchinson's triad (deafness, saddle-nose deformity, and interstitial keratitis) often occurs in addition to mental retardation, papillomacular rash, anemia and hepatosplenomegaly, and failure to thrive.

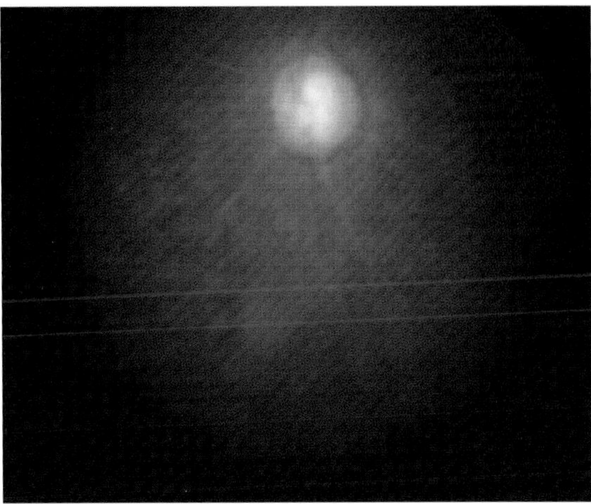

FIGURE 6.3.1 Syphilitic retinitis.

- Acquired: primary disease consists of a chancre (genital, labial, oral) and painless lymphadenopathy 1 week after exposure. Conjunctivitis and a rare eyelid or conjunctival chancre may occur.
- Secondary disease may occur from 3 weeks to 6 months after primary infection and consist of skin rash on palm and soles, fever, weight loss, arthralgias, general lymphadenopathy, and hair loss. Ocular findings consist of granulomatous or nongranulomatous iridocyclitis, roseola iritis (diffuse iris hyperemia lasting for a few days), iritis papulosa (nodules near pupillary margin lasting for several weeks with residual atrophy), syphilids (white, painless nodules on conjunctiva or sclera), episcleritis or scleritis, dacryoadenitis, monocular interstitial keratitis, multifocal or focal chorioretinitis, peripapillary and periarteriolar exudates, and neuroretinitis with papillitis.
- Tertiary disease consists of neurosyphilis, tabes dorsalis, aortitis, and gumma. Ocular findings consist of Argyll Robertson pupil (small, unequal, irregular pupils that constrict in response to light but not accommodation), chorioretinitis (present in 50% of cases; 50% bilateral),

vitritis, cotton-wool spots; flame hemorrhages with fibrosis may be found in addition to other secondary disease findings.
- In patients with AIDS, the normal rates of progression of syphilis are greatly increased, and previously treated disease may reactivate.

Management VDRL and FTA-ABS testing. The level of VDRL or RPR reactivity represents disease activity and decreases with treatment. The FTA-ABS or MHA-TP is a measure of disease exposure and remains positive throughout life.

- A positive FTA and a nonreactive VDRL should be treated only if no previous treatment was administered. A positive VDRL and positive FTA-ABS represents latent disease that may have existed for years to decades with no clinical symptoms. A lumbar puncture should then be performed to rule out neurosyphilis. HIV, chlamydia, and gonorrhea tests should be considered. Remember that false-positive VDRL may occur in pregnancy, increased age, mononucleosis, and leprosy. A false-positive result may occur in primary or latent disease. A false-positive FTA-ABS may occur with rheumatoid arthritis, SLE, or Lyme disease.
- Treat inflammation or active interstitial keratitis with topical steroids and cycloplegics. Syphilitic uveitis should be treated as neurosyphilis. Treatment for acquired syphilis of less than 1 year's duration with a normal CSF includes benzathine penicillin G (2.4 million units IM) or tetracycline or erythromycin (500 mg PO qid) for 15 days. Topical steroids and cycloplegics are used for anterior segment inflammation.

6.3.2 Sarcoidosis

6.3.2 Sarcoidosis—a chronic systemic granulomatous disease of unknown etiology, most commonly affecting the lungs, eyes, and skin.

Presentation more commonly found in African-American women, 20 to 50 years of age.

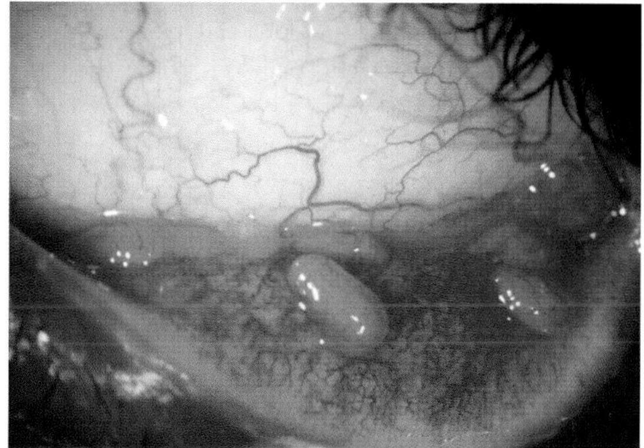

FIGURE 6.3.2 Palpebral conjunctival nodules due to sarcoidosis.

- Ocular findings are present in 25 to 50% of all disease. There may be varying degrees of pain, photophobia, and decreased visual acuity. Granulomas can occur in the orbit, lid, palpebral and bulbar conjunctiva, and lacrimal gland. Anterior segment involvement is more common than posterior segment inflammation. Findings may include dacryoadenitis (50% of cases), chronic granulomatous uveitis with mutton-fat keratic precipitates and Koeppe and Busacca nodules, intermediate uveitis, vitritis with fluffy opacities, retinal and choroidal nodules, "candle-wax drippings," retinal neovascularization, cystoid macular edema, and optic nerve head granulomas or edema. Secondary glaucoma and cataract may be present.
- Systemic findings include all organ systems; lung involvement with hilar adenopathy, cranial and peripheral neuropathy, aseptic meningitis, cardiac arrhythmias and pericarditis, arthritis and myositis secondary to immune-complex deposition, erythema nodosa (tender nodules commonly on the anterior tibia), renal involvement with hepatosplenomegaly, and bone marrow infiltration. When bilateral lacrimal gland inflammation is associated with salivary or parotid gland swelling, it is called Mikulicz's syndrome.

Management positive serum ACE and lysozyme levels and CXR can be suggestive of sarcoidosis. Negative laboratory test results do not rule out the diagnosis. ACE levels correlate with disease activity and decrease with steroid treatment. Biopsy of conjunctival, lacrimal, skin, or hilar lesions may lead to a definitive diagnosis. A gallium scan of the head, neck, and mediastinum can aid in diagnosis but involves radiation exposure. Topical, periocular, and systemic steroids are used to control the inflammation, and topical cycloplegics can help prevent synechiae formation. Joint management with an internist or pulmonologist is helpful, especially if systemic findings are present.

6.3.3 Tuberculosis

6.3.3 Tuberculosis—infection caused by *Mycobacterium tuberculosis* (rarely other species) via inhalation with lymphatic or hematogenous spread.

Presentation varying degrees of pain, photophobia, and decreased vision.

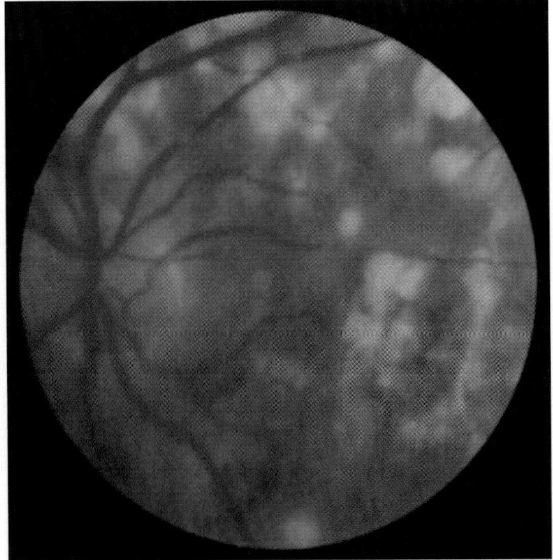

FIGURE 6.3.3 Disseminated choroiditis due to tuberculosis.

- Ocular findings may include granulomatous or non-granulomatous anterior uveitis with or without an accompanying interstitial keratitis. The classic posterior segment findings are multifocal, yellow-white choroidal nodules with indistinct borders or a large choroidal mass. Conjunctivitis, phylectenule formation, scleritis, vitritis with opacities, papillitis, endophthalmitis, necrotizing retinochoroiditis, retinal vascular occlusion, and cystoid macular edema can occur. The ocular disease is usually not associated with active pulmonary tuberculosis.
- Systemic findings include changes in the lungs (especially the apices and hilum), lymph nodes, pleura, urogenital tract, bones, joints, meninges, and the peritoneum.

Management CXR and PPD. Remember that PPD may be false positive after BCG vaccination. As with all chronic inflammation, other causes, such as syphilis, should be ruled out. A trial of isoniazid (300 mg PO qd for 2 weeks) with unequivocal improvement of inflammation is considered diagnostic. Once a diagnosis is made, two or three antitubercular agents should be used because of the rise of multidrug resistance. The agents include isoniazid with pyridoxine (10 mg PO qd) given to prevent neurotoxicity, rifampin, pyrazinamide, and ethambutol. Second-line agents include streptomycin, ciprofloxacin, ofloxacin, kanamycin, ethionamide, cycloserine, paraaminosalicylic acid, and clofazimine. Treatment is required for 6 to 12 months. Steroids should be started only in conjunction with antitubercular agents.

6.3.4 Phacoantigenic Uveitis—an immune response to lens proteins released by traumatic or surgical injury of the lens capsule.

Presentation abrupt onset of pain and photophobia with dense cell and flare in the anterior chamber. Granulomatous keratic precipitates, congested iris vessels, elevated IOP, - posterior synechiae, and a cyclitic membrane may be present.

Management careful history of trauma or surgery. Must rule out infectious endophthalmitis. Diagnosis may be confirmed by anterior and vitreous paracentesis and culture. Treatment options consist of topical and systemic steroids, cycloplegics, and timely, surgical removal of lens material.

6.4 Intermediate Uveitis/Pars Planitis

inflammatory exudate over the pars plana, often of unknown etiology.

Presentation may be asymptomatic and present as an incidental finding, or blurred vision, photophobia, and floaters may be present. The eye is usually quiet, with a small anterior chamber reaction. The pars plana exudate is usually more pronounced inferiorly and is described as a "snowbank."

- Ocular findings include vitreal cells and opacities and patchy, peripheral retinal periphlebitis. Complications include band keratopathy, cataract, glaucoma, peripapillary and cystoid macular edema, vitreous hemorrhage from vitreous base neovascularization and retinal detachment.
- Systemic findings include arthralgias, especially knee symptoms.

Differential Diagnosis sarcoidosis, syphilis, TB, multiple sclerosis, trauma, severe iridocyclitis, toxoplasmosis, Lyme disease, peripheral toxocariasis, AIDS, candidiasis, rheumatoid arthritis, masquerade syndromes (i.e., tumors), retinal detachment and tears, Irvine-Gass syndrome, Whipple's disease, and Behçet's syndrome.

Management the laboratory workup is similar to that of anterior uveitis, with the addition of a Lyme titer. Treatment is necessary for patients with VA of less than 20/40. Topical, sub-Tenon's, or oral steroids may be used on a chronic basis. More advanced disease may require systemic therapy such as cyclosporin A, and pars plana vitrectomy may be used for unresponsive cases to remove vitreous veils, traction, and hemorrhage.

6.5 Posterior Uveitis

inflammation involving the vitreous, retina, and/or choroid.

Presentation

blurred vision, floaters, scotomas; vitritis possibly associated with various retinal and choroidal lesions and a varying degree of anterior segment inflammation. Complications include cataract, secondary glaucoma, cystoid macular edema, retinal or choroidal neovascularization, and retinal detachment.

Differential Diagnosis

- Bacterial agents: TB, syphilis, Lyme, Whipple's disease, brucellosis.
- Fungal agents: any metastatic cause.
- Viral agents: CMV, HSV and HZV, ARN, rubella, measles and mumps, subacute sclerosing panencephalitis, EBV, rickettsia, HTLV-1, nonspecific viral syndromes.
- Protozoal agents: toxoplasmosis, pneumocystis, *Giardia,* amoebiasis, malaris, trypanosomiasis.
- Insect: ophthalmomyiasis.
- Autoimmune: SLE, Behçet's disease, relapsing polychondritis, IBD, Wegener's granulomatosis, polyarteritis nodosa, dermatomyositis, postvaccination, Sjögren's syndrome, Buerger's disease, scleroderma, cryoglobulinemia, multiple sclerosis, sarcoidosis, antiphospholipid antibody syndrome.
- Multifocal inflammation: MEWDS, AMPPE, POHS, punctate inner choroidopathy, multifocal choroiditis, serpiginous chorioretinopathy, embolic retinitis, birdshot retinochoroiditis, acute macular neuroretinitis, Leber's stellate neuroretinitis, cat-scratch neuroretinitis, postviral inflammation.

- Other: posterior scleritis, sympathetic ophthalmia, VKH syndrome, radiation vasculitis, retained foreign body, masquerade syndromes.

Management complete medical history; laboratory tests similar to anterior uveitis workup, including toxoplasma titers. Further tests should be directed toward suspected entities. Cultures and titers for suspected organisms, lumbar puncture, and fluorescein angiography can be helpful. Diagnostic vitrectomy may be performed with antibody titers, culture, and cytology.

6.5.1 Toxoplasmosis—a congenital or acquired infection caused by *Toxoplasma gondii,* a feline intestinal parasite; the most common cause of posterior uveitis.

Presentation blurred vision, floaters, scotoma.

- Ocular findings include the characteristic whitish, yellow, minimally raised, fuzzy lesion that is often found adjacent to an old chorioretinal scar. Dense vitritis and perivasculitis are commonly associated. The active lesion in primary toxoplasmosis infection is often described as "a headlight in the fog." Other manifestations include papillitis, papilledema (ruptured intracerebral cysts with increased intracranial pressure), glaucoma, microphthalmos, strabismus, nystagmus, cystoid macular edema, retinal artery or vein occlusion, and rhegmatogenous retinal detachment.
- Systemic disease is divided into congenital and acquired types.
- Congenital disease is most common and is transmitted transplacentally. Findings include hydrocephalus, necrotizing encephalitis with scattered cerebral calcification, neonatal jaundice, mental retardation, convulsions, microcephaly, and hepatosplenomegaly.
- Acquired disease is mostly subclinical. Lymphadenopathy is the most common finding, but polymyositis, encephalitis, and skin rash may occur.

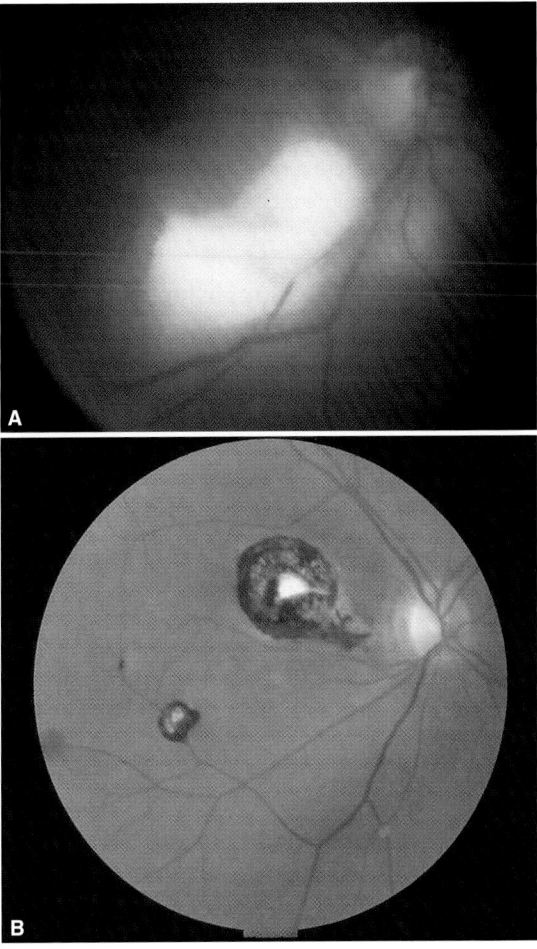

FIGURE 6.5.1a Acute toxoplasmosis: "headlight in a fog" lesion.
FIGURE 6.5.1b Chorioretinal scarring due to inactive toxoplasmosis.

Management

dietary habits, pets, HIV risk factors, and immunocompromised state are all essential to a complete history. Antibody titers may be extremely low, but a negative titer rules out infection. This is a self-limited disease, and treatment may not be necessary if the macula or optic nerve are not threatened. The 6-week antibiotic regimen is bactrim DS (1 tablet PO bid) and clindamycin (300 mg PO qid), or pyrimethamine (25 mg PO qd) plus folinic acid (5 mg PO qod), and sulfadiazine (1 g qid). Oral steroids (prednisone, 1 mg/kg) are begun after a few days of antibiotics when the optic nerve or macula are threatened.

6.5.2 Presumed Ocular Histoplasmosis Syndrome—a retinal disease believed to be caused by systemic infection with *Histoplasma capsulatum*. Patients live in endemic areas, usually in the Ohio–Mississippi River Valley.

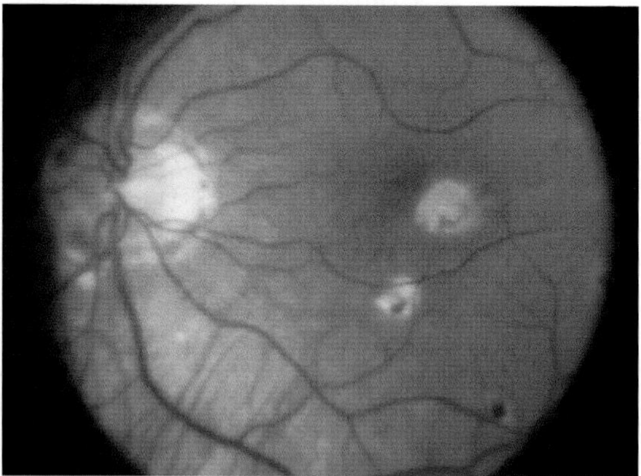

FIGURE 6.5.2 POHS: note the peripapillary atrophy and "punched-out" histo spots.

Presentation patients are usually in the 20- to 50-year age range. Infection may have been mild or subclinical. Findings include any of the following in the absence of vitreous or aqueous inflammatory cells: small, yellow-white punched-out round spots deep to the retina ("histo" spots), peripapillary atrophy, exudative maculopathy including CNV and disciform macular scar, linear chorioretinal atrophy, concentric to the disc, in the midperipheral retina.

Differential Diagnosis multifocal choroiditis, high myopia, angioid streaks, AMD, pseudoxanthoma elasticum.

Management there is a high incidence of HLA-DR2. Amsler's grid testing and FA may be helpful in detecting CNV. Laser photocoagulation has been proven effective for juxtafoveal and extrafoveal CNV. Subfoveal CNV should not be treated, because vision is often good, and treatment may cause loss of vision. Patients have a 12% chance of developing symptoms in the other eye in 5 years.

6.5.3 White Dot Syndromes—various inflammatory diseases that cause a "white dot" appearance to the retina or choroid.

Differential Diagnosis MEWDS, AMPPE, multifocal choroiditis, serpiginious choroiditis, birdshot chorioretinitis, punctate inner choroidopathy, POHS, diffuse unilateral subacute neuroretinitis, subretinal fibrosis and uveitis syndrome, unilateral acute idiopathic maculopathy, acute retinal pigment epitheliitis, sarcoidosis, syphilis or Lyme disease, miliary TB, multifocal choriocapillaris occlusion (e.g., eclampsia, hypertension, giant cell arteritis, disseminated intravascular coagulopathy, sickle cell disease, Goodpasture's syndrome, intraocular lymphoma), fundus albipunctatus, retinitis punctata albescens, Stargardt's disease, familial drusen, Bietti's crystalline retinopathy, pattern dystrophy, macular degeneration, pseudoxanthoma elasticum, crystalline retinopathy.

6.5.3.1 Multifocal Choroiditis—a progressive RPE and choroidal inflammatory disorder with multiple relapses.

Presentation in 80% of cases, bilateral with 3 : 2 female–male ratio; associated with myopia; possible viral prodrome associated with EBV-specific antibodies. The median age of patients is 33 years, but it can occur in children. Blurred vision, floaters, and scotomas may be present. There is anterior uveitis in 50%, vitritis, acute diffuse, yellow and gray, cho-

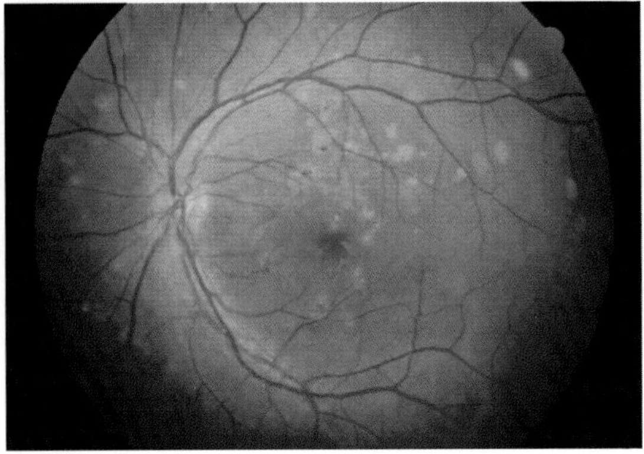

FIGURE 6.5.3.1 Multifocal choroiditis.

roidal or RPE lesions. CME, choroidal neovascularization, and subretinal fibrosis may occur. Vitritis differentiates this disease from POHS.

Management FA shows early hyperfluorescence consistent with RPE window defects. ERG is subnormal in 50%. Lesions quiesce with oral corticosteroid treatment.

6.5.3.2 Multiple Evanescent White Dot Syndrome—an acute, multifocal retinopathy, primarily involving the RPE and outer retina.

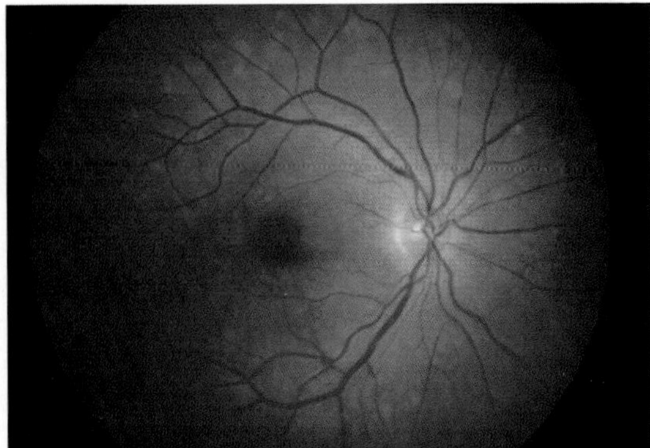

FIGURE 6.5.3.2 MEWDS: white dots near the vascular arcades.

Presentation usually unilateral in young women with a prodromal flu-like syndrome; recurrent cases reported; decreased visual acuity with acute onset of temporal or paracentral scotoma in one eye accompanied by photopsias. APD, vitritis, and characteristic fundus lesion: multiple small, round, slightly indistinct, white or yellow-white spots scattered over the posterior retina, concentrating toward the optic nerve and vascular arcade. There is mild optic disc swelling and a granular appearance to the macula. Enlarged blind spot syndrome is a variant with absent white spots.

Management the visual field may show an enlarged blind spot. FA shows focal areas of early punctate hyperfluorescence corresponding to the white dots and intervening areas. There is staining of the optic disc and leakage from deep retinal capillaries and RPE. ERG is acutely subnormal and elevated IgM has been reported. The natural course of this disease is self-limited. White dots fade and disappear in 4 to 6 weeks, and the vision and ERG return to normal. The enlarged blind spot may persist.

6.5.3.3 Acute Multifocal Posterior Placoid Pigment Epitheliopathy—multifocal inflammatory disorder with yellow-white-gray posterior, circumscribed flat lesions at the level of the RPE and choroid.

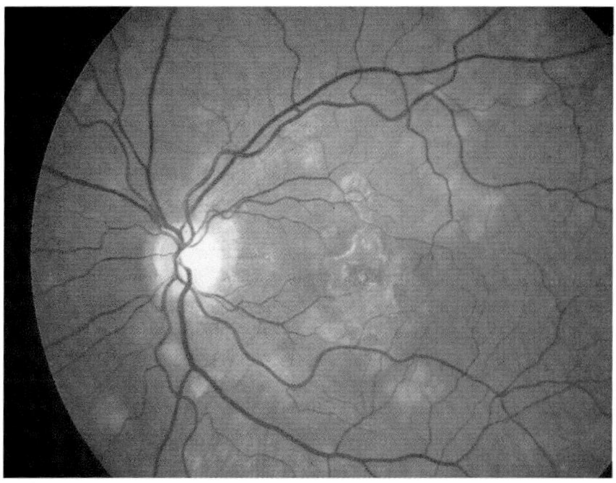

FIGURE 6.5.3.3 AMPPE: large scattered placoid lesions.

Presentation age range, 15 to 42 years. There is a bilateral, often sequential, painless visual loss over several days with preceding viral illness. Patients may complain of headache; beware of cerebral vasculitis. APD, anterior and posterior uveitis, episcleritis, retinal vasculitis, optic neuritis, and a serous RD may occur. Placoid lesions at the level of the RPE and choroid are larger than in MEWDS.

Management FA shows lesions with early blockage and late, diffuse staining. There is spontaneous resolution over several months. The spots fade, leaving partially depigmented RPE behind. The visual prognosis is good if the fovea is uninvolved (usually >20/30). No treatment is therefore necessary unless cerebral vasculitis and/or severe foveal disease is present. Cerebral vasculitis workup includes MRI or MRA, and treatment with high-dose steroids and possibly long-term systemic immunosuppressives. Recurrence is rare.

6.5.3.4 Serpiginous Choroiditis—a bilateral, recurrent, inflammatory disease of the RPE and choroid.

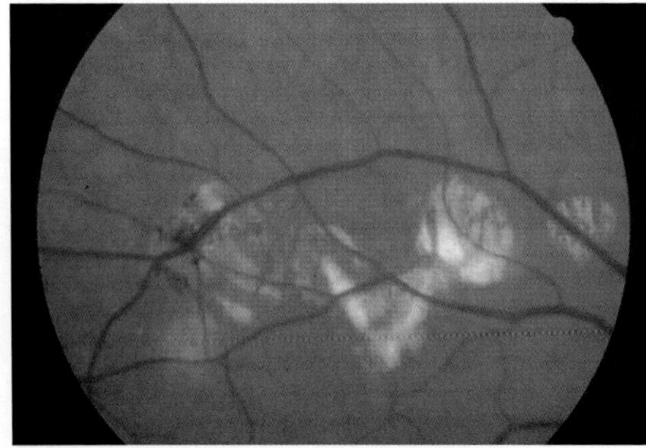

FIGURE 6.5.3.4 Serpiginious choroiditis.

Presentation age range, 30 to 70 years. Patients complain of blurred vision, metamorphopsia, and central scotoma and have anterior and posterior uveitis, with hazy, pale, gray-white lesions with ill-defined margins, beginning adjacent to the optic nerve head and progressing toward the macula in a helicoid manner. Acute lesions appear at the edge of chronic lesions, sometimes appearing as satellite lesions. There is also characteristic RPE and choriocapillaris atrophy. Other possible findings include CNV, retinal vasculitis, papillitis, neovascularization of the disc, sensory retinal detachment, BRVO, or BRAO.

Management there is an increased incidence of HLA-B7. The visual field shows an absolute or relative scotoma corresponding to lesions. FA during active disease shows early hypofluorescence with late hyperfluorescence of lesions. FA during inactive disease shows central areas of hypofluorescence with a border of hyperfluorescence. Oral steroid treatment is indicated; triple therapy with prednisone, azathioprine, and cyclosporine may be needed.

6.5.3.5 Birdshot Chorioretinitis (Vitiliginous Chorioretinitis)—a bilateral, inflammatory disease with multiple oval yellow-white spots in the deep retina and choroid with a vascular predilection for the posterior fundus.

Presentation occurs in the fifth to seventh decades, with a 2 : 1 female–male ratio. There is no visual loss initially. Then, patients

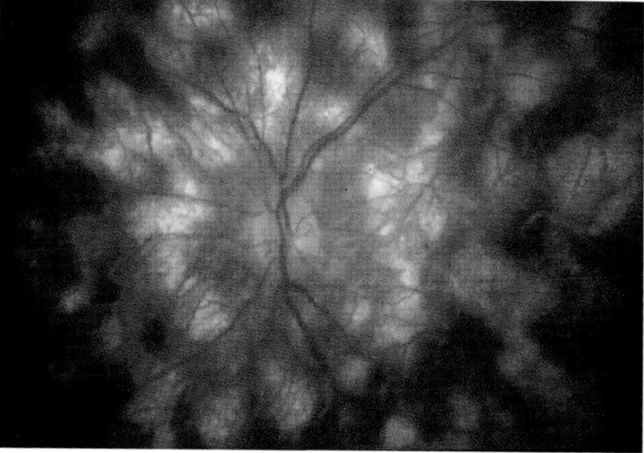

FIGURE 6.5.3.5 Birdshot chorioretinitis.

complain of blurred vision, floaters, photopsias, night blindness, and decreased color vision. There is occasionally an anterior uveitis with multiple, discrete, depigmented, or cream-colored spots, at the level of the RPE, with chronic vitritis and debris. CME, CNV, and papillitis may occur.

Management HLA-B29.2 is present in almost all cases. Exacerbation and remission with progressive atrophic changes are common. FA may show early hypofluorescence and late hyperfluorescence of spots or may be normal. ERG is abnormal in 90% of cases. Treatment consists of low-dose corticosteroids, cyclosporine, and immunosuppressives.

6.5.4 Cytomegalovirus Retinitis—a hemorrhagic, viral retinitis occurring in immunocompromised patients with CD4 counts generally less than 100.

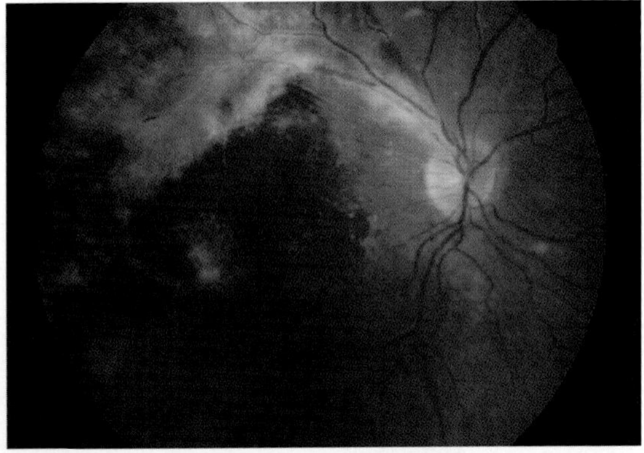

FIGURE 6.5.4 Hemorrhagic and necrotic retinitis due to CMV.

Presentation floaters and loss of vision. Findings include hemorrhages, necrotic retinitis (white, granular, irregularly shaped perivascular areas) that progresses to total retinal destruction and blindness if left untreated. Mild vitritis may be present, and papillitis may accompany the retinitis. "Frosted-branch" angiitis may be present, and exudative and rhegmatogenous detachments may occur.

Differential Diagnosis AIDS retinopathy (cotton-wool spots, flame and dot hemorrhages, microaneurysms), severe hypertension, sarcoidosis, diabetes, retinal vein occlusion, choroidal metastasis, ARN, PORN, toxoplasmosis, syphilis, HSV, varicella-zoster, candida, and cryptococci.

Management susceptible individuals have a 20% risk per year of developing CMV retinitis. Treat with 14-day induction therapy of IV ganciclovir (5 mg/kg q12h) or IV foscarnet (60 mg/kg q8h). Ganciclovir may cause neutropenia, whereas foscarnet may be toxic to the kidneys. Examine the retina at the end of the induction phase, and consider maintenance therapy to prevent disease reactivation. If there is still active disease, consider further treatment with the same agent if there is no toxicity or consider switching from one agent to the other. Cidofovir is a newly approved antiviral with a longer half-life. Intravitreal injections, drug reservoir implants, and Cytovene (oral ganciclovir) are available; however, it is important to treat systemic disease to prolong longevity.

6.5.5 Acute Retinal Necrosis Syndrome

—a rare unilateral or bilateral syndrome in typically healthy adolescents and older adults caused by herpes virus.

Presentation a mild to severe anterior inflammation followed by vitreous cell, pain, and loss of vision due to a rapidly progressive occlusive retinal vasculitis, scleritis, and optic neuritis. Retinal whitening begins in multifocal areas in the peripheral retina, spreading circumferentially, and becoming confluent as the disease progresses. The posterior pole is usually spared, and there is a sharp demarcation between involved and normal retina. Periphlebitis and hemorrhage are present. Retinal detachment is common (70%), and glaucoma may be present.

Management the diagnosis is based on clinical appearance and course, and progression is rapid without antiviral treatment. Treat with IV acyclovir (1500 mg/mm²/day, divided into 3 doses, for 7 to 10 days) and then oral acyclovir (400 to 600 mg 5 times per day). Newer antivirals, such as valacyclovir, may be effective. Cycloplegics may be used, and oral prednisone is begun 2 to 3 days after acyclovir. Aspirin, heparin, or coumadin are used for anticoagulation. Therapy is continued until all signs of ARN have disappeared. Laser photocoagulation is used prophylactically or to wall off an early retinal detachment. In addition, trans–pars plana vitrectomy may be indicated.

6.6 Vogt-Koyanagi-Harada Syndrome

an autoimmune, bilateral panuveitis with multifocal serous retinal detachments, associated with vitiligo, alopecia, poliosis, CNS involvement, and deafness.

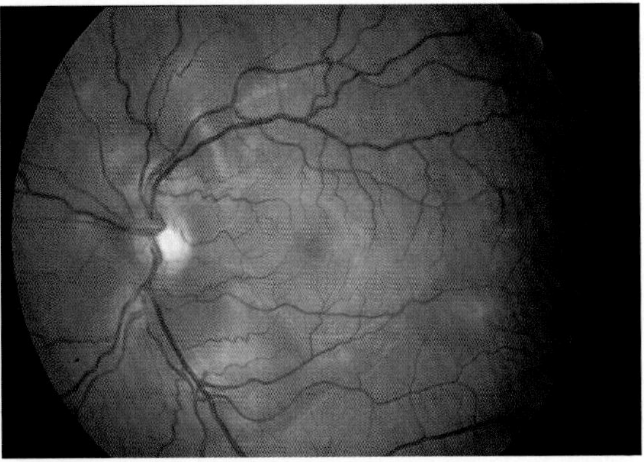

FIGURE 6.6 Multifocal serous detachments due to VKH syndrome.

Presentation commonly occurs in Asians and American Indians, usually 20 to 50 years old. Three of four findings must be present for diagnosis: (1) bilateral chronic iridocyclitis; (2) posterior uveitis with exudative retinal detachment, disc hyperemia or edema, "sunset glow" fundus; (3) neurologic signs such as tinnitus, cranial nerve palsies; (4) cutaneous signs such as poliosis, alopecia, and vitiligo. There is no history of ocular trauma or surgery. The syndrome is characterized by four phases:

- Prodromal phase: headache, nausea, vertigo, fever, meningismus, orbital pain, and photophobia.
- Uveitic phase: bilateral panuveitis with acute decrease in vision.
- Convalescent phase: depigmentation of skin and choroid ("sunset-glow" fundus). Sugiura's sign of limbal vitiligo is considered pathognomonic. Dalen-Fuchs–like nodules are seen as white lesions in the deep retina and choroid.
- Chronic, recurrent phase: iris nodules and other complications of chronic inflammation, such as posterior synechiae, cataract, glaucoma, and SRN membranes.

Differential Diagnosis sympathetic ophthalmia, intraocular lymphoma, sarcoidosis, syphilis, TB, AMPPE, MEWDS, bilateral diffuse melanocytic hyperplasia, lupus choroidopathy, uveal effusion syndrome, posterior scleritis, central serous chorioretinopathy, and other systemic disorders.

Management workup as for anterior uveitis plus fluorescein angiography (multiple focal, early leakage), B-scan (diffuse choroidal thickening), lumbar puncture (pleocytosis), and MRI if there is CNS involvement. Treat with cycloplegics; topical, periocular, or systemic steroids; and/or immunosuppressive agents. With aggressive treatment, 66% of patients will have a visual outcome of 20/40 or better. Poor prognostic signs are increased age at time of onset, chronic ocular inflammation, and CNV membranes.

6.7 Behçet's Disease

a triad of ocular inflammation and oral and genital ulcers of unknown etiology with highest incidence in countries along the Silk Road (Mediterranean Sea to Japan).

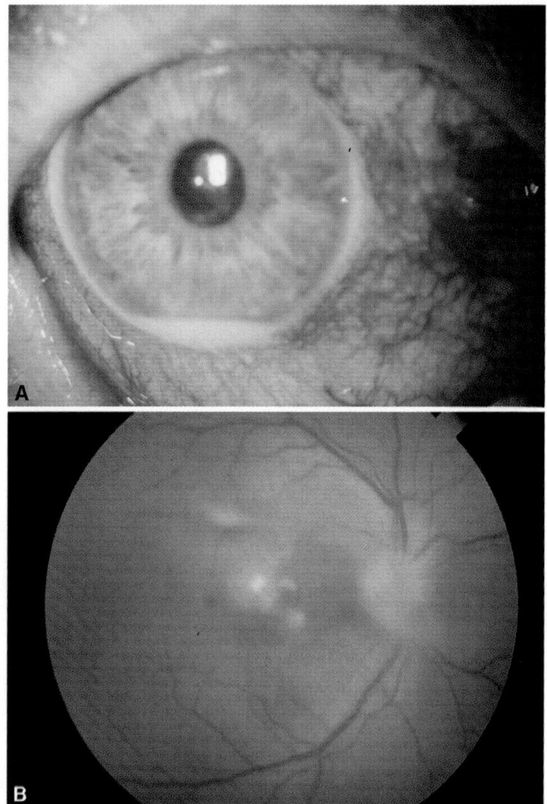

FIGURE 6.7a Hypopyon uveitis due to Behçet's disease.
FIGURE 6.7b Posterior uveitis due to Behçet's disease.

Presentation

- Ocular findings are present in 75% of cases and include conjunctivitis; subconjunctival hemorrhage; episcleritis; scleritis; iridocyclitis, with or without hypopyon (usually bilateral); vitritis; papillitis; retinal hemorrhage, edema, and serous detachment; branch and central retinal vein occlusion; choroiditis; and myositis.
- Systemic findings include oral and genital ulcers, erythema nodosa, vesiculopapular eruptions, arthritis, thrombophlebitis, GI symptoms, epididymitis, and CNS findings of meningitis and seizures.

Differential Diagnosis sarcoidosis, multiple sclerosis, encephalitis, Stevens-Johnson syndrome.

Management genetic influence with HLA-B51 prevalence. Treatment includes oral steroids, azathioprine, chlorambucil, cyclophosphamide, and other immunosuppressives.

6.8 Sympathetic Ophthalmia

a rare bilateral panuveitis 5 days to decades following penetrating trauma or surgery.

Presentation decreased visual acuity and accommodation, photophobia, pain, and epiphora. Bilateral granulomatous panuveitis with Dalen-Fuchs nodules (small yellowish, yellow-red, or white elevated granulomas between Bruch's membrane and the RPE), peripheral depigmentation, exudative retinal detachment, and optic neuritis. Complications include cataract formation, glaucoma, and optic atrophy.

Differential Diagnosis VKH syndrome, lens-induced uveitis, other granulomatous uveitis, toxoplasmosis, Behçet's disease, birdshot chorioretinopathy, serpiginous choroiditis.

Management most cases occur 4 to 8 weeks after insult, and 20% of cases are associated with phacoantigenic uveitis. Diagnosis is based on history and clinical examination, with the exclusion of other causes of granulomatous uveitis. FA reveals late hyperfluorescence of nodules with possible initial hypofluorescence (an appearance similar to VKH) and possible window defects. ERG and EOG have decreased amplitudes. Treatment consists of topical, periocular, and/or systemic steroids and nonsteroidals. Immunosuppressives such as azathioprine, methotrexate, chlorambucil, or cyclosporine are required. The course is often chronic with frequent exacerbations.

6.9 Endophthalmitis

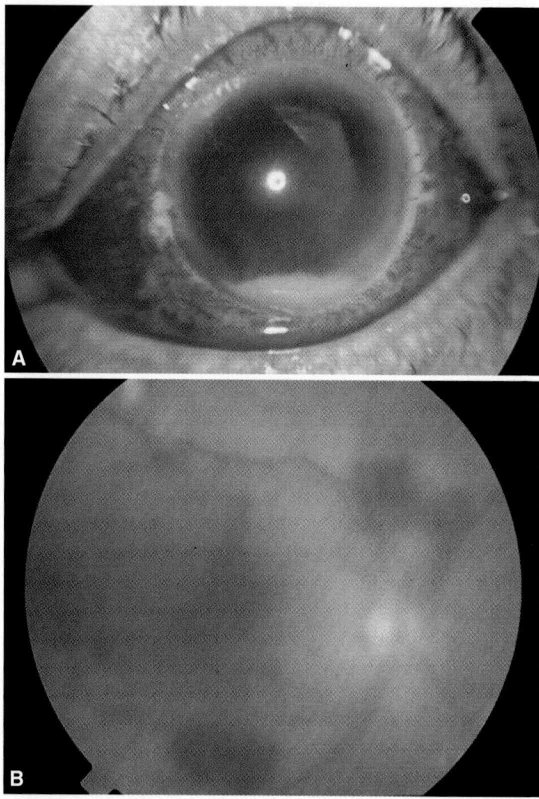

FIGURE 6.9a Hypopyon and scleral injection in endophthalmitis.
FIGURE 6.9b Fundus of endophthalmitis eye.

6.9.1 Traumatic Endophthalmitis—an inflammatory and infectious complication of penetrating ocular injuries.

Presentation pain, photophobia, and visual loss weeks, months, or years following penetrating ocular injuries. The pain is often worse with eye movement. Anterior uveitis, often with hypopyon, and vitritis are present. There may be eyelid edema and erythema, chemosis, corneal edema and infiltrate, and retinal periphlebitis and hemorrhage.

Management risk factors include retained foreign body and delay of treatment following injury. After initial management of penetrating injury, aqueous and vitreous cultures are drawn. If endophthalmitis is suspected, consider using intravitreal antibiotics: vancomycin hydrochloride (1 mg in 0.1 ml) and amikacin (0.4 mg in 0.1 ml) or ceftazidime (2.25 mg in 0.1 ml). The routine use of intravitreal antibiotics with penetrating trauma is controversial, and subconjunctival and topical fortified antibiotics may be used. Intravitreal, subconjunctival, topical, and oral steroids may also be used. *Staphylococcus, Streptococcus,* and *Bacillus* species are the most common isolates. *Bacillus* from soil-contaminated injuries has a rapid course associated with a poor outcome. Vitrectomy is indicated for foreign-body or fulminant infection.

6.9.2 Postoperative Endophthalmitis—postoperative infection.

Presentation intraocular inflammation greater than expected usually beginning within the first week after an operation. In most cases, the pain is often greater than expected. An anterior uveitis often with hypopyon and vitritis are present. There may be eyelid edema and erythema, chemosis, corneal edema and infiltrate, retinal periphlebitis and hemorrhage.

Differential Diagnosis

- Sterile or toxic endophthalmitis (inflammation 1 to 4 days postoperatively from retained lens material, foreign body, or iatrogenically used chemicals)
- Idiopathic endophthalmitis, with an excessive inflammatory response to surgical trauma by some individuals.

Management diabetics and other immunosuppressed individuals are predisposed. Nearly 75% of aqueous and vitreous cultures are positive, with *S. epidermidis* being the most common isolate, followed by *S. aureus,* and gram-negative rods, such as *Serratia marcescens, Proteus,* and *Pseudomonas* species. A poor prognosis is associated with rapid development. *Proprionobacterium acnes,* which causes a low-grade endophthalmitis, has been reported more than 1 year postoperatively. Bleb-related endophthalmitis after trabeculectomy occurs late, usually after several months to years, but has been reported up to 60 years later. The majority are culture positive, caused by *Streptococcus* species, *Haemophilus influenzae,* and *Staphylococcus* species. The prognosis for all cases is poor.

- Obtain aqueous sample and vitreous biopsy sample from eyes with vision better than light perception.
- Intravitreal antibiotics: vancomycin (1.0 mg in 0.1 ml) and amikacin (0.4 mg in 0.1 ml) or ceftazidime (2.25 mg in 0.1 ml).
- Subconjunctival antibiotics: vancomycin (25 mg in 0.5 ml) and ceftazidime (100 mg in 0.5 ml) or amikacin (25 mg in 0.5 ml).
- Topical fortified antibiotics: vancomycin (50 mg/ml) and amikacin (20 mg/ml), alternating every 1 to 4 hours.
- Corticosteroids: topical, subconjunctival (dexamethasone sodium phosphate, 6 mg in 0.25 ml), oral (prednisone 30 mg PO bid for 5 to 10 days), or intravitreal (controversial).
- Topical cycloplegics.
- Intravenous or oral antibiotics have been shown not to effect outcome.
- Trans–pars plana vitrectomy for cases with light-perception vision or worse has been shown to improve visual outcome.

6.9.3 Endogenous Endophthalmitis—ocular infection from hematogenous seeding from a remote source.

Presentation immunosuppressives, invasive procedures, broad-spectrum antibiotic use, corticosteroids, antibody deficiencies, neonates, antimetabolites, hyperalimentation, and chronic debilitating diseases, such as diabetes, malignancies, renal failure, cardiac disease, and stroke, are predisposing factors. There is a wide range of initial presentation, either a focal process or panophthalmitis, with decreased visual acuity and floaters. Aqueous and vitreous inflammation, hypopyon, corneal opacification, white nodules of the iris, choroid, or retina, white-centered retinal hemorrhages, retinal vascular occlusions, periorbital edema, proptosis, and decreased motility may occur. Fungal infection, which may present with yellow-white retinal lesions with fluffy borders that can exude into the vitreous, has a more indolent course.

Management

both bacteria and fungus are etiologic organisms.

- Bacterial isolates commonly include *Streptococcus* species, *Staphylococcus* species, *Listeria monocytogenes, Clostridia* species, *Bacillus* species, *Escherichia coli, Klebsiella pneumoniae, Haemophilus influenzae, Serratia marscescens, Pseudomonas aeruginosa, Neisseria meningitidis, Actinobacillus* species, *Salmonella* species, *Proteus* species, *Nocardia asteroides,* and *Mycobacterium tuberculosis.*
- Fungal isolates commonly include *Candida* species (75% of fungal cases), *Aspergillus fumigatus, Geotrichum candidum, Cryptococcus neoformans, Histoplasma capsulatum, Sporotrichum schenckii* (Gardener's syndrome), *Blastomyces dermatidis, Mucor rarmosus,* and *Fusarium* species.

Management includes:

- Cultures of the aqueous, vitreous, blood, urine, and CSF.
- Intravenous or oral antibiotic or antifungal agents, preferably directed against suspected organism(s).
- Intravitreal antibiotics include vancomycin (1 mg in 0.1 ml) and amikacin (0.4 mg in 0.1 ml) or ceftazidime (2.25 mg in 0.1 ml).
- Topical and periocular antibiotic or antifungal agents may be used.
- Cycloplegia is recommended.

Overall prognosis depends on the virulence of the infective organism, premorbid condition of the patient, and timing of diagnosis and treatment. Vitrectomy is controversial and depends on the overall assessment.

6.10 Masquerade Syndromes

conditions that mimic uveitis, including retinitis pigmentosa, amyloidosis, lymphomas, reactive lymphoid hyperplasia, leukemia, tumors (e.g., retinoblastoma, melanoma, metastasis), retinal detachment (Schwartz-Jampel syndrome), phacolytic glaucoma, pigment dispersion syndromes, inherited vitreoretinopathies, radiation retinopathy, orbital pseudotumor, juvenile xanthogranuloma, intraocular foreign body, vitreous hemorrhage, ocular ischemia, and asteroid hyalosis.

6.10.1 Lymphoma—usually presents in older adults. CNS lymphoma more commonly has ocular involvement than does visceral lymphoma. B-cell tumors more common. Should be considered in all cases of vitritis in older individuals, especially if refractory to treatment. May show initial response to steroids.

6.10.2 Intraocular Leukemia—ocular involvement is more common in acute leukemia than in chronic leukemia, and more common with myeloid than lymphoid types. Ocular findings occur in the majority of cases at some point in the course of the disease: vitritis, intraretinal, preretinal, and vitreous hemorrhages, papillitis, and serous retinal detachment. CNS symptoms can occur (see Section 11.1.7, Leukemic Iris Nodules).

6.10.3 Retinoblastoma—must be considered in children under age 3 years who present with ocular inflammation. Ocular findings include pseudohypopyon, retinal lesions, and vitreous seeding.

6.10.4 Choroidal Melanoma—may present with inflammation, vitreous hemorrhage, and a black hypopyon (see Section 11.3.2, Choroidal Melanoma).

6.10.5 Intraocular Foreign Body—small, high-velocity, steel fragments that penetrate the globe may present with anterior and local inflammation, heterochromia, other signs of siderosis (brown stromal and anterior lens capsule discoloration, vitreous opacities) or chalcosis (Kayser-Fleisher ring, sunflower cataract, red vitreous opacities).

6.10.6 Schwartz-Jampel Syndrome—anterior chamber reaction and glaucoma with rhegmatogenous retinal detachment. The inflammation consists mainly of retinal photoreceptors and pigment granules (Shafer's sign).

6.10.7 Juvenile Xanthogranuloma—oculocutaneous disorder presenting with unilateral iridocyclitis, fleshy brown iris or ciliary-body lesion, spontaneous hyphema, heterochromia, unilateral glaucoma, posterior scleritis, small yellowish-orange lesions of the skin, cornea, and orbit (see Section 11.1.5, Juvenile Xanthogranuloma).

6.10.8 Anterior Ischemic Syndrome—presents in patients with carotid occlusive disease, aortic arch syndrome, or after recti muscle or retinal surgery. Patients complain of decreased visual acuity and pain without photophobia. Findings include chemosis, episcleral injection without ciliary flush, corneal edema, large keratic precipitates, Descemet's folds, anterior inflammation, iris atrophy, hypotony, cataract, asymmetric retinopathy, microaneurysms, midperipheral hemorrhages, retinal or disc neovascularization, and decreased ipsilateral ophthalmodynametry. Carotid bruit and a history of amaurosis fugax or transient ischemic attacks are common.

6.10.9 Paraneoplastic Syndromes—carcinoma-related (especially small cell lung carcinoma) autoantibodies that cross-react with retinal antigens. Patients present with retinitis, without vitritis, and a decreased ERG.

Chapter 7
LENS AND CATARACT

Jessica Lattman, Jack M. Dodick, Norman B. Medow

7.1 Congenital Lens Defects

7.1.1 Congenital Aphakia—absence of the lens, which is very rare. Primary aphakia results from failure of the lens plate to form; it occurs concurrently with other anterior and posterior segment anomalies. Secondary aphakia occurs when the developing lens is spontaneously absorbed. Often only a wrinkled capsule remains.

Presentation absent lens in a newborn, microphthalmia, other anterior and posterior segment anomalies.

Differential Diagnosis subluxated lens.

7.1.2 Lenticonus and Lentiglobus—ectasias in the anterior or posterior lens capsule. Lenticonus is a conical bulge, and lentiglobus is a spherical deformation.

Presentation retinoscopy through the center of the lens produces a distorted and myopic reflex. On retroillumination, the deformity appears as an "oil droplet." This malformation is often progressive, with development of a subcapsular lens opacity. Amblyopia often develops as a result of anisometropia induced by lenticular myopia, astigmatism, or increasing lens opacity. Anterior lenticonus may be associated with Alport's syndrome (autosomal dominant hearing loss, renal failure, maculopathy).

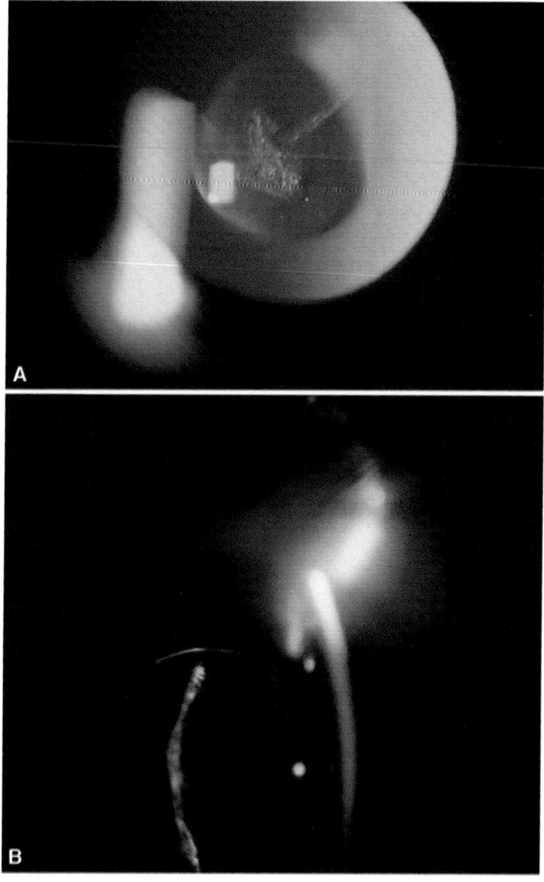

FIGURE 7.1.2a Lenticonus.
FIGURE 7.1.2b "Oil droplet" sign on retroillumination.

7.1.3 Lens Coloboma—an anomaly of lens shape with flattening or notching of the lens periphery. It is often associated with abnormal zonular attachments in the region of the coloboma.

Presentation

- Primary coloboma: Wedge-shaped defect of the lens periphery.

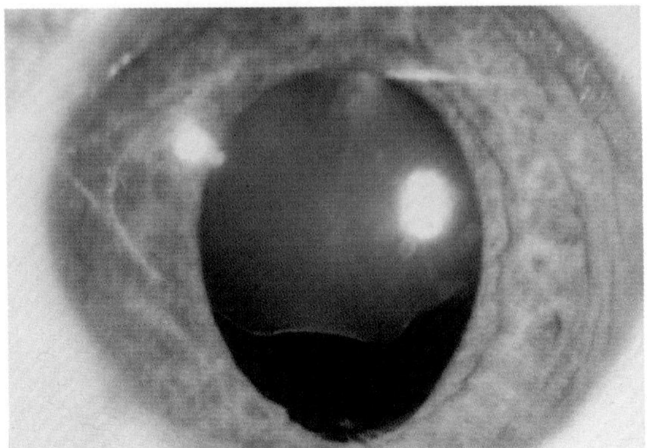

FIGURE 7.1.3 Inferior lens and zonular coloboma.

- Secondary coloboma: flattening or indentation in the lens periphery secondary to the lack of zonular or ciliary body development. The defect is often inferonasal in position.
- Other colobomatous malformations of the eye may be present.

7.2 Congenital Cataracts

a lens opacity present at birth. One-third of congenital cataracts are inherited, one-third are associated with systemic or ocular disease, and one-third are idiopathic.

Presentation a white reflex (leukocoria) or abnormal eye movements (nystagmus). One or both eyes may be affected. If visually insignificant, congenital cataracts may be an incidental finding.

7.2.1 Polar Cataract—a congenital opacity of the subcapsular cortex and lens capsule either in the anterior or posterior pole of the lens. In general, posterior polar cataracts produce more visual impairment than anterior polar cataracts.

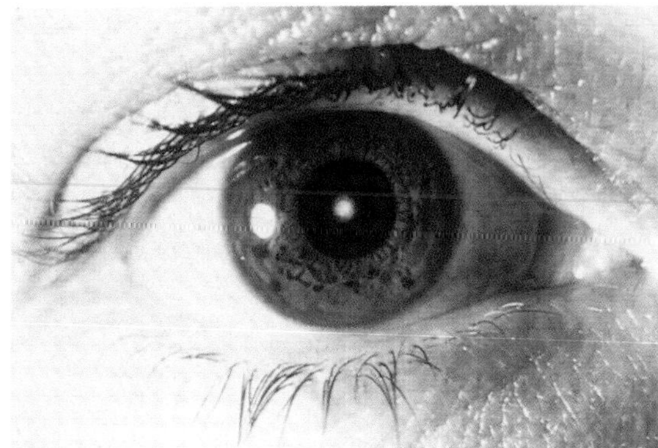

FIGURE 7.2.1 Anterior polar cataract.

7.2.2 Sutural Cataract—an opacification of the fetal nuclear Y-shaped sutures. It rarely impairs vision.

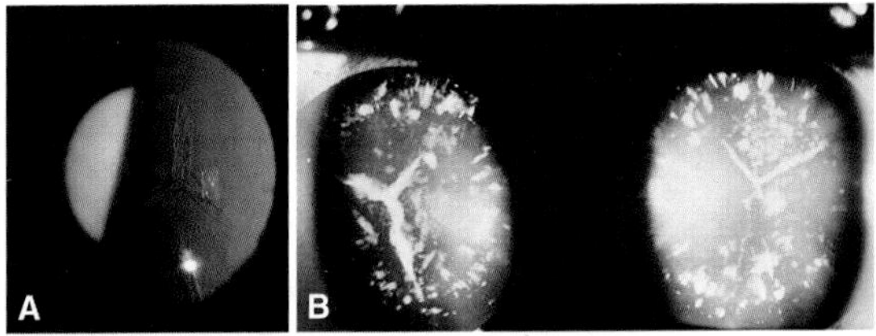

FIGURE 7.2.2a Sutural cataract on retroillumination.
FIGURE 7.2.2b Bilateral sutural cataracts.

7.2.3 Complete (Total) Cataract—congenital cataract involving the entire lens. Complete cataracts are usually bilateral and white, allowing no view of the retina. Maternal rubella infection, especially in the first trimester, can cause complete congenital cataracts. Cataract extraction in congenital rubella may cause release of live virus from the lens and excessive inflammation (see Congenital Rubella in Chapter 15). Metabolic causes include diabetes and galactosemia.

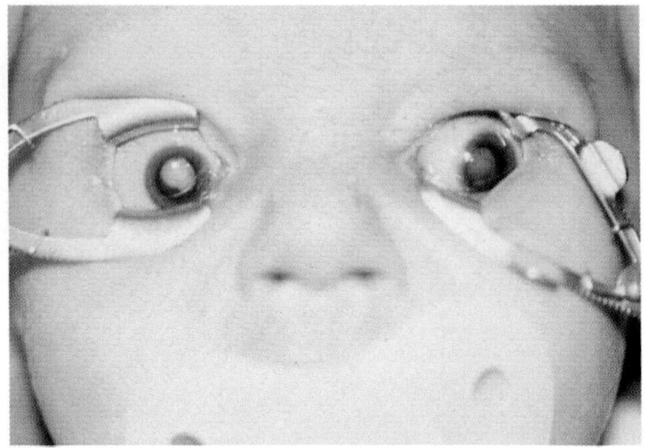

FIGURE 7.2.3 Complete congenital cataracts in rubella syndrome.

7.2.4 Lamellar (Zonular) Cataract—a congenital opacity of discrete layers of the lens. Lamellar cataracts are thought to be due to transient insults during development, where the exposed lens fibers are opacified while surrounding fibers are normal. Examination reveals a number of "riders," or linear projections from the surface of the cataract into the clear peripheral cortex. Usually bilateral and symmetric, their impact on visual acuity depends on the size and density of the opacification.

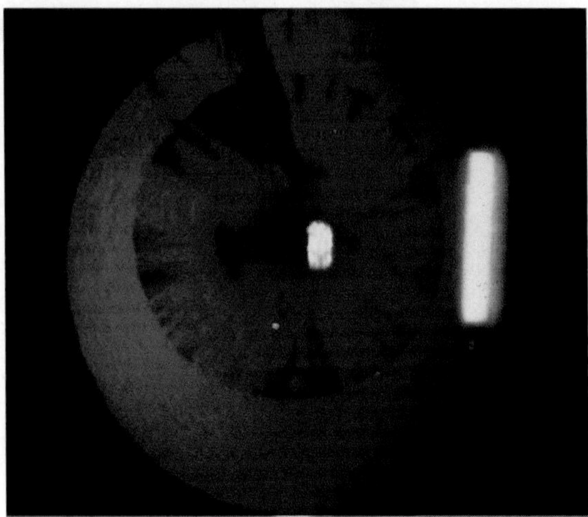

FIGURE 7.2.4 Lamellar cataract.

7.2.5 Membranous Cataract—occurs when lens proteins are resorbed from the lens, allowing the anterior and posterior lens capsules to fuse and opacify. Membranous cataracts are dense white opacities and cause significant visual impairment. The condition is usually unilateral and may be associated with other ocular abnormalities such as persistent hyperplastic primary vitreous.

Differential Diagnosis traumatic cataract.

7.2.6 Mittendorf's Dot—a punctate opacity located inferior and nasal to the central capsule. It is a common remnant of the posterior capsule of the tunica vasculosa lentis, a network of vessels that surrounds the lens during embryogenesis. Anterior remnants of the vascular tunic include persistent pupillary membranes and epicapsular stars.

7.2.7 Persistent Hyperplastic Primary Vitreous—a malformation of the eye with a broad range of severity. The mildest presentation may include prominent hyaloid vessel remnants with a large Mittendorf's dot. PHPV is usually unilateral. Often a retrolental white fibrous membrane is seen with posterior cortical opacification of the lens. Severely affected eyes show cataract formation from fibrovascular invasion of the lens through a defect in the posterior lens capsule with shallowing of the anterior chamber and angle-closure glaucoma. Other findings include elongation of the ciliary processes, prominent radial iris vessels, and a smaller involved eye than the normal one.

Differential Diagnosis see Leukocoria, in Section 12.2.

Management of Congenital Cataracts

- History: congenital infection (rubella, cytomegalovirus, varicella, syphilis, toxoplasmosis); family history of congenital cataract or genetic or metabolic disease; exposure to corticosteroids or radiation; trauma.
- Assess vision and ocular alignment.
- Determine visual significance of cataract. Evaluate size, location, and density.

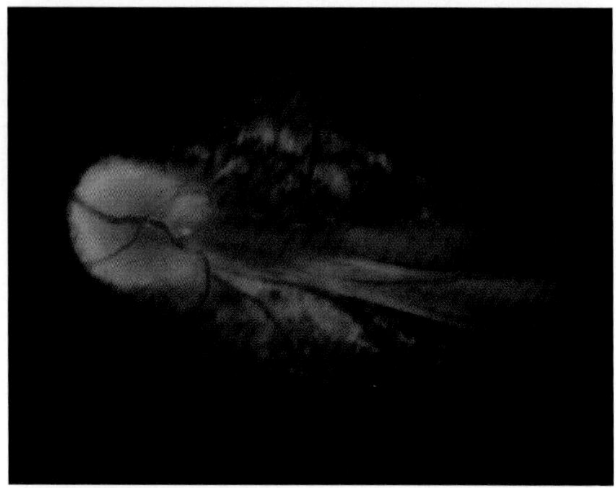

FIGURE 7.2.7 PHPV.

- Complete ocular examination, noting signs of associated glaucoma, retinal pathology, or other ocular anomalies (aniridia, anterior segment dysgenesis). B-scan ultrasonography if fundus view is obscured.
- Physical examination by a pediatrician to tailor workup.
- Blood tests: galactokinase levels, RBC galactose 1-phosphate uridylyltransferase activity (galactosemia); calcium, phosphorus (hypocalcemia, hypoparathyroidism); glucose (hypoglycemia, diabetes mellitus).
- Urine tests: sodium nitroprusside test (homocystinuria), blood and protein (Alport's syndrome), amino acid content (Lowe syndrome—oculocerebrorenal syndrome), copper level (Wilson's disease).
- Antibody titers (rubella, mumps, toxoplasmosis, herpes, syphilis).
- Young infants who do not undergo surgery (visually insignificant lens opacities) must be followed closely for cataract progression and amblyopia.
- Cataract extraction is indicated for visually significant lens opacities and possibly PHPV when progression is associated with poor prognosis (i.e., angle-closure glaucoma).
- Postoperative care involves correction of aphakia, preferably with a contact lens. (Intraocular lens implan-

tation is controversial before age 3 years). Glaucoma is common. Treat amblyopia with patching of the better eye.

7.3 Senile Cataracts

lens opacities associated with aging.

Presentation slowly progressive decrease in visual acuity, over months to years, often with associated glare and decreased color discrimination. May affect one or both eyes. Symptoms are closely related to the proximity of the cataract to the visual axis.

7.3.1 Senile Nuclear Sclerotic Cataract—common, progressive yellowing of the nucleus. An excessive amount is considered a senile nuclear sclerotic cataract. They tend to progress slowly, are bilateral, and produce more impairment of distance vision than of near vision. There may be an increase in the refractive power (myopic shift), causing new ability to read without reading glasses. A very advanced nuclear cataract becomes opaque and brown and is called a brunescent nuclear cataract.

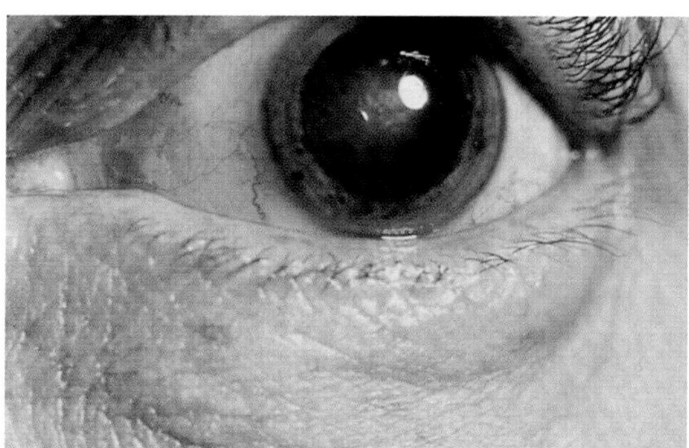

FIGURE 7.3.1 Senile nuclear sclerotic cataract.

7.3.2 Cortical Cataract—changes in the ionic composition of the lens cortex and subsequent hydration changes of the lens fibers lead to cortical opacifications. They are usually bilateral and cause glare. Ef-

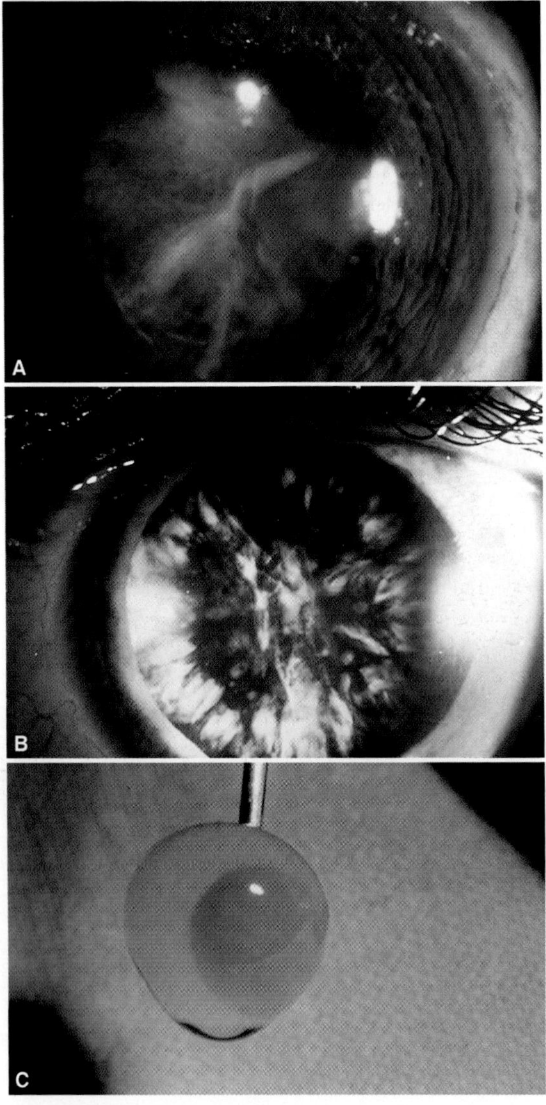

FIGURE 7.3.2a Cortical cataract.
FIGURE 7.3.2b Cortical spoking.
FIGURE 7.3.2c Morgagnian cataract after intracapsular extraction.

fect on vision depends on involvement of the visual axis. "Cortical spokes" or wedge-shaped opacities are seen in the periphery of the lens. Vacuoles are seen on retroillumination. The stages of cortical cataracts are as follows:

- Intumescent: swollen capsule from hydration of the cortex.
- Mature: the entire cortex from the capsule to the nucleus is white and opaque.
- Hypermature: shrunken, wrinkled capsule due to leakage of degenerated lens material.
- Morgagnian: liquefaction of the cortex with free-floating or sunken brown nucleus within the capsular bag.

7.3.3 Posterior Subcapsular Cataract—located in the posterior cortical layer, usually axial. Subcapsular cataracts produce glare, poor vision in bright lights, and reduced near vision more than distance. Granular or plaquelike deposits in the posterior subcapsular cortex are often seen well by retroillumination.

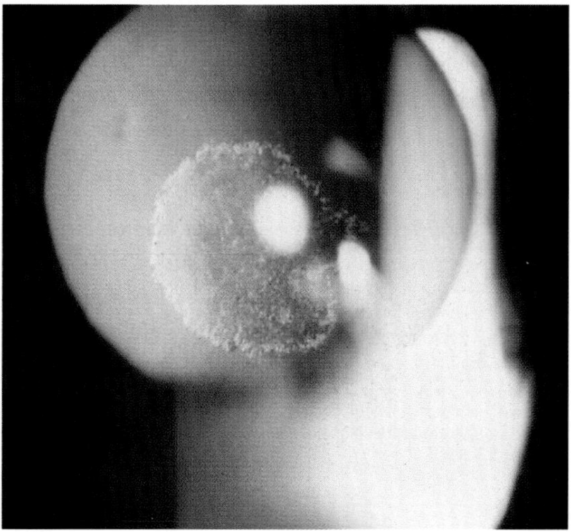

FIGURE 7.3.3 Posterior subcapsular cataract.

Differential Diagnosis of Senile Cataract

trauma, steroid use (topical or systemic), other medications (steroids, phenothiazines, phospholine iodide, amiodarone), environmental exposure (radiation, infrared/glassblower, ultraviolet, alkali injury, electric shock), intraocular inflammation, intraocular tumor, degenerative diseases (e.g., retinitis pigmentosa), systemic disease (diabetes, galactosemia, Wilson's disease, hypocalcemia, atopy), Hoeve's syndrome (blue sclera, brittle bones, deafness), Hallermann-Streiff syndrome (oculomandibulofacial dyscephaly), Marfan syndrome, Turner's syndrome.

Management of Senile Cataract

- History to determine etiology of the cataract.
- Complete ocular examination to assess whether the cataract is responsible for the decreased vision. Assess visual acuity in light and dark.
- B-scan ultrasound when the fundus is not visualized secondary to a dense cataract.
- Visual potential may be estimated using the potential acuity meter. However, the potential acuity meter may be unreliable with a dense lens or with coexistent macular pathology.
- Assess visual complaints and visual needs of the patient.
- If surgery is planned, keratometry and A-scan ultrasound are needed to determine the power of the intraocular lens. The corneal endothelium is also evaluated; occasionally an endothelial cell count is helpful in assessing need for concomitant penetrating keratoplasty.
- Cataract surgery is indicated to improve visual function in patients with symptomatic visual disability, treat ocular disease (lens-related glaucoma or uveitis), and provide visualization of the posterior structural for management of vitreoretinal or optic nerve disease.

- If surgery is postponed or declined, a trial of mydriasis may improve visual symptoms in some patients.

7.4 Systemic Disease and Cataract

7.4.1 Diabetes Mellitus—variations in hydration of the lens with labile blood sugar levels lead to refractive shifts. Cataracts occur at a younger age and are frequently advanced cortical or posterior subcapsular. Snowflake cataracts occur in uncontrolled diabetes and are quickly progressing bilateral subcapsular changes.

7.4.2 Myotonic Dystrophy—approximately 90% of patients with myotonic dystrophy develop bilateral presenile cataracts. The characteristic "Christmas tree" cataract is due to iridescent crystals that accumulate in the subcapsular area (see Chapter 15).

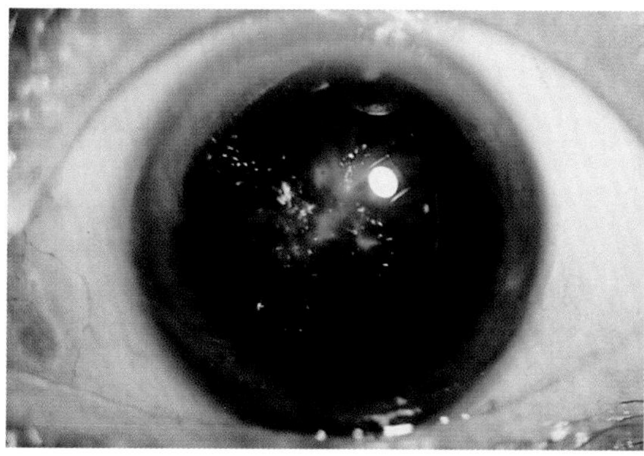

FIGURE 7.4.2 "Christmas tree" cataract in a patient with myotonic dystrophy.

7.4.3 Wilson's Disease—in addition to the well-recognized deposition of copper in the cornea (Kayser-Fleischer ring), copper deposition in the anterior subcapsular cortex is known as a sunflower cataract (see Chapter 15).

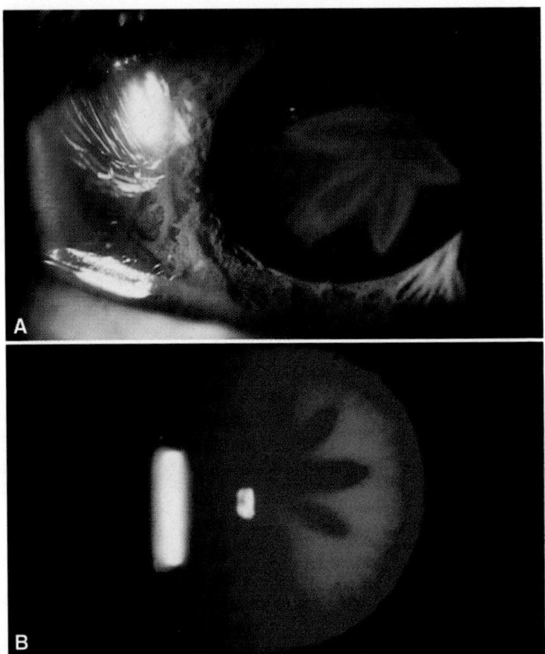

FIGURE 7.4.3a Sunflower cataract in Wilson's disease.
FIGURE 7.4.3b Sunflower cataract on retroillumination.

7.4.4 Dermatogenous Cataract—several skin diseases are associated with cataract. Atopic dermatitis is the most common. About 10% of adults with severe atopic dermatitis develop anterior subcapsular opacifications, which tend to thicken with time and distort the anterior capsule. Bloch-Sulzberger syndrome (incontinentia pigmenti), which consists of patchy skin pigmentation, dental anomalies, and alopecia, is also frequently associated with cataracts.

7.5 Drug-Induced Cataract

many drugs and chemicals have been shown to cause lens changes.

Presentation posterior subcapsular cataract (corticosteroids), pigmented deposits in the anterior lens epithelium (phenothiazines), small vacuoles within and posterior to the anterior lens capsule (long-acting anticholinesterase inhibitors), stellate anterior axial pigment deposition (amiodarone).

Management

- History of drug use: corticosteroids, phenothiazines, echothiophate iodide, demecarium bromide, amiodarone.
- If possible, discontinue drug or reduce dosage.
- If visually significant, consider cataract extraction.

7.6 Traumatic Cataract

characteristic traumatic lens damage may be caused by blunt trauma, radiation, or electrical or penetrating injury.

Presentation

- Vossius' ring: during blunt trauma, pigment from the pupillary ruff may be imprinted on the anterior lens capsule in a ring shape.
- Contusion cataract: initially presents as a stellate or rosette-shaped opacification involving the posterior lens capsule, usually axial in location. May progress to involve the entire lens. In cases of rupture of the lens capsule, opacification occurs rapidly with hydration of the lens fibers.
- Subluxated or dislocated lens.

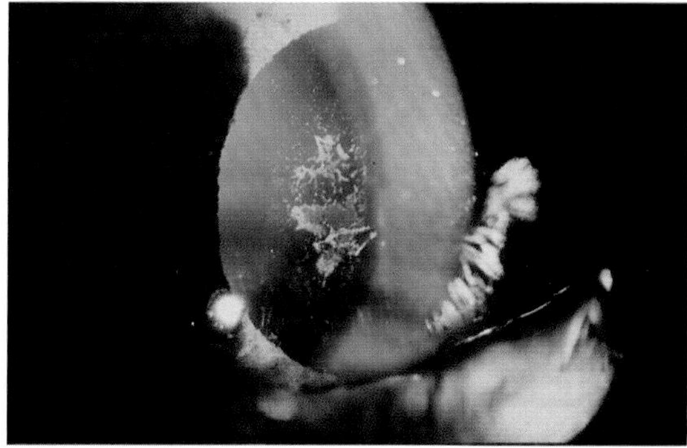

FIGURE 7.6.1 Vossius' ring.

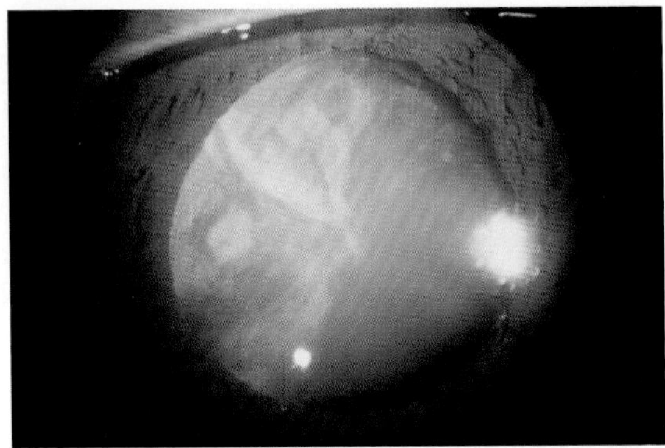

FIGURE 7.6.2 Contusion cataract.

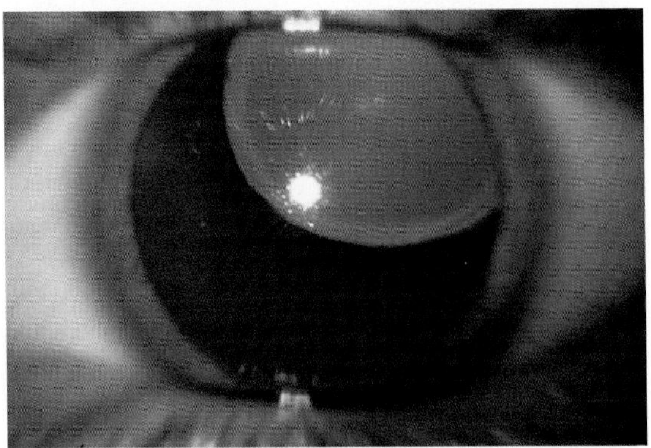

FIGURE 7.6.3 Subluxated lens.

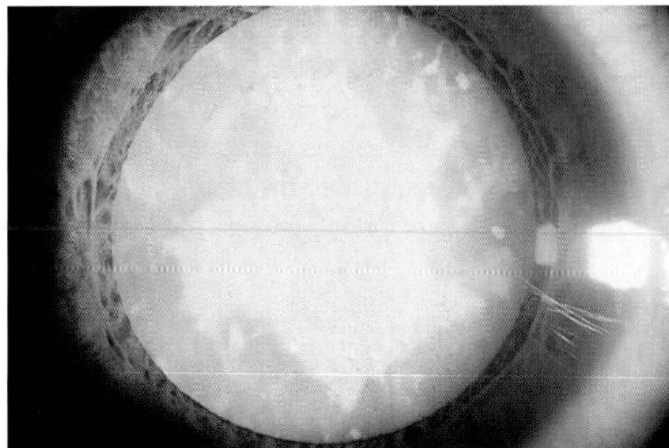

FIGURE 7.6.4 Electrical injury.

- Electrical injury causes coagulation of the lens proteins and irreversible lens opacification. The cataract is usually unilateral, on the side proximal to the point of contact.
- Radiation cataract: cataracts often occur after exposure to high-dose radiation. Glassblowers' cataract has been reported in individuals with lifelong exposure to intense and prolonged levels of infrared radiation. Posterior subcapsular cataracts are seen with splitting of the layers of the anterior capsule. This "splitting" is called true exfoliation, as distinguished from the pseudoexfoliation syndrome.

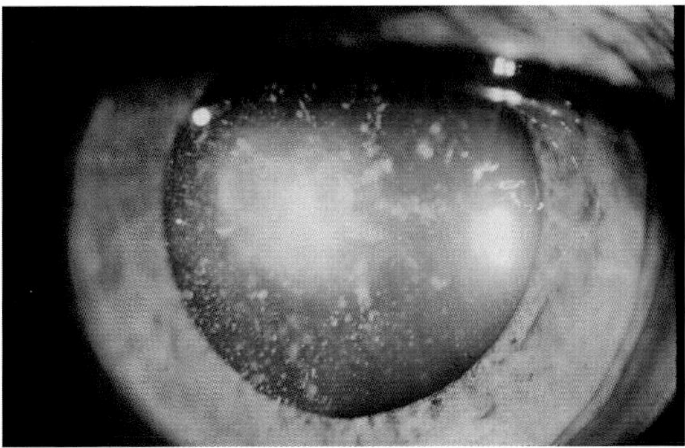

FIGURE 7.6.5 Radiation cataract.

Management

- History: mechanism of injury.
- Complete ocular examination. Subluxated or dislocated lenses are removed if visually significant. Traumatic capsular ruptures are treated with corticosteroids and antiglaucoma medications, if necessary. Delaying surgery for 3 to 6 weeks is preferred to emergent surgery.

7.7 Ectopia Lentis

a displacement of the lens, which may be congenital, developmental, or acquired. With *dislocation,* there is complete disruption of zonular fibers, and the lens is out of the pupillary aperture. With *subluxation,* there is partial disruption of zonular fibers, and the lens remains decentered in the pupillary aperture.

Presentation

fluctuation of vision, impaired accommodation, monocular diplopia, high astigmatism, hyperopia when the lens is out of visual axis, angle-closure glaucoma as a result of pupillary block, asymmetry of the anterior chambers. Iridodonesis or phakodonesis may also be present.

Differential Diagnosis

- Trauma is the most common cause of acquired ectopia lentis.
- Marfan syndrome (see Section 15.14): increased zonular elasticity causes bilateral lens subluxation, usually superotemporally.
- Homocystinuria (see Section 15.15): subluxation usually inferiorly and nasally.
- Weill-Marchesani syndrome (see Section 15.16): microspherical lens causes high myopia and possibly pupillary block.
- Others: sulfite oxidase deficiency, congenital ectopia lentis, Ehler-Danlos syndrome, hyperlysinemia.

Management

- History: trauma, family history, systemic disease.
- Complete ocular examination.

- Physical examination, referral to internist.
- Dislocated into the anterior chamber: reposition of the lens by dilating the pupil and positioning the patient face-down. After the lens is back in position, treat with pilocarpine 0.50 to 1.0 %. Remove the lens surgically if attempts to reposition fail or if there is lens-corneal touch.
- Dislocated into the posterior chamber: if there are no signs of inflammation and the lens capsule appears intact, observe. If the lens capsule is broken and there is a lens-induced uveitis, consider lensectomy.
- Subluxated lens: if asymptomatic, observe. If there are visual symptoms (monocular diplopia, high uncorrectable astigmatism), try careful refraction. If not improved, consider lens extraction. There are increased rates of vitreous loss and complications for removal of subluxated lenses.
- Pupillary block: treat as if aphakic pupillary block (see Chapter 8).

7.8 Complications of Cataract Extraction and Intraocular Lenses

7.8.1 Corneal Edema after Cataract Extraction—usually transient and thought to be the result of intraoperative hydration of the cornea, temporary decreased endothelial cell function, and/or acute rises in IOP. Corneal edema may also become chronic and is one of the most common visually disabling complications of cataract surgery.

Presentation decreased vision, pain, photophobia. Vision may be worse in the morning and improve during the day. Findings include stromal edema, Descemet's folds, and microcystic edema.

Differential Diagnosis

- Sudden endothelial cell death from mechanical, heat, and toxic trauma of surgery, or increased IOP, or epithelial defect.
- Chronic: ABK, PBK.

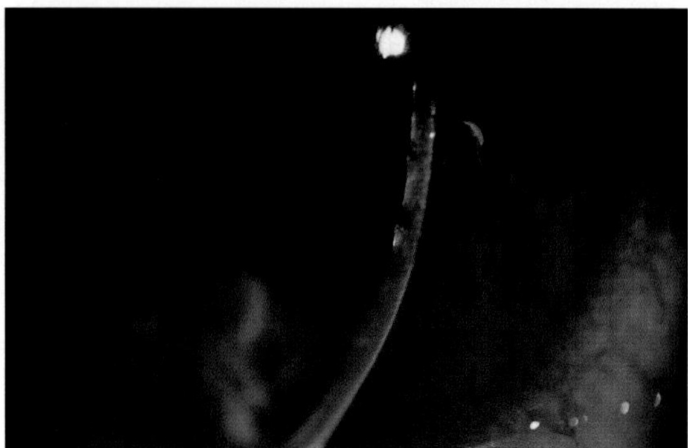

FIGURE 7.8.1 Moderate corneal edema after cataract extraction.

Management

- History: date of lens extraction, preexisting or contralateral corneal dystrophy or guttata.
- Slit-lamp examination with fluorescein to identify denuded epithelium. Check position of intraocular lens. Look for vitreous in the anterior chamber and its proximity to the corneal endothelium. Note any anterior chamber inflammation.
- Measure intraocular pressure.
- Treat all underlying ocular disease: suppress anterior chamber and ciliary body inflammation with prednisolone acetate 1% q 2 to 4h. Lower elevated IOP with antiglaucoma medications.
- Treat stromal edema: topical sodium chloride 2% or 5% drops qid or ointment hs.
- A bandage lens may be used to manage pain secondary to ruptured epithelial bullae.
- For chronic corneal edema, intraocular lens exchange or penetrating keratoplasty may be considered.

7.8.2 Hypotony and Wound Leak after Cataract Extraction

7.8.2 Hypotony and Wound Leak after Cataract Extraction—occurs secondary to poor surgical closure, poor wound healing, or trauma.

Presentation asymptomatic or mild pain with decreased vision, low IOP (usually <6 mm Hg), corneal folds, shallow or flat anterior chamber, chorioretinal folds, choroidal detachment.

Differential Diagnosis angle-closure glaucoma with pupillary block, choroidal detachment.

Management

- Check IOP.
- Examine wound with a strip of fluorescein to identify a leak (Seidel's sign). If the wound is draining under the conjunctiva, the Seidel's sign will be negative. In this case, look for a conjunctival filtering bleb.
- Full ocular examination including dilated fundus examination or B-scan to rule out choroidal detachment.
- Large wound leaks with flat anterior chamber: surgical repair.
- Small wound leaks with shallow anterior chamber: pressure patch with antibiotic ointment to allow the wound to close spontaneously. Usually a carbonic anhydrase inhibitor (acetazolamide, 500 mg bid) and a topical β-blocker (timolol 0.5%) are given if patching is attempted. Consider reforming anterior chamber with BSS or viscoelastic or with surgical repair.
- Wound leaks under a conjunctival flap are repaired only if hypotony is affecting vision or causing a flat anterior chamber.

7.8.3 Elevated Intraocular Pressure after Cataract Extraction—see Chapter 8.

7.8.4 Cystoid Macular Edema after Cataract Extraction—see Chapter 9.

7.8.5 Retinal Detachment, Suprachoroidal Hemorrhage/Effusion after Cataract Extraction—see Chapter 10.

7.8.6 Endophthalmitis after Cataract Extraction—see Chapter 6.

Chapter 8
GLAUCOMA

Michael Levine, Maurice Luntz,
Raymond Harrison

8.1 Primary Open-Angle Glaucoma

optic nerve head atrophy and characteristic cupping due to retinal ganglion cell death associated with typical glaucomatous visual field changes.

Presentation risk factors include high IOP, family history, and black race. Currently there is controversy as to whether myopia, diabetes, hypertension, and other vasculopathies are risk factors for glaucoma. Patients are typically asymptomatic. Examination may reveal elevated IOP (at least 21 mm Hg on at least one occasion), a large C/D ratio, C/D asymmetry, localized areas of neural rim thinning (notching), and peripapillary flame hemorrhages. Red-free examination of the fundus may reveal nerve fiber layer dropout. Gonioscopy is normal. Visual fields reveal scotomas including arcuate, nasal step, paracentral, and temporal wedge defects.

Differential Diagnosis congenitally enlarged C/D ratio (especially in African Americans and Hispanics), low-tension glaucoma, fluctuating IOP (angle-closure glaucoma, Posner-Schlossman syndrome, uveitis), secondary open-angle glaucoma, optic nerve atrophy (ischemic optic neuropathy, compressive lesions, syphilis), congenital optic nerve anomalies (myopic discs, coloboma, optic nerve pits), ocular hypertension.

Management assessment of IOP, C/D appearance, risk factors, and visual fields as is necessary for management. Multiple IOP measurements at different times of the day can be helpful.

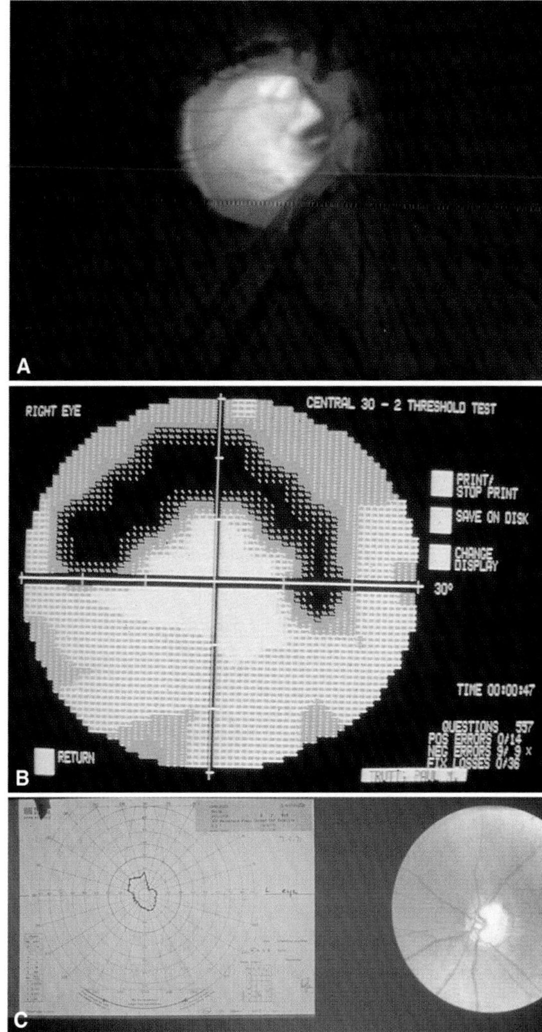

FIGURE 8.1a Glaucomatous cupping.

FIGURE 8.1b Superior arcuate visual field defect detected by static perimetry.

FIGURE 8.1c End-stage primary open-angle glaucoma.

The patient's C/D ratio should be followed with stereo disc photographs. Multiple automated visual field tests should be obtained for an accurate baseline field and for monitoring visual field loss. Patients who fit the criteria for the diagnosis of POAG should be treated. See Chapter 14 for dosages and contraindications.

- First-line therapy includes topical medications: β-blockers (timolol, levobunolol, betaxolol), topical carbonic anhydrase inhibitors (dorzolamide), possibly prostaglandin analogues (latanoprost).
- Second-line agents include topical and oral medications: parasympathomimetics (pilocarpine, echothiophate iodide), epinephrine compounds (dipivefrin, epinephrine), α_2 agonists (apraclonidine, brominidine), oral carbonic anhydrase inhibitors (methazolamide, acetazolamide).
- Argon laser trabeculoplasty should be considered if one medicine is inadequate or if compliance is in question.
- Surgical intervention (trabeculectomy, filtering implants) is performed for progression of visual fields or optic discs or for inadequate IOP control or compliance on medical therapy.

8.1.1 Glaucoma Suspect—a patient with elevated IOP or optic nerve head changes with normal or questionable visual field changes.

Presentation a positive family history, black race, and older age raise suspicion. Glaucoma is likely with the findings of elevated IOP (>21 mm Hg), optic disc asymmetry (C/D ratio difference of >0.1), a C/D ratio equal to or greater than 0.5, deep cupping of the nerve head, or neural rim thinning of the optic disc. Elevated IOP in the absence of optic nerve or visual field changes is termed ocular hypertension.

Differential Diagnosis ocular hypertension, congenitally enlarged C/D ratio, POAG.

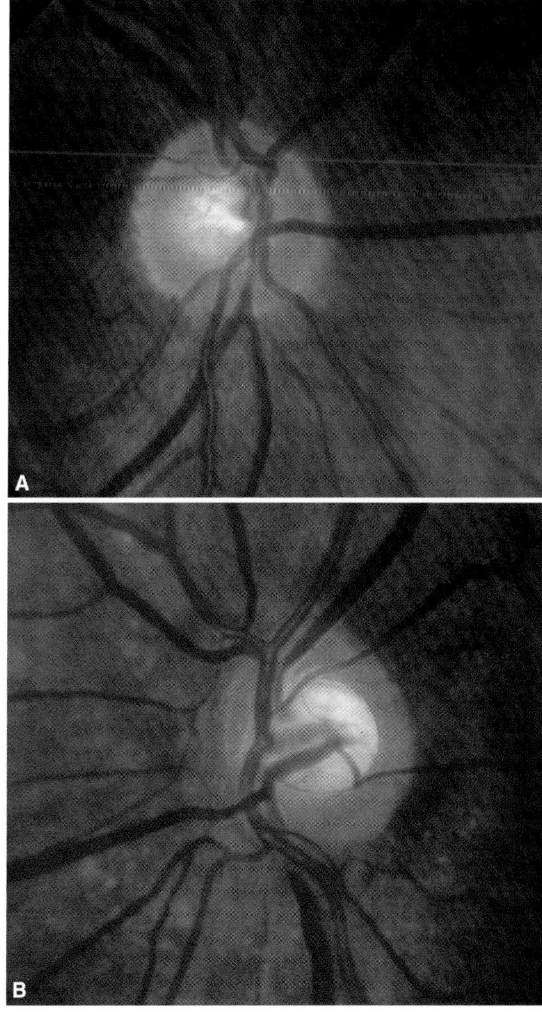

FIGURE 8.1.1a Glaucoma suspect with 0.3 C/D ratio and IOP of 28mm.

FIGURE 8.1.1b Glaucoma suspect with 0.55 C/D ratio and increased excavation of disc but normal visual field.

Management patients without risk factors and an elevated IOP can be followed with optic nerve photographs and repeated visual fields. Some clinicians empirically treat when the IOP is greater than 28 mm Hg because of increased risk and for protection against retinal vein occlusions. Patients with risk factors are often treated at lower IOPs and should be followed more closely. If optic nerve head progression or glaucomatous visual field changes are documented, a diagnosis of POAG is confirmed, and treatment is then initiated.

8.2 Normal-Tension (or Low-Tension) Glaucoma

glaucomatous optic nerve head with visual field changes similar to those of POAG, but with ocular tensions within the normal range. This disorder may result from increased optic nerve susceptibility to IOP or a vasculopathic process.

Presentation suspicious optic nerve head (C/D ratio >0.5) or disc asymmetry. Glaucomatous visual field changes such as paracentral scotoma or arcuate defects. No documented IOP above 21 mm Hg. The patient often has systemic illnesses such as diabetes, heart disease, or vasculospastic disorders (e.g., migraine, Raynaud's phenomenon). The diagnosis is one of exclusion.

Differential Diagnosis POAG, previous or intermittent increase in IOP (previous uveitis, previous topical steroid use, Posner-Schlossman syndrome, angle-closure attacks), optic nerve atrophy (ischemic optic neuropathy, trauma, compressive lesions, syphilis), congenital optic nerve anomalies (myopic discs, coloboma, optic nerve pits).

Management

- Stereo optic nerve head photographs, gonioscopy, baseline visual fields, and a diurnal curve. Systemic illness must be ruled out: history of hypotensive events such as shock or myocardial infarction, carotid occlusive disease (previous history of cerebrovascular accident), vasculopathies (diabetes, temporal arteritis), vasculospastic disorders (migraine headaches, Raynaud's phenomenon), anemia, syphilis, other autoimmune disorders.

- The workup includes complete physical examination, including neurologic evaluation; serologic tests (complete blood count, chemistries, erythrocyte sedimentation rate, FTA-ABS, antinuclear antibodies, folate, vitamin B_{12}); CT imaging of orbits, optic nerves, and brain; carotid ultrasound and transcranial Doppler studies.
- Any systemic disease should be treated. Management includes lowering of the "normal" IOP to levels around the 10- to 12-mm Hg range, especially if C/D enlargement or progressing visual field changes are observed. Treatment is the same as for POAG. Some advocate the use of calcium channel blockers (e.g., nifedipine), although the efficacy of this treatment is unclear.

8.3 Secondary Open-Angle Glaucoma

glaucomatous optic neuropathy with typical visual field changes and elevated IOP that can be associated with a specific etiologic factor.

8.3.1 Pigmentary Dispersion Glaucoma

8.3.1 Pigmentary Dispersion Glaucoma—deposition of iris pigment in the anterior chamber, which may result in glaucoma by mechanical obstruction of aqueous outflow through the trabecular meshwork. Iris pigment is thought to be liberated by zonular contact with the posterior iris, especially in myopes. Liberation of pigment and characteristic findings without glaucoma is called pigmentary dispersion syndrome.

Presentation the typical patient is a young, male myope. Pigment may be found on the corneal endothelium (Krukenberg's spindle), on the lens capsule surface, or in a heavily pigmented trabecular meshwork on gonioscopy. Transillumination of the iris may reveal midperipheral pigment loss in a spoke-like pattern. Pigment release may follow vigorous exercise or pupillary dilation, leading to intermittently elevated IOPs, pain, halos, and decreased visual acuity.

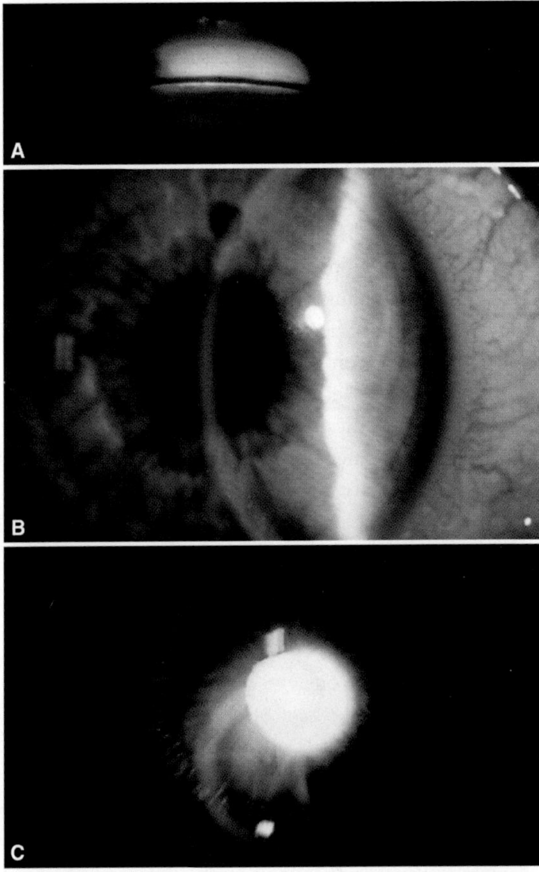

FIGURE 8.3.1a Gonioscopic view of anterior chamber angle in a patient with pigmentary dispersion glaucoma. Note the heavily pigmented trabecular meshwork.
FIGURE 8.3.1b Krukenberg's spindle.
FIGURE 8.3.1c Transillumination defects.

Differential Diagnosis pseudoexfoliation, uveitis, intraocular melanoma.

Management approximately 25 to 50% of patients with pigment dispersion syndrome develop glaucoma. Slit-lamp examination including gonioscopy and IOP assessment, stereo optic nerve head photographs, and a baseline visual field should be done. Treatment is usually topical medications such as β-blockers or carbon anhydrase inhibitors at first. Some recommend miotics to fix the iris, thereby preventing its chafing over the zonules. Miotics are poorly tolerated by young adults, however, although a low concentration (e.g., pilocarpine 1%) or a continuous delivery system (i.e., Ocuserts) may be helpful. If a lower IOP is needed, argon laser trabeculoplasty is often successful. Laser peripheral iridectomy may favorably alter iris configuration and cure this condition in some patients.

8.3.2 Pseudoexfoliation Syndrome—deposition of white fibrillar material of unknown origin in the anterior segment of the eye and the trabecular meshwork, sometimes resulting in secondary open-angle glaucoma. This condition is more common in people of Scandinavian, Eastern European, and Mediterranean origin, suggesting a genetic predisposition.

Presentation most often an asymptomatic, lightly pigmented individual, often with elevated IOP and characteristic findings in one or both eyes. There is a deposition of white, fibrillar material on the pupillary margin. On dilation, the same material is found on the anterior capsule of the lens, often with a cleared ring area where the movement of the iris has brushed away the material. Gonioscopy may reveal a heavily pigmented trabecular meshwork with deposition of pigment anterior to Schwalbe's line called Sampaolesi's line. Of note, affected eyes may have weaker zonular support, which may complicate cataract extraction.

Differential Diagnosis true exfoliation (patients exposed to infrared radiation, typically glassblowers, rare), anterior capsular changes from trauma, uveitis, pigmentary glaucoma, amyloidosis.

Management full examination including slit-lamp examination with IOP, gonioscopy, C/D assessment. Optic nerve head photographs and visual fields if suspicion of nerve damage.

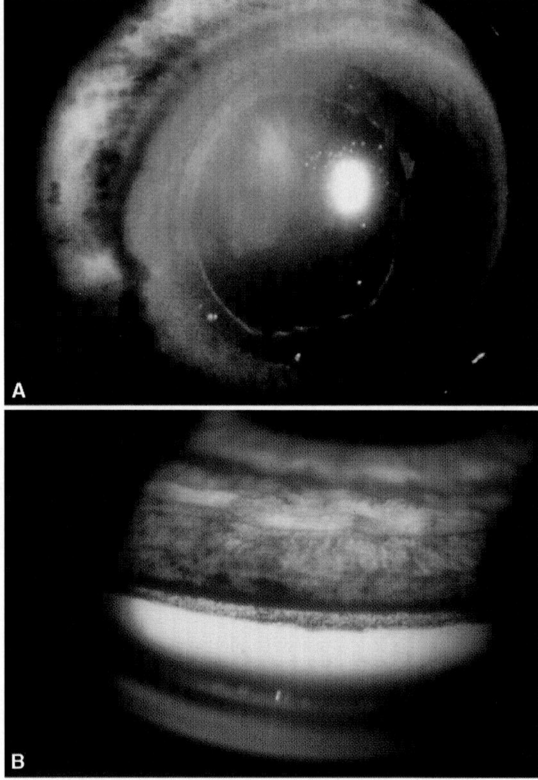

FIGURE 8.3.2a Deposition of fibrillar material on the anterior lens capsule in pseudoexfoliation glaucoma.
FIGURE 8.3.2b Sampaolesi's line.

- Treat as POAG, although the IOP may be higher and harder to control with pseudoexfoliative glaucoma.
- Argon laser trabeculoplasty is often successful, but the results may diminish rapidly.

8.3.3 Lens-Induced Glaucoma—there are three distinct types of glaucoma caused by lens materials and inflammation.

Presentation all lead to marked inflammation, pain, and elevated IOP due to obstruction of outflow by inflammatory materials.

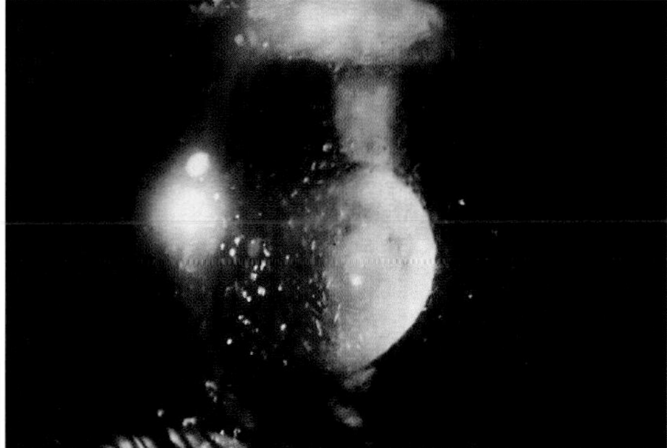

FIGURE 8.3.3 Mature cataract leaking lens protein.

- Phacolytic glaucoma: leakage of lens protein from a mature cataract through a clinically intact capsule; macrophages block aqueous outflow.
- Lens-particle glaucoma: leakage of lens proteins through a disrupted lens capsule as a result of trauma or recent surgery with retained lens material.
- Phacoanaphylactic glaucoma: hypersensitivity to lens material after surgery, after penetrating ocular injury, or from a hypermature lens causing a granulomatous inflammation. Note: Phacomorphic glaucoma is a lens induced pupillary block or angle-closure glaucoma (see Section 8.4, Angle-Closure Glaucoma).

Differential Diagnosis

uveitic glaucoma, Posner-Schlossman syndrome (see Uveitic Glaucoma), endophthalmitis, angle-closure glaucoma.

Management

careful history regarding surgery and trauma. Slit-lamp examination with attention to the crystalline lens and IOP assessment. Control of inflammation with steroids (e.g., prednisolone acetate q1h), prevention of posterior synechiae with mydriatics (e.g., cyclogyl 1% tid), and control of IOP are important. Oral hyperosmotic agents or mannitol may be necessary in addition to control IOP in urgent situations.

- Phacolytic glaucoma: cataract extraction is the definitive therapy. Topical steroids and antiglaucoma medications are used to quiet the eye prior to surgery.
- Lens-particle and phacoanaphylactic glaucoma: Medical management is attempted until material is resorbed. Evacuation of lens material may be necessary if medical management fails.

8.3.4 Uveitic Glaucoma—secondary open-angle glaucoma resulting from inflammatory cells mechanically obstructing outflow through the trabecular meshwork.

Presentation patients may complain of pain and photophobia or may be relatively asymptomatic. Examination reveals anterior chamber inflammation and sequelae (keratic precipitates, peripheral anterior synechiae, posterior synechiae, cataract) and elevated IOP.

Differential Diagnosis anterior uveitis without glaucoma, glaucomatocyclitic crisis or Posner-Schlossman syndrome (unilateral cyclic attacks of elevated IOP accompanied by mild anterior chamber reaction), Fuchs' heterochromic iridocyclitis, steroid response elevated IOP, lens-related glaucoma.

Management complete history including previous ocular trauma, angle-closure attacks, and prior episodes of uveitis. Slit-lamp examination for stigmata of previous uveitic processes and IOP assessment. Gonioscopy and optic nerve evaluation. Treatment consists of topical steroids, mydriatics, and IOP-lowering medications. Miotics are avoided, because they exacerbate inflammation and facilitate the formation of posterior synechiae. Prostaglandin analogues may increase inflammation.

8.3.5 Elevated Episcleral Venous Pressure—raised episcleral venous pressure from impeded outflow of blood from the eye, resulting in elevated IOP.

Presentation elevated IOP on slit-lamp examination, large C/D ratio. Careful examination of the trabecular meshwork by gonioscopy may reveal RBCs in the trabecular meshwork resulting from venous congestion. There may be dilated episcleral veins.

Differential Diagnosis POAG.

Management rule out and treat possible etiologic conditions:

- Retrobulbar tumor: Exophthalmometry, dilated examination for retinal folds or subretinal mass. Consider B-scan, CT, or MRI.
- Vascular pathology: Sturge-Weber syndrome (fundus photography may reveal diffuse choroidal hemangioma), carotid or dural fistulas (ocular bruit, exophthalmometry), orbital fistulas.
- Thyroid eye disease: see Chapter 3.

Treatment includes topical and oral pressure-lowering medications. Medications such as topical β-blockers, apraclonidine, and dorzolamide, which decrease aqueous production, can be used.

8.3.6 Steroid Response—elevated IOP associated with the concomitant use of topical or systemic corticosteroids administration.

Presentation elevated IOP in a patient, usually using topical corticosteroids. Steroid response can take place in days to months but most commonly occurs in the first few weeks after initiation of therapy. Patients with a family history of glaucoma, diabetics, or POAG are more likely to be "steroid responders."

Differential Diagnosis inflammatory glaucoma, Cushing's syndrome.

Management

- Taper off the steroid or decrease the frequency of the dosage.

- Change a topical steroid to one with less hypertensive effects, such as fluorometholone or prednisolone 0.12%. Rimexolone, a synthetic corticosteroid, is reported to be as efficacious as prednisolone 1% in controlling inflammation with less pressure-elevating effects.

8.4 Angle-Closure Glaucoma

elevated IOP secondary to mechanical obstruction of the trabecular meshwork by an anteriorly displaced iris.

8.4.1 Acute-Angle Closure Glaucoma

8.4.1 Acute-Angle Closure Glaucoma—an ophthalmic emergency; acutely elevated IOP due to angle closure.

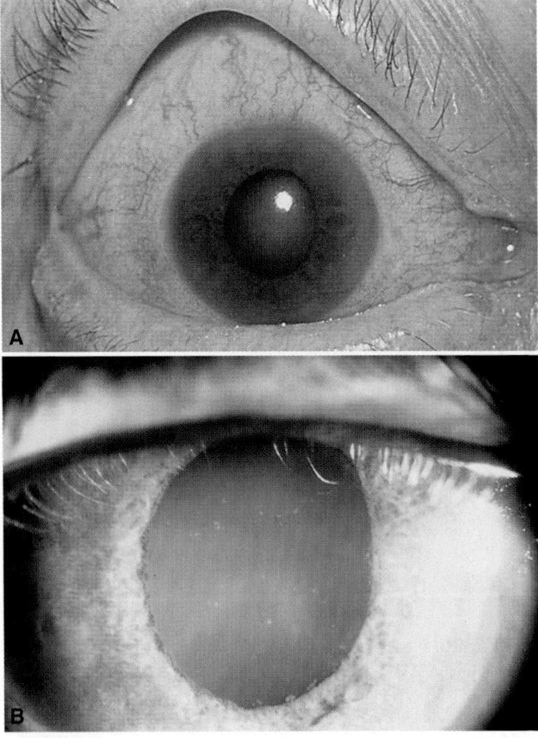

FIGURE 8.4.1a Fixed, middilated pupil of angle-closure glaucoma.
FIGURE 8.4.1b Glaukomflecken.

Presentation risk factors include age (larger crystalline lens), hyperopia, and white or Asian race. Acute attacks cause marked pain, redness, headache, nausea/vomiting, decreased visual acuity, and halos. Microcystic corneal edema, a mid-dilated and nonreactive pupil, anterior chamber inflammation, and elevated IOP are also present. The fellow eye has a shallow anterior chamber and a narrow angle. There may be a history of intermittent attacks occurring in the dark. Mechanisms include the following:

- Pupillary block: most common; increased posterior chamber pressure due to restricted flow through the pupil causes iris bombé and anatomic narrowing of the angle.
- Plateau iris.
- Phacomorphic glaucoma: enlarged cataractous lens plugs the pupillary aperture.
- Aphakia/pseudophakia: intraocular lens—iris capture or anterior hyaloid face obstruction of the pupil and peripheral iridectomy.
- Choroidal effusion (after panretinal photocoagulation, scleral buckle, or intraocular surgery) anteriorly displaces the lens–iris diaphragm.
- Iris pulled forward: neovascularization of iris, peripheral anterior synechiae, ICE syndrome.

Differential Diagnosis uveitis, inflammatory glaucoma, malignant glaucoma, neovascular glaucoma, conjunctivitis.

Management initial management includes emergent reduction of IOP to prevent optic nerve damage and gonioscopy with glycerin to clear microcystic edema to determine whether the angle is closed.

- Control medically: topical β-blocker q30min, apraclonidine 1% q30min, prednisolone acetate q30min to control inflammation, oral or carbonic anhydrase inhibitor (dorzolamide q30min or acetazolamide, 500 mg), oral or intravenous hyperosmotic agent (isosorbide, glycerol, or mannitol—see Section 14.14.1).

- Pilocarpine 4% q15min when pressure begins to decrease. Iris ischemia prevents miosis at high IOP. When the crystalline lens is not present, mydriatics should be used.
- Systemic analgesia and antiemetics may be necessary.
- Laser peripheral iridectomy is definitive therapy as soon as cornea is sufficiently clear. Pilocarpine (1 to 2% qid) should be used in the interim to prevent attack in both eyes.
- Gonioscopy for fellow eye. Consider prophylactic laser peripheral iridectomy of fellow eye if occludable angle.

8.4.2 Chronic Angle-Closure Glaucoma—angle-closure glaucoma secondary to narrow angles and peripheral anterior synechiae with gradual rise in IOP.

Presentation symptoms and signs of intermittent angle-closure glaucoma. Elevated IOP, narrow angles with broad peripheral anterior synechiae. Stigmata of previous inflammation, mature cataract or subluxated lens, and iris bombé may be present.

Differential Diagnosis inflammatory glaucoma, mixed mechanism glaucoma (a combination of angle-closure and open-angle glaucoma, with elevated IOP despite laser peripheral iridectomy), POAG.

Management laser peripheral iridectomy: More than one iridectomy may be necessary away from peripheral anterior synechiae, with special attention to prevent IOP spikes. Medically treat similar to POAG, avoiding miotics and argon laser trabeculoplasty, which exacerbate peripheral anterior synechiae formation and angle closure. Mydriatics may be helpful also. Filtering surgery may be necessary.

8.4.3 Plateau Iris—angle-closure glaucoma resulting from iris configuration that obstructs the trabecular meshwork outflow.

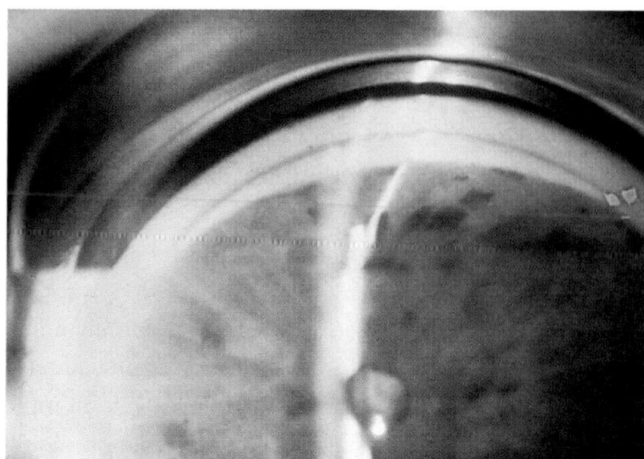

FIGURE 8.4.3 Plateau iris with obscuration of angle structures and a deep anterior chamber.

Presentation symptomatology similar to acute angle-closure glaucoma. Deep anterior chamber with occluded angle on gonioscopy. The iris appears flat.

Differential Diagnosis pupillary block glaucoma, malignant glaucoma.

Management initial treatment is the same as for acute angle-closure glaucoma. Laser peripheral iridectomy is the definitive treatment. However, these patients are still at some risk of an acute attack of angle closure even with patent peripheral iridectomies. Laser gonioplasty of peripheral anterior synechiae may be considered if contributing to angle closure. High-frequency ultrasound can confirm the plateau iris.

8.4.4 Neovascular Glaucoma—neovascularization of the iris and trabecular meshwork associated with peripheral anterior synechiae and consequent angle closure.

Presentation patients often have a history of retinal hypoxia, often from diabetic retinopathy or central retinal vein occlusion. Complains include pain and decreased vision. Examination reveals an elevated IOP, neovascularization of the iris, and trabecular meshwork on gonioscopy.

Differential Diagnosis uveitic glaucoma, acute angle-closure glaucoma.

Management initial management includes medical treatment of the elevated IOP and inflammation. Control pressure with topical medications, oral carbonic anhydrase inhibitors, oral or intravenous hyperosmotic agents, and mydriatics (atropine 1% tid). Control inflammation with topical corticosteroids. Panretinal photocoagulation should be performed as soon as possible. If the fundus cannot be visualized, cryotherapy may be applied to the peripheral retina. Filtering procedures such as trabeculectomy and seton valves may be used for pressure control once the neovascular process is stabilized. If the IOP remains elevated, the patient continues to experience pain, and little useful vision is present, YAG, diode, or CO_2 cyclophotocoagulation can be performed. Neovascular glaucoma often results in a blind, painful eye.

8.5 Blind, Painful Eye

a painful eye that has no light perception and no chance for visual rehabilitation. Pain is usually from elevated IOP but may also be due to inflammation and surface breakdown.

Presentation the patient has a history of a blind eye due to any number of etiologies including perforating corneal ulcer, retinal detachment, uveitis, multiple surgical procedures, and neovascular glaucoma.

Management complete ocular examination including fluorescein staining of the cornea, IOP, and fundus examination, if possible. It is common for the cornea to be opacified obstructing visualization of the ocular anatomy. If possible, examine the anterior segment to evaluate for presence of neovascularization of the iris and anterior chamber reac-

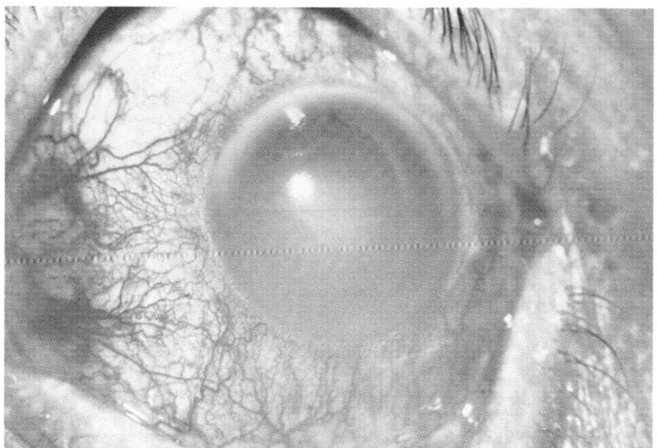

FIGURE 8.5 Blind, painful eye.

tion. B-scan ultrasonography of the posterior segment may be necessary for evaluation.

- Standard treatment includes prednisolone acetate 1% qid and atropine 1% bid.
- If a large corneal epithelial defect is present, a topical antibiotic and cycloplegic should be used. Aggressive lubrication and tarsorrhaphy are considered.
- Standard glaucoma medications may be used for IOP control but are not necessary if pain and cornea status are improved, even in presence of high pressures.
- If elevated IOP is not controlled with topical medications and the pain persists, YAG, diode, or CO_2 cyclophotocoagulation of the ciliary body may be performed to lower IOP. Retrobulbar injection of alcohol and enucleation are offered as final options.

8.6 ICE (Iridocorneal Endothelial) Syndrome

corneal endothelial downgrowth over the anterior chamber and iris resulting in obstructed trabecular meshwork outflow with consequent elevation of IOP. The ICE syndromes are believed to be a spectrum of separate disease entities.

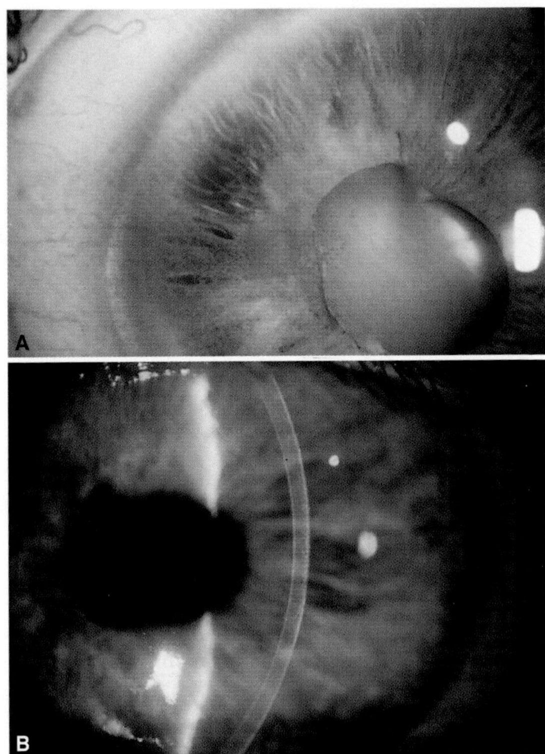

FIGURE 8.6a Essential iris atrophy with atrophic iris holes.
FIGURE 8.6b Chandler's syndrome with mild endothelial changes.

Presentation

patients may complain of an abnormal pupil, blurred vision, or pain. Most often unilateral and more common in women. Atrophic iris, corectopia, corneal endothelial changes with or without edema, ectropion uveae, and peripheral anterior synechiae. The optic nerve may show glaucomatous change.

- Essential iris atrophy: characterized by marked iris atrophy, atrophic iris holes, corectopia, and angle-closure glaucoma.
- Chandler's syndrome: abnormal corneal endothelium ("beaten metal" appearance), often with resultant

corneal edema at normal IOP. Atrophic iris changes and corectopia are minimal.

- Cogan-Reese syndrome: also known as iris–nevus syndrome. Characterized by excessive pigmentation of the anterior iris surface in the form of nodules or nevi. Degree of atrophic iris changes is variable.

Differential Diagnosis previous ocular trauma, corneal guttata or Fuchs' endothelial dystrophy, anterior chamber cleavage syndromes (i.e., Peter's anomaly, Axenfeld-Rieger syndrome), iris melanoma, posterior polymorphous dystrophy.

Management control of IOP and glaucoma management. Medical management includes topical pressure-lowering medications and hypertonic preparations to control corneal edema if present. Surgical management includes trabeculectomy for control of advanced disease. If corneal edema from dysfunctional endothelial cells impedes vision, penetrating keratoplasty may be necessary.

8.7 Malignant Glaucoma

misdirected aqueous flow into the posterior segment resulting in an anteriorly displaced ciliary body and lens–iris diaphragm, with consequent narrowing of the angle. This complication occurs in postsurgical patients with narrow angles.

Presentation painful, red eye that occurs during the early postoperative period, elevated IOP, corneal edema, shallow anterior chamber, and anterior inflammation. Causes include recent cataract extraction, surgical iridectomy, and glaucoma surgery.

Differential Diagnosis angle-closure glaucoma, inflammatory glaucoma, choroidal hemorrhage or effusion, retained viscoelastic, failed trabeculectomy, hyphema, endophthalmitis.

Management initial management should include gonioscopy to determine whether the angle is open. If the patient does not have a peripheral iridectomy or the present one is obstructed with vitreous, another peripheral iridectomy should be performed emergently. Dilated funduscopic examination or B-scan ultrasonography to rule out choroidal hemorrhage should be done. Medical management includes mydriatics (atropine 1% tid), topical pressure-lowering drugs, oral carbonic anhydrase inhibitors, and oral or intravenous hyperosmotic agents. Nd:YAG laser can be utilized in aphakic and pseudophakic patients to disrupt the vitreous face. Vitrectomy may be necessary to remove anterior vitreous and displaced aqueous to restore normal aqueous flow to the anterior chamber.

8.8 Complications of Trabeculectomy Surgery

8.8.1 Blebitis or Wound Infection—microbial infestation of the surgical wound or bleb, which most often occurs during the immediate postoperative period. A nonhealing wound from antimetabolites predisposes to wound infection.

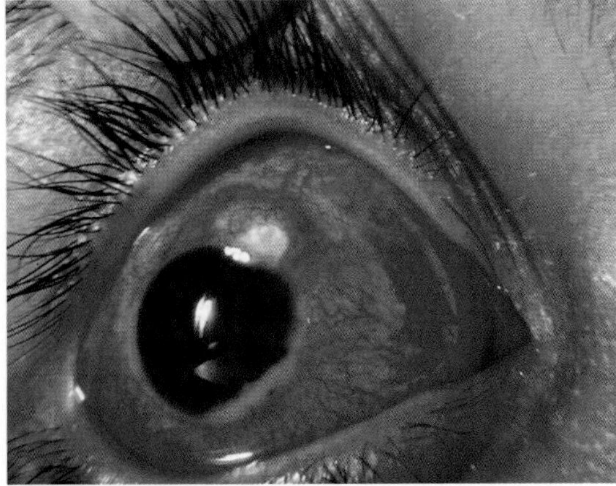

FIGURE 8.8.1 Infected bleb with hypopyon.

Presentation pain, decreased vision, and photophobia in postoperative period. There is infiltrate or purulence at the wound margins or in the bleb, and a hypopyon may be present. There may be progression to frank endophthalmitis.

Differential Diagnosis reaction from cautery, postoperative inflammation, frank endophthalmitis.

Management topical antibiotics (fluoroquinolone q1h or fortified vancomycin or cephalosporin and tobramycin) to cover major pathogens such as streptococci and staphylococci. Intravitreal antibiotics may be necessary if endophthalmitis is suspected (see Section 6.9, Endophthalmitis).

8.8.2 Wound or Bleb Leaks—result from poor conjunctival closure, wound dehiscence, or bleb leakage. The use of antimetabolites has increased the rate of these complications.

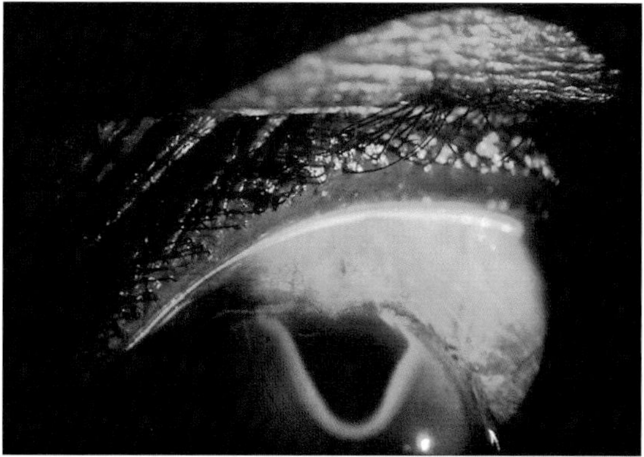

FIGURE 8.8.2 Leaking bleb. Positive Seidel's sign is demonstrated by fluorescein staining of leaking aqueous.

Presentation bleb leaks can occur during the immediate postoperative period or may occur years later. The diagnosis is made by observing a stream of aqueous with the aid of fluorescein from the leaking site (Seidel's sign).

Management revision of conjunctival sutures if inadequate, broken, or removed too early. More sutures can be added at the slit lamp or the operating room. If the bleb itself is leaking, a bullet patch can be tried first. If leakage continues, a large-diameter bandage contact lens and symblepharon ring may be used to slow aqueous flow through the hole. Aqueous suppressants such as β-blockers, apraclonodine, and topical or oral carbonic anhydrase inhibitors can be used to slow aqueous production as well. Another treatment for bleb leaks includes autologous blood injections into and around the leaking bleb.

8.8.3 Hypotony—intraocular tension that is low enough to endanger ocular anatomy and function, often the result of an overfiltering bleb; also caused by penetrating trauma, leaking surgical wounds, and vitreoretinal surgery.

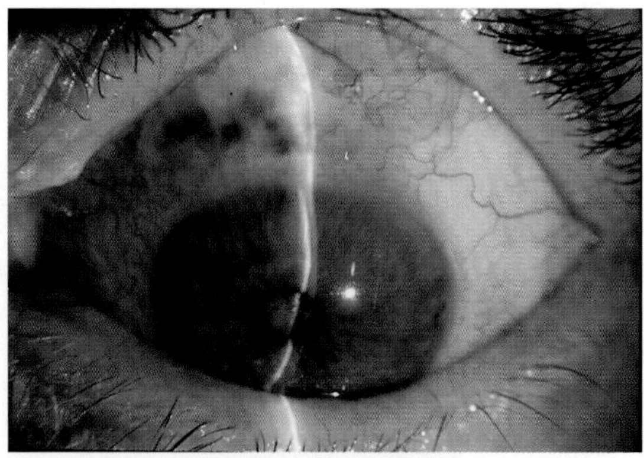

FIGURE 8.8.3 Excessively filtering bleb resulting in hypotony.

Presentation IOP is usually below 5 mm Hg. Choroidal effusions may be present on funduscopic examination or B-scan. Hypotensive maculopathy with chorioretinal folds and decreased vision may be present.

Management treatment includes close observation if the anterior chamber is formed and there are no choroidal hemorrhages on funduscopic examination. If the anterior chamber appears shallow, viscoelastic may be injected to reform the anterior chamber. Aqueous suppressants can decrease flow and enhance closure. As the bleb and scleral flap begin to heal, the IOP will most often rise to acceptable levels.

8.8.4 Bleb Failure—elevated IOP occurring in the postoperative period as a result of bleb scarification and excessive wound healing. Patients at greater risk for bleb failure include the young and those with a history of keloid formation.

Presentation absence of a bleb or a localized encapsulated bleb, vascularization of bleb, increased IOP, possible closure or iris obstruction of sclerostomy.

Differential Diagnosis malignant glaucoma, retained viscoelastic.

Management the use of antimetabolites in trabeculectomies has greatly decreased the rate of bleb failure. A failing bleb may be treated with local injections of an antimetabolite (5-fluorouracil) in an attempt to impede scarification. Needling of the bleb can be performed for encapsulation. Nd:YAG or needle suture lysis may increase filtration. Medical therapy may be adequate despite surgical failure, but reoperation is frequently necessary.

Chapter 9
MEDICAL RETINA

Belinda Shirkey, David Guyer,
Lawrence Yannuzzi

9.1 Hypertensive Retinopathy

a retinal vasculopathy due to systemic hypertension that can be acute or chronic.

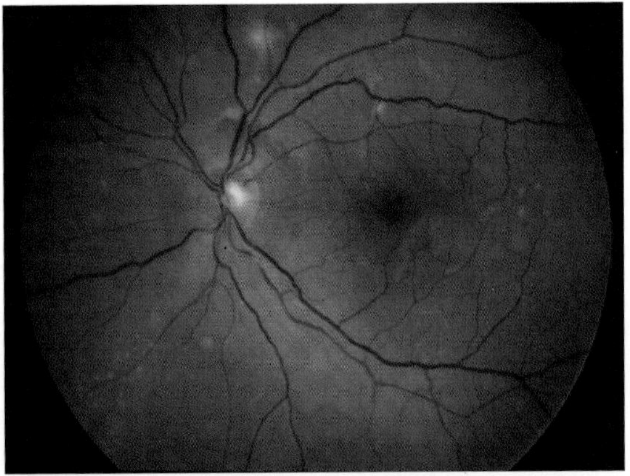

FIGURE 9.1 Choroidal ischemia due to HTN with Siegrist's streaks and Elschnig's spots.

Presentation

- Chronic: patients are usually asymptomatic and have chronic essential hypertension (blood pressure: systolic >140 mm Hg and/or diastolic >90 mm Hg). Findings include retinal arteriolar sclerosis and narrowing (copper or silver wiring), AV crossing, and increased tortuosity. Siegrist's streaks, linear pattern of hyperpigmentation, may develop over choroidal arteries. Long-term complications include venous and arterial occlusions and macroaneurysms.

- Acute: patients are more likely to be younger, black, and to have a secondary cause of hypertension (pre-eclampsia/eclampsia, pheochromocytoma, hyperthyroidism, renal vascular or parenchymal disease, adrenal disease, Cushing's syndrome, alcohol withdrawal, or coarctation of the aorta). Blurred vision and headache are common. There may be mental status changes, chest pain, and renal failure. Findings include cotton-wool spots, hard exudates, and flame-shaped retinal hemorrhages. Sclerotic changes may be absent. Choroidal ischemia causes pale patches of the retina (Elschnig's spots, serous detachments, and retinal edema. Optic neuropathy with bilateral disc edema, congested veins, and exudate in a macular star pattern may be present.

Differential Diagnosis

includes diabetic retinopathy, collagen vascular disease, anemia, radiation retinopathy, CRVO or BRVO, ischemic optic neuropathy. Macular star may be seen in hypertension, acute febrile illnesses like cat-scratch fever, Behçet's disease, chronic infections such as TB or syphilis, cilioretinal artery occlusion, papilledema due to increased intracranial pressure, papillitis, and ocular trauma.

Management

if the patient is asymptomatic and the blood pressure is moderately elevated, referral to an internist is appropriate. If the patient has symptoms of end-organ damage, including headache, chest pain, difficulty breathing, confusion, or blurred vision with optic disc swelling and retinal hemorrhages, the patient requires immediate medical attention.

9.2 Diabetic Retinopathy

retinal vasculopathy affecting about 25% of diabetics, with increased incidence proportional to severity and duration of diabetes. This leading cause of blindness tends to occur in the posterior pole.

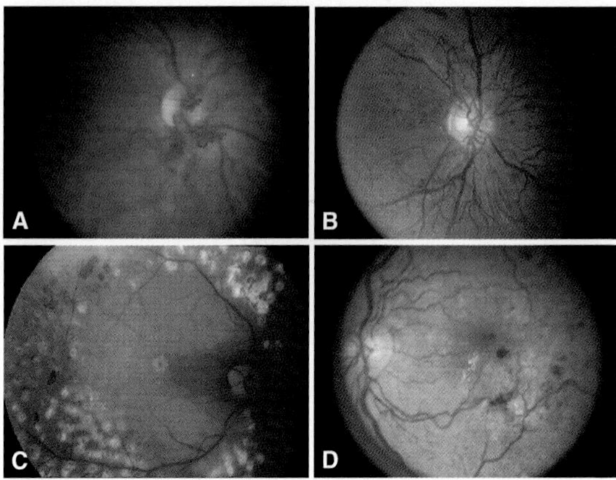

FIGURE 9.2a Disc neovascularization.
FIGURE 9.2b Retinal neovascularization.
FIGURE 9.2c PRP.
FIGURE 9.2d Diabetic macular edema.

Presentation

- NPDR, or background diabetic retinopathy, is characterized by bilateral dot and blot intraretinal hemorrhages, lipid exudates, microaneurysms, and areas of capillary nonperfusion. Flame-shaped nerve fiber layer hemorrhages and mild cotton-wool spots may be present. More severe disease causes venous beading, IRMA, and widespread capillary nonperfusion and cotton-wool spots.
- PDR carries a 70% risk of total blindness if not treated. Findings are the same as above with in the presence of fibrovascular proliferation along the posterior surface of the vitreous and adherent to the retina, which may cause tractional retinal detachment and VH. This neovascularization can occur on or within 1 disc diameter of the optic disc (NVD), on the iris (NVI), or elsewhere in the retina (NVE).
- Diabetic macular edema is the major cause of visual loss in both diabetic retinopathy. Findings include hard exudate and focal or diffuse retinal edema (or thicken-

ing), which may be cystic. Microaneurysms are frequently associated.

- Diabetic macular ischemia causes profound visual loss. Findings include capillary dropout by FA and atrophy of the macula.

Differential Diagnosis

- NPDR: CRVO and BRVO, ocular ischemic syndrome, hypertensive retinopathy, radiation retinopathy.
- PDR: neovascularization secondary to vein occlusion, sickle cell retinopathy, embolization from IV drug abuse, sarcoidosis.
- Macular edema: neuroretinitis, juxtafoveal retinal telangiectasis, vein occlusion, macroaneurysm.

Management

demands early detection of NVI, NVD, or NVE is the key to maintain vision. Meticulous blood control has been shown to decrease the incidence and progression of diabetic retinopathy. Concurrent hypertension should also be aggressively treated. Patients should have a DFE every 6 months for NPDR and every 3 months if any PDR is seen.

- FA may be helpful in directing focal laser treatment and confirming macular edema, early neovascularization, and macular ischemia. B-scan may be required to rule out tractional detachment of the macula in eyes with a dense VH obscuring a view of the fundus.
- Focal or grid laser treatment for CSME, by contact lens or 90-D examination, defined as

1. Retinal thickening (edema) within 500 μm (one-third of disc diameter) of the center of the fovea.
2. Hard exudates within 500 μm of the center of the macula, associated with retinal thickening.
3. Retinal thickening greater than 1 disc area in size, part of which is within 1 disc diameter of the center of the fovea.

- PRP laser is indicated for any one of the following high-risk characteristics:

1. NVD greater than one-fourth to one-third of the disc area in size.
2. Any degree of NVD with preretinal hemorrhage or VH.
3. NVE greater than one-half of the disc area when associated with preretinal hemorrhage or VH.
4. Significant NVI, especially with increased IOP.

(Some clinicians perform PRP for high-risk NPDR, such as poorly compliant patients, poor sugar control, or PDR in the contralateral eye.)
See Section 10.7, Proliferative Diabetic Retinopathy, for surgical indications.

9.3 Branch Retinal Vein Occlusion

blockage of a sectoral retinal vein, usually due to thrombosis at a site of the vein crossing a sclerotic arteriole. Hypertension (75%), arteriosclerosis, and diabetes are common associations.

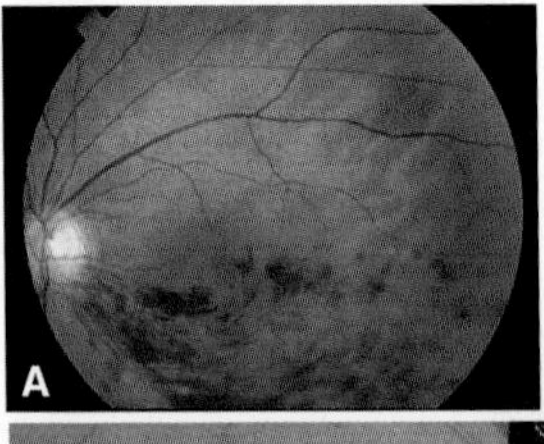

FIGURE 9.3a BRVO.
FIGURE 9.3b Vein occlusion with FA.

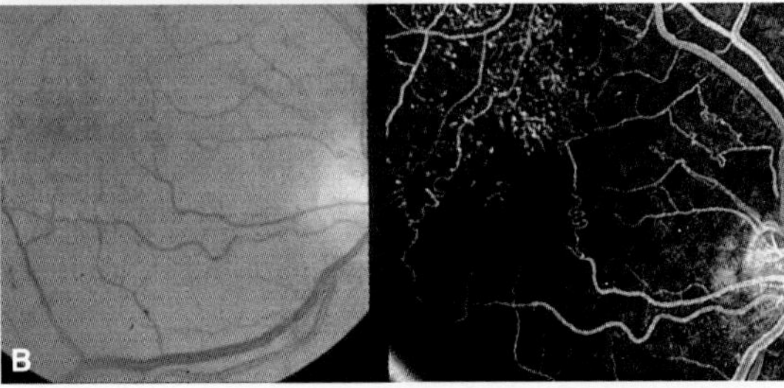

Presentation

a unilateral shadow in the visual field or decreased visual acuity is the usual patient complaint. Nasal vein occlusions may be asymptomatic and may go undetected. Findings are superficial retinal hemorrhages in a sector of the retina along a dilated and tortuous retinal vein. Cotton-wool spots, retinal edema, narrowing and sheathing of the adjacent artery, retinal neovascularization (about 28%, usually NVE or NVD), and VH are associated findings. Macular edema is the source of persistent visual loss.

Differential Diagnosis

vascular disease secondary to hypertension, arteriosclerosis, and/or diabetes.

Management

- Systemic history and physical examination to rule out hypertension, diabetes, and arteriosclerotic disease are warranted.
- Complete ophthalmic examination for neovascularization or macular edema. FA after hemorrhages have cleared may help to detect early neovascularization.
- Observation. Follow-up is every 1 to 2 months then every 3 to 12 months to check for neovascularization and macular edema. Retinal hemorrhages resolve over weeks. In one-half of patients, macular edema resolves spontaneously and vision returns to 20/40 or better in 6 months.
- Chronic macular edema (3 to 6 months): laser macular grid photocoagulation for vision below 20/40 in the absence of macular capillary nonperfusion.
- Neovascularization: consider sector panretinal photocoagulation in the retinal area of capillary nonperfusion as delineated by FA.
- Atypical cases (no systemic disease, multiple BRVO, age <50 years) should undergo a workup for a hypercoagulable state or vasculitis (protein S and C, serum viscosity, CBC, PT, PTT, ESR, ANA, FTA, VDRL, chest radiography).

9.4 Central Retinal Vein Occlusion

blockage of the central retinal vein, which drains the entire inner retina. Etiology is usually a thrombosis posterior to the lamina cribosa of the optic nerve. Causes include ocular hypertension or glaucoma (the most commonly associated ocular disease), arterosclerosis of the adjacent central retinal artery, hypertension, optic disc edema, optic disc drusen, hypercoagulable state (polycythemia, lymphoma, leukemia, sickle cell disease, multiple myeloma, cryoglobulinemia, Waldenstrom's macroglobulinemia, antiphospholipid syndrome), vasculitis (sarcoid, syphilis, SLE), drugs (oral contraceptives, diuretics), abnormal platelet function (mitral valve prolapse), retrobulbar external compression (thyroid disease, orbital tumors), and migraine.

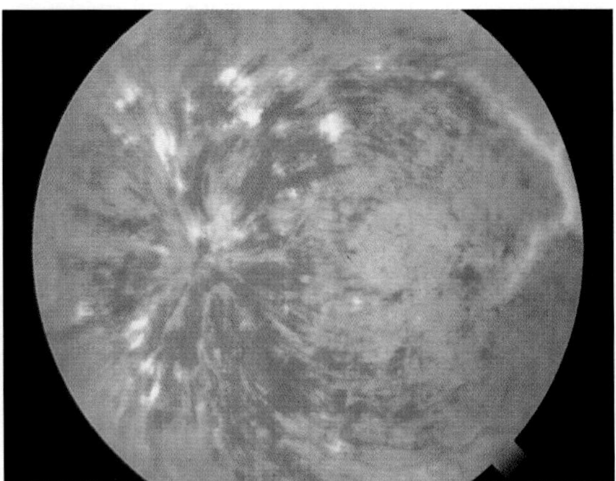

FIGURE 9.4 Ischemic CRVO.

Presentation

unilateral, painless loss of vision is the presenting symptom. Findings include diffuse retinal hemorrhages in all quadrants of the retina, dilated and tortuous retinal veins, cotton-wool spots, retinal edema, disc edema, and disc hemorrhages. Optociliary shunt vessels on the disc may develop.

- Nonischemic CRVO: the findings, as just listed, are mild. Visual acuity is usually better than 20/200. No APD is found.
- Ischemic CRVO: often, an APD is present, and acuity is 20/200 or worse. More extensive retinal hemorrhage, more cotton-wool spots (usually >10), and widespread capillary nonperfusion on FA are seen. Neovascularization of the anterior segment, optic disc, or retina may ensue. NVI and neovascularization of the angle are most common and may cause neovascular glaucoma, with a peak incidence in 90 days (called "90-day glaucoma").

Differential Diagnosis

diabetic retinopathy, acute hypertensive retinopathy, ocular ischemic syndrome, papilledema, radiation retinopathy.

Management

a medical evaluation to rule out cardiovascular disease is recommended, as is an ophthalmic examination to rule out ocular hypertension or glaucoma. If the IOP is elevated over 25 mm Hg in either eye, antiglaucoma agents may be considered. Some clinicians recommend aspirin for anticoagulation.

- Nonischemic CRVO: Cases should be followed every month for 6 months to detect the deterioration into the ischemic category (around 20% incidence).
- Ischemic CRVO: Ischemic CRVO eyes are at risk for neovascularization proportional to the area of capillary nonperfusion. These cases should be followed every 2 to 3 weeks for the first 6 months to detect neovascularization. Gonioscopy is crucial to detect neovascularization of the angle.

Scatter PRP is performed if 2 or more clock hours of NVI exist or any degree of neovascularization of the angle, or in cases of poor follow-up and severe ischemia. Macular grid photocoagulation for persistent macular edema does not improve vision.

- Atypical cases (no systemic disease, bilateral, age <50 years) should undergo a workup for a hypercoagulable state or vasculitis (physical examination, CBC with differential, FTA-VDRL, PT, PTT, ESR, ANA, lipid profile, antiphospholipid antibodies, serum electrophoresis, chest radiography).

9.5 Central Retinal Artery Occlusion/ Ophthalmic Artery Occlusion

occlusion of central retinal artery after it branches from the ophthalmic artery, causing ischemia of only the inner retina. Ophthalmic artery occlusion affects both inner and outer retinal circulation, as well as the anterior segment. The cause is usually arteriosclerosis of the carotid, ophthalmic, or central retinal arteries and secondary thrombus or embolism. Emboli may be from numerous sources: disease, metastatic tumors, sepsis, or fractured long bones. In a younger patient, consider atrial myxoma, talc emboli, and oral contraceptives. Other causes are markedly increased IOP after surgery, collagen vascular disease (SLE, polyarteritis nodosa), hypercoagulation disorders (oral contraceptives, polycythemia, antiphospholipid syndrome), migraine, Behçet's disease, syphilis, sickle cell disease, and trauma.

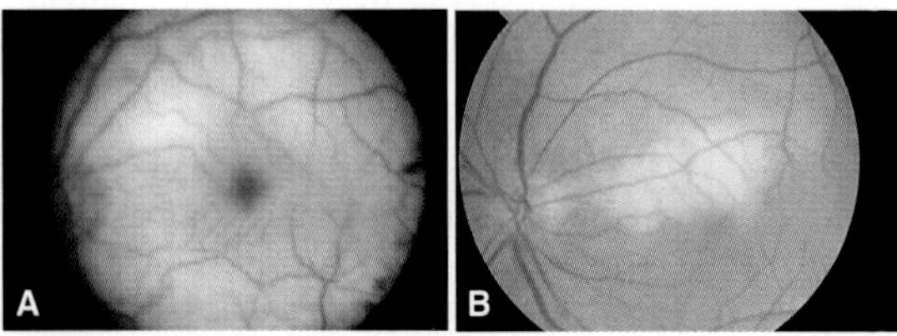

FIGURE 9.5a CRAO with "cherry-red spot."
FIGURE 9.5b CRAO.

Presentation

- CRAO: unilateral, painless, acute loss of vision occurs usually over seconds. An APD is present, and visual loss is profound unless there is a patent cilioretinal artery (a

variant in anatomy, present in 20% of population). Many patients will give a history of previous visual obscurations. Fundus findings include retinal edema (opaque, thickened, and pale retina) in the posterior pole, with a "cherry-red spot" in the fovea, narrowed retinal arterioles, "boxcarring" of blood in the arterioles, and retinal arteriolar emboli. Temporal GCA causes 1 to 2% of CRAOs. An APD, pale optic disc swelling, and a markedly elevated ESR are seen with this systemic disease (see Section 13.4.6, Arteritic Ischemic Optic Neuropathy [Giant Cell Arteritis]).
- Ophthalmic artery occlusion: vision is very poor (LP or NLP), ischemic optic neuropathy may be present, and no cherry red spot is seen. Cause is usually carotid artery disease, and ocular ischemic syndrome is common.

Differential Diagnosis arteritic ischemic optic neuropathy (occurs with and without CRVO), inadvertent intraocular injection of gentamicin, severe trauma. Of cherry-red spot: Tay-Sachs disease and other sphingolipidoses, quinine toxicity, macular hemorrhage, hypertension, Hurler's syndrome, macular hole, steroid injection, traumatic retinal edema.

Management the following may be useful if CRAO has been present less than 24 hours:

- Anterior chamber paracentesis. The IOP is checked. A drop of antibiotic [e.g., Polytrim (trimethoprim sulfate and polymyxin B sulfate)]. and anesthetic are given. Using a 30-gauge needle and a tuberculin syringe with the plunger removed, a limbal corneal entry into the anterior chamber is made. The bevel is kept toward the clinician, and the needle is kept over the iris. A few drops (0.1 to 0.2 ml) are extracted. Antibiotic is placed, and IOP is rechecked. May be repeated if the IOP is still greater than 10 mm Hg.
- Digital ocular massage. May also be performed with a fundus contact lens while watching for dislodgement of an embolus and/or reperfusion.

- Acetazolamide (500 mg IV or PO), topical drops to lower the IOP (i.e., timolol 0.5%, iopidine 1%, latanoprost).
- Consider carbogen (95% oxygen, 5% carbon dioxide) inhalation therapy, 10 minutes every 2 hours around the clock for 48 hours. The patient must be monitored for blood pressure, pulse, and mental status changes.

In patients older than age 55, immediately determine the ESR to rule out GCA. Cardiac and carotid artery evaluation are needed to rule out an embolic source. NVI or NVD develops in 20% of patients at a mean of 4 weeks after onset. Eye examination is repeated in 1 to 2 weeks. If neovascularization develops, PRP should be performed to deter subsequent neovascular glaucoma.

9.6 Branch Retinal Artery Occlusion

similar in etiology to CRAO, but affecting only a sector of the inner arterial circulation.

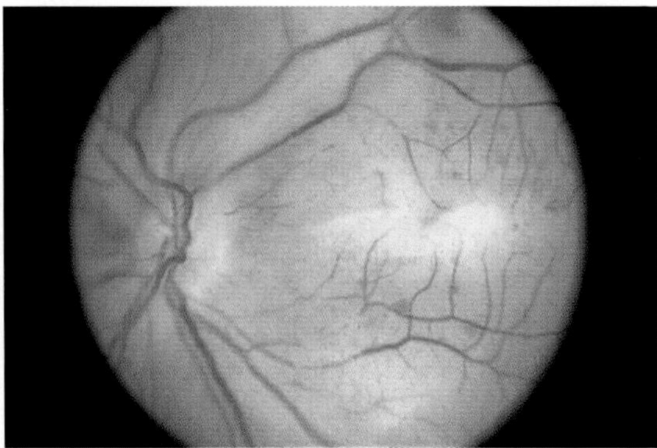

FIGURE 9.6 BRAO.

Presentation unilateral, painless, abrupt loss of partial visual field. Visual acuity is usually good. A history of transient visual loss may be elicited. Fundus findings may be absent acutely. Within hours, retinal edema is seen along the distribution of the involved branch retinal artery. Narrowed branch retinal artery, boxcarring, cotton-wool spots, and emboli may be seen. Hollenhorst's plaque is a cholesterol embolus appearing as bright, reflective crystal, generally at a vessel bifurcation.

Differential Diagnosis retinal vasculitis.

Management no immediate ocular therapy is of proven value. Conservative treatment as for CRAO (see above) may be tried, especially for immediate presentation. Conduct a medical workup as for CRAO and reevaluate every 3 to 6 months.

9.7 Ocular Ischemic Syndrome

decreased blood supply to the entire eye. Occurs usually when carotid stenosis is less than 90%.

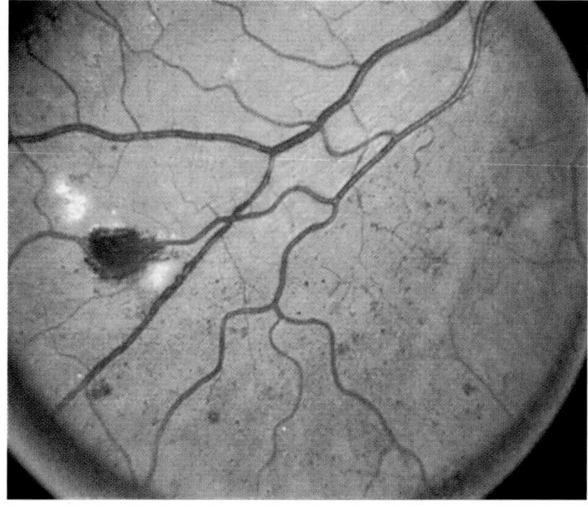

FIGURE 9.7 Midperipheral intraretinal heme in ocular ischemic syndrome.

Presentation the eye may be painful due to anterior segment or orbital ischemia, or neovascular glaucoma. Visual obscurations may precede permanent visual loss due to CRAO or ophthalmic artery occlusion, neovascular glaucoma, or optic neuropathy. An ipsilateral carotid bruit or decreased pulsation may be present. Anterior findings include ciliary and conjunctival injection, anterior chamber cells and flare, cataract, and neovascularization. Retinal findings include large round intraretinal hemorrhages in the midperipheral retina.

Differential Diagnosis partial CRVO, diabetic retinopathy, panuveitis, and vasculitis.

Management includes workup for an embolic source. Ophthalmodynamometry reveals low retinal artery pressure, in contrast to CRVO.

9.8 Macroaneurysm

a saccular dilatation of arteriolar walls in the retina, usually acquired from weakening due to hypertension or arteriosclerosis in elderly women. Other causes are radiation retinopathy, venous occlusive disease, sickle cell, and diabetes.

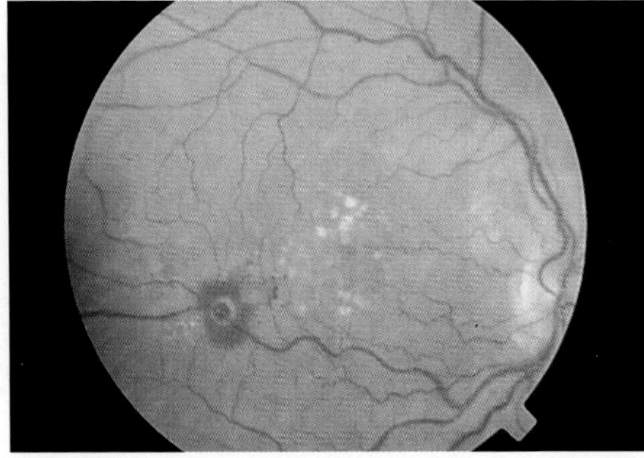

FIGURE 9.8 Macroaneurysm with lipid exudation.

Presentation decreased vision due to vitreous hemorrhage, retinal hemorrhage, or lipid exudate into the macula.

Differential Diagnosis parafoveal telangiectasis, diabetic maculopathy, retinal capillary hemangioma.

Management a medical evaluation for hypertension and cardiovascular disease is warranted. Spontaneous resolution is the natural course. Lipid exudate that is threatening the fovea may be treated with argon laser or yellow-dye laser applied around the aneurysm. Complications include hemorrhage and occlusion of the arteriole.

9.9 Vitreous Hemorrhage

bleeding of native or neovascular vessels into vitreous cavity. Causes include diabetic retinopathy, retinal break, hypertension PVD, retinal vein occlusion, AMD, sickle cell disease, trauma, intraocular tumor, Terson's syndrome (subarachnoid or subdural hemorrhage). Even more rare causes are retinal capillary angioma, Eales' disease, congenital prepapillary vascular loop, radiation retinopathy, anterior segment hemorrhage because of an IOL, bleeding diathesis. The causes of VH in infancy are birth trauma, shaken-baby syndrome, ROP, and juvenile X-linked retinoschisis.

Presentation sudden painless loss of vision or sudden appearance of black spots with flashing lights are common symptoms. Red fundus reflex may be absent, and the view to the fundus obscured. Chronic VH has a yellow-ochre appearance secondary to the breakdown of hemoglobin.

Differential Diagnosis uveitis (dense vitritis can simulate hemorrhage), retinal detachment, Coats' disease.

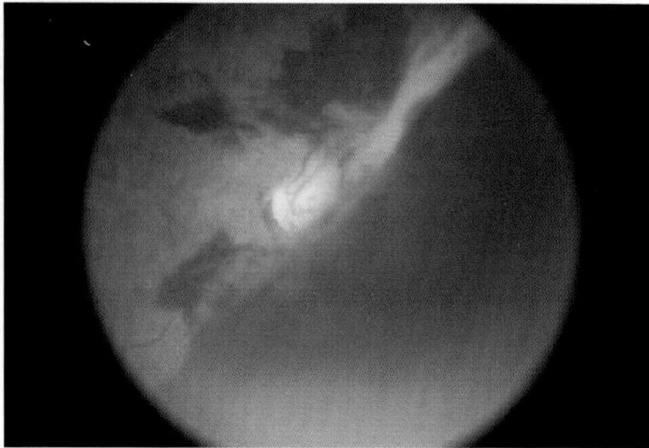

FIGURE 9.9 Vitreous and subhyaloid hemorrhage secondary to diabetes mellitus.

Management detailed history of ocular and systemic disease, trauma; examination of the fellow eye to assess the presence of diabetic retinopathy, macular pathology, peripheral retinal neovascularization; B-scan to rule out retinal tear, detachment, tumor, vitreoretinal traction as in diabetes, posterior vitreous detachment. Treatment includes the following:

- Bedrest, with the head of the bed elevated 30° to 45° to allow hemorrhage to settle inferiorly.
- No aspirin or NSAIDs (unless medically indicated for anticoagulation).
- Serial B-scans to rule out retinal detachment.
- For diabetic retinopathy: Initiate PRP as the view clears, with close follow-up. If tractional macular detachment or bilateral VH, consider vitrectomy (see Tractional Retinal Detachment).
- For retinal break: laser photocoagulation or cryotherapy when hemorrhage clears.
- For retinal detachment: vitrectomy with or without scleral buckle.
- For an unknown cause: with a normal B-scan, observation; vitrectomy considered in 6 months if VH is nonclearing.

9.10 Angioid Streaks

breaks in Bruch's membrane so called because of an appearance similar to blood vessels. The majority are idiopathic. Associated systemic disease PXE, Ehlers-Danlos syndrome, Paget's disease, sickle cell disease, acromegaly, and Marfan syndrome.

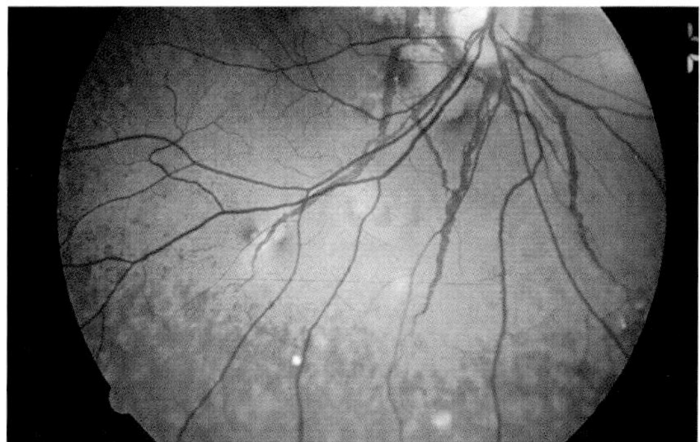

FIGURE 9.10 Angioid streaks with *peau d'orange* in PXE.

Presentation

asymptomatic, unless CNV of the macula causes decreased vision. The lesions are reddish brown and radiate in branches from the optic disc. PXE is associated with a *peau d'orange,* mottled background fundus appearance, focal fine exudates in the midperipheral retina, and drusen of the optic disc. Loose skin folds and plaquelike lesions in the neck ("chicken skin") and on flexor aspects of joints are present. Increased risk of cardiovascular complications and GI bleeds are associated.

Differential Diagnosis

myopic lacquer cracks, choroidal rupture.

Management angioid streaks may develop CNV, which may endanger vision. Patients should be advised that even mild ocular trauma may cause choroidal rupture and subretinal hemorrhages. In select cases, extrafoveal CNV membranes may be treated with photoablation.

- For suspected PXE: skin biopsy, cardiovascular evaluation.
- For suspected Paget's disease: serum alkaline phosphatase and urine calcium.
- For suspected sickle cell disease: sickle cell preparation.

9.11 Degenerative Myopia

choroidal degeneration associated with myopia greater than −6.0 D and axial length greater than 26 mm. However, progressive choroidal degeneration in the posterior pole and vision loss from lacquer cracks (breaks in Bruch's membrane) and CNV may occur in any degree of myopia.

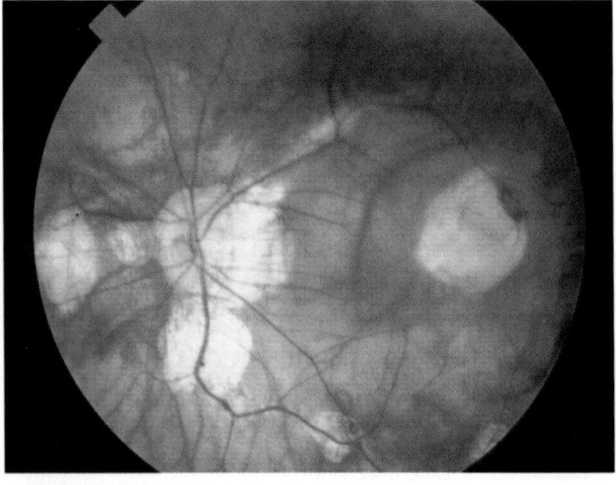

FIGURE 9.11 Myopic degeneration with macular staphyloma.

Presentation with decreased best-corrected visual acuity, usually beyond the fifth decade. Findings include a temporal crescent of peripapillary atrophy, an obliquely inserted optic nerve, posterior staphylomata, RPE abnormalities, and Fuchs' spot (dark area caused by CNV). Risk for rhegmatogenous retinal detachment is increased, especially with concurrent lattice degeneration.

Differential Diagnosis AMD, ocular histoplasmosis, gyrate atrophy.

Management the fundus should be carefully examined every 6 months to detect CNV and retinal breaks. Glaucoma may be associated with myopia and difficult to diagnose due to oblique insertion of the optic nerve. Symptomatic retinal breaks are treated with laser photocoagulation, cryotherapy, or scleral-buckling surgery. Treatment of asymptomatic retinal breaks should be considered when there is no surrounding pigmentation or demarcation line. Extrafoveal or juxtafoveal CNV may need laser photocoagulation.

9.12 Central Serous Chorioretinopathy

a serous detachment of neurosensory retina in the macula due to alteration of the RPE and choroidal circulation.

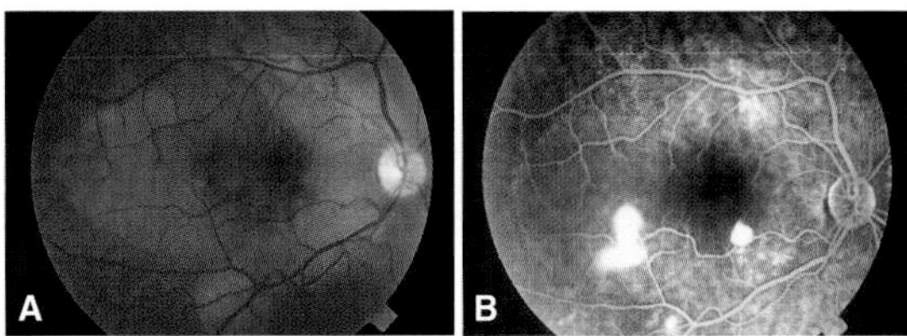

FIGURE 9.12a CSC with blisterlike sensory elevation in the macula.
FIGURE 9.12b FA with "smokestack" sign.

Presentation the typical patient is a male with type-A personality, age 25 to 50 years, with central blurring of vision, micropsia (objects appear smaller), mild acquired hyperopia, and altered color vision. CSC has been seen in the elderly, in pregnant women, and in some Hispanic and Asian populations. Findings include a yellow, blister-like elevation of sensory retina in the macula. Visual acuity ranges from 20/20 to 20/80, and Amsler's grid testing reveals distortion of straight lines often with a scotoma. FA shows a classic pinpoint area of leakage ("smokestack" sign) within the subretinal blister. Subretinal fibrin, CNV RPE pigmentation, or atrophy may be associated.

Differential Diagnosis macular hole with detachment (especially in myopes), optic pit with serous detachment, Harada's disease, causes of CNV (AMD, POHS, others), choroidal tumor or metastasis, idiopathic choroidal effusion.

Management prognosis for spontaneous recovery is excellent. Patients should be examined every 6 to 8 weeks. Photocoagulation may be considered if persistence of a serous detachment is beyond 4 to 6 months, if permanent visual deficit was sustained from a previous episode in the eye or contralateral eye, and if the patient requires prompt restoration of vision because of an occupational requirement.

9.13 Cystoid Macular Edema

perifoveal capillary leakage causing intraretinal accumulation of fluid within the macula. Etiology includes uveitis, postoperative complication, diabetic maculopathy, AMD, retinal vein occlusions, RP, vitreomacular traction, topical epinephrine (or dipivefrin) drops, retinal vasculitis, choroidal neovascularization, retinal telangiectactic diseases, nicotinic acid, intraocular tumors, juvenile retinoschisis.

Presentation decreased vision and metamorphopsia. Findings include decreased foveal light reflex and foveal thickening, with or without small intraretinal cysts. Optic nerve swelling and vitreous cells can appear in severe cases. A foveal cyst, or a lamellar macular hole causing permanent visual loss, may

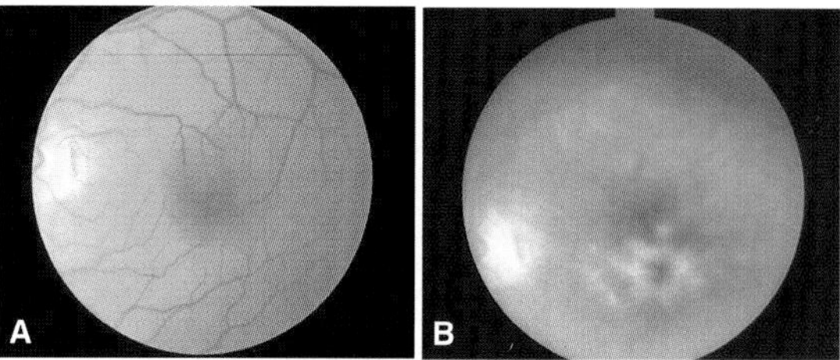

FIGURE 9.13a CME.
FIGURE 9.13b FA of CME with classic petaloid pattern.

develop. Irvine-Gass syndrome is CME occurring after cataract surgery, with peak incidence in 6 to 10 weeks often are found vitreous to the wound, iris prolapse, and vitreous loss. FA shows early leakage out of perifoveal capillaries and late macular staining, classically in a petaloid or spoke-wheel pattern. The optic nerve may also demonstrate leakage and late staining. Leakage is characteristically absent in nicotinic acid maculopathy.

Differential Diagnosis

phototoxic injury, foreal cyst, CNV.

Management

- Postoperative: spontaneous resolution occurs within 6 months in 75% of eyes. Treatment may include topical NSAIDs (flurbiprofen or ketorolac, qid) and topical steroids (prednisolone acetate, 1% qid). Persistent cases may benefit from periocular steroid (methylprednisolone, 80 mg/ml, 0.5 ml).
- Macular edema in the presence of vitreous incarceration in a surgical wound may be improved by anterior vitrectomy or YAG-laser lysis of the vitreous strand.
- Uveitic: topical steroid and systemic or periocular steroid to control inflammation.
- RP: may benefit from oral carbonic anhydrase inhibitor (Diamox [acetazolamide], 500 mg bid).
- BRVO-related macular edema persisting for 3 to 6 months with vision below 20/40 may improve with laser photocoagulation.

9.14 Age-Related Macular Degeneration

a heredetodegenerative disease of the macula.

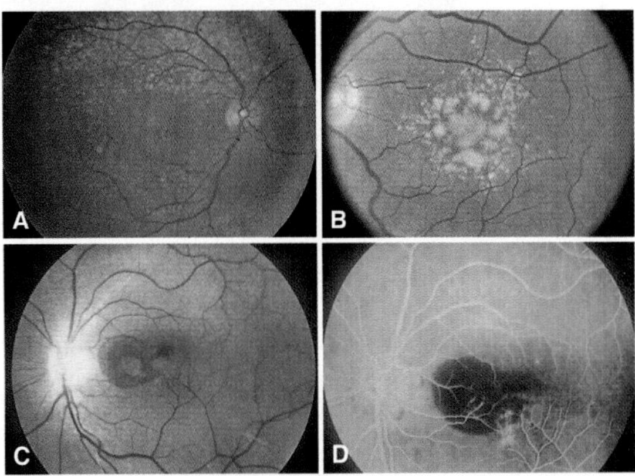

FIGURE 9.14a AMD with drusen and RPE hypertrophy secondary to RPE rip.
FIGURE 9.14b AMD with soft, confluent drusen in the macula.
FIGURE 9.14c Subretinal heme secondary to choroidal neovascularization from AMD.
FIGURE 9.14d FA of subretinal heme secondary to occult choroidal neovascularization.

Presentation age usually above 50 years, with decreased vision, metamorphopsia. Findings include bilateral macular drusen, or yellow deposits at the level of the RPE and Bruch's membrane. Drusen may be "hard" (small, distinct, calcific lesions) or "soft" (large, indistinct, sometimes confluent). Atrophy and hyperpigmentation of the RPE may be seen. "Dry" or nonexudative AMD has a better visual prognosis. "Wet" or exudative AMD refers to serous exudate or hemorrhage due to choroidal neovascularization (CNV), which appears as a gray-green subretinal mass. Causes of CNV include presumed ocular histoplasmosis syndrome, angioid streaks, high myopia, traumatic choroidal rupture, photocoagulation scars, inflammatory chorioretinal lesions, and idiopathic.

Management

visual acuity and Amsler's grid self-monitoring. With reading correction, one eye is occluded and fixated on the central dot. Any change in waviness, blurriness, or absence of part of the grid warrants urgent follow-up to rule out CNV. Hemorrhage, subretinal fluid, and clinical suspicion for CNV also warrant urgent follow-up to rule out CNV by FA and possibly indocyanine green angiography.

- Nonexudative: no treatment is available.
- Exudative: early CNV may be photocoagulated to reduce the risk of severe visual loss under the guidelines of the Macular Photocoagulation Study. Cases should be followed for CNV every 4 to 6 months. No medical therapy (including nutritional supplements) has been proven effective.

9.15 Stargardt's Disease and Fundus Flavimaculatus

a usually autosomal recessive macular disorder. These two disorders are now known to be different presentations of the same disease.

Presentation

decrease in central vision is often out of proportion to the relatively normal-appearing fundus. Yellow-white fleck-like deposits may be seen at the RPE level, usually in a pisciform (fish-tail) configuration. Atrophic macular degeneration may be seen as bull's eye or beaten-metal appearance.

Differential Diagnosis

- Of flecks: fundus albipunctatus, retinitis punctata albescens, familial drusen, Bietti's crystalline retinopathy, pattern dystrophy, RP inversus, macular degeneration, PXE, crystalline retinopathy, histo spots.

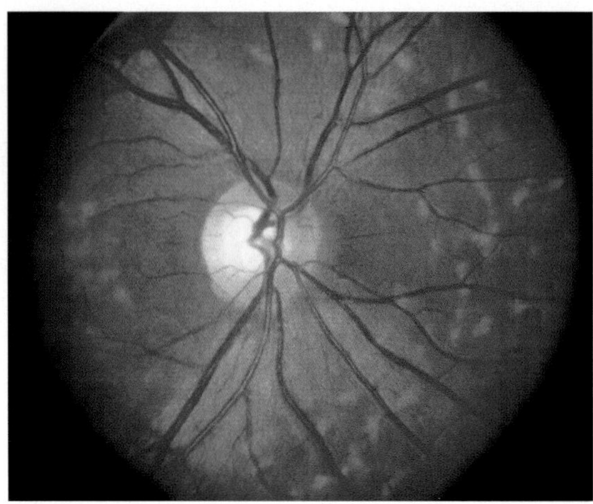

FIGURE 9.15 Stargardt's disease with pisciform deposits.

- Of bull's eye maculopathy: cone–rod dystrophy, chloroquine or hydroxychloroquine maculopathy, AMD.

Management FA shows a blockage of choroidal fluorescence producing a "silent choroid" or as a result of increased lipofuscin in the RPE cells. ERG is typically normal but may become abnormal in the late stage of disease. EOG is normal. No treatment is available.

9.16 Fundus Albipunctatus

autosomal recessive form of congenital stationary night blindness.

Presentation patients may be asymptomatic or night blind. Diffuse, white, discrete dots in the midperipheral fundus, not the fovea, are typical.

Differential Diagnosis retinitis punctata albescens (progressive, behaves like RP), birdshot chorioretinitis, Stargardt's disease, familial drusen,

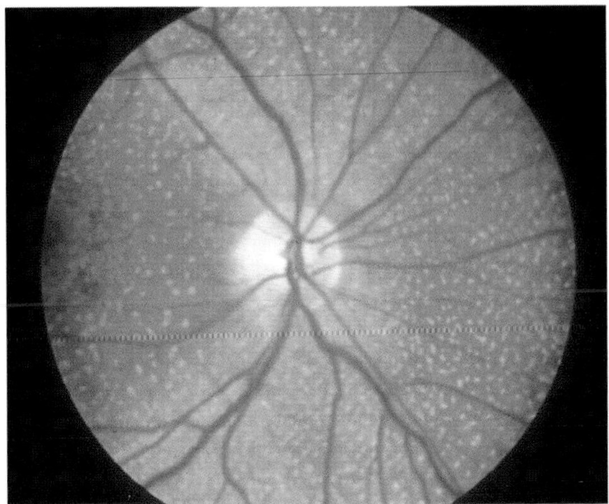

FIGURE 9.16 Fundus albipunctatus.

Bietti's crystalline retinopathy, pattern dystrophy, RP inversus, macular degeneration, PXE, crystalline retinopathy, histo spots.

Management vision and fields remain normal.

9.17 Best's Disease: Vitelliform Macular Dystrophy

autosomal dominant (variable penetrance) degenerative maculopathy.

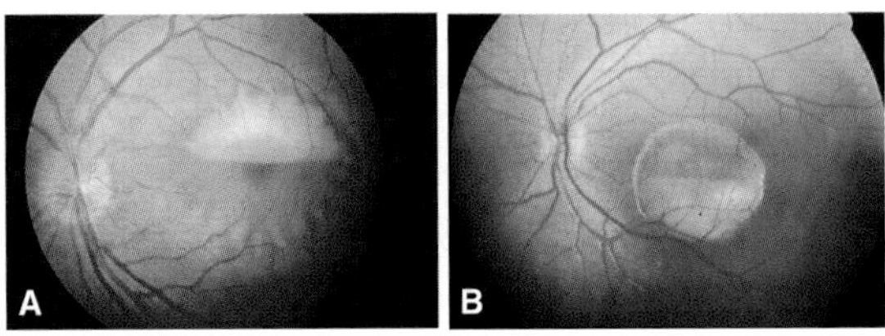

FIGURE 9.17a Best's disease with pseudohypopyon.
FIGURE 9.17b Best's disease.

Presentation onset is at birth, but patients may not be detected for years. Foveal lesions are bilateral, yellow, round, and approximately 1 to 2 disc areas in size. Vision may be better than expected from macular appearance but declines later in life. The lesions have been described as an egg yolk or pseudohypopyon; they may degenerate and macular CNV, hemorrhage, and disciform scar may develop.

Differential Diagnosis the late scar stage is difficult to distinguish from AMD.

Management the EOG is diminished, while the ERG is normal. There is no known treatment. Cases should be followed with an Amsler's grid for early detection of CNV.

9.18 Retinal Drug Toxicity

9.18.1 Thioridazine (Mellaril)—antipsychotic, used especially for chronic schizophrenia.

Presentation patients taking more than 700 mg/day may present with blurred vision, brown vision, nyctalopia; retinal toxicity

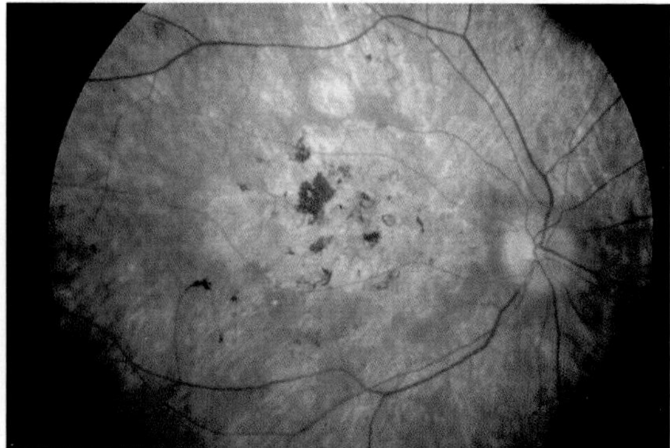

FIGURE 9.18.1 Mellaril (thioridazine) toxicity. (With permission from Yannuzzi L, Guyer D in The Retina Atlas, Mosby, 1995)

(seen as pigment clumps between the posterior pole and the equator), retinal depigmentation and atrophy, retinal edema, visual field abnormalities, central scotoma and general constriction, a depressed or extinguished ERG.

Differential Diagnosis pigment clumping may be seen in RP, syphilitic chorioretinopathy, viral chorioretinitis, choroideremia, Bietti's crystalline dystrophy, retinal detachment, and ocular trauma.

Management mellaril (thioridazine) should be discontinued promptly to reverse fundus abnormalities if still in the early stage. However, retinopathy may still progress. Baseline studies and follow-up of patients are needed: VA, fundus photographs, visual fields, ERG, and color vision testing (Farnsworth-Munsell 100-hue test).

9.18.2 Chlorpromazine (Thorazine)—antipsychotic, used especially for chronic schizophrenia.

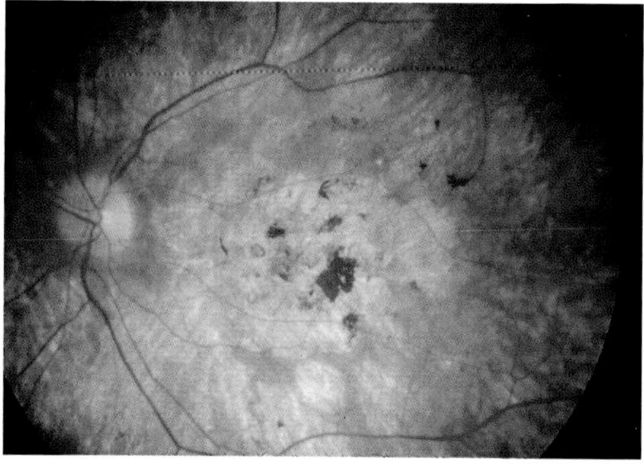

FIGURE 9.18.2 Thorazine (chlorpromazine) toxicity.

Presentation patients may be asymptomatic or present with blurred vision. Findings in this pigment retinopathy include abnormal pigmentation of the eyelids, cornea, conjunctiva (especially within the palpebral fissure), anterior lens capsule, and subcapsular cataract. Dose required is 1200 to 2400 mg/day for longer than 12 months.

Differential Diagnosis same as thioridazine toxicity.

Management monitor visual field and ERG changes. Discontinue medication.

9.18.3 Chloroquine or Hydroxychloroquine (Plaquenil) Toxicity

Toxicity—antimalarials, used chronically for connective tissue disorders such as lupus.

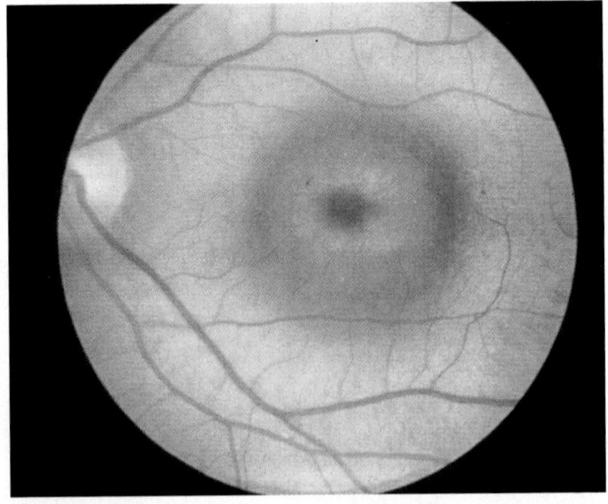

FIGURE 9.18.3 Hydroxychloroquine toxicity with bull's eye maculopathy.

Presentation patients may have difficulty adjusting to darkness. There is a loss of the foveal reflex in this bull's eye maculopathy. Whorl-like corneal changes may occur and are almost always present in chloroquine retinopathy. Dose required for retinopathy:

- Chloroquine, > 300 g total cumulative dose.
- Hydroxychloroquine, more than 750 mg/day for months to years.

Differential Diagnosis bull's eye macula may be seen in AMD, cone dystrophy, Stargardt's disease, and Spielmeyer-Vogt syndrome.

Management follow-up every 6 to 12 months when the patient is using medication. Obtain visual field, color vision testing, and possibly EOG. Medication should be discontinued on appearance of retinopathy, which may still progress.

9.18.4 Drug-Related Crystalline Retinopathy—crystallin retinal deposits due to various drug usage.

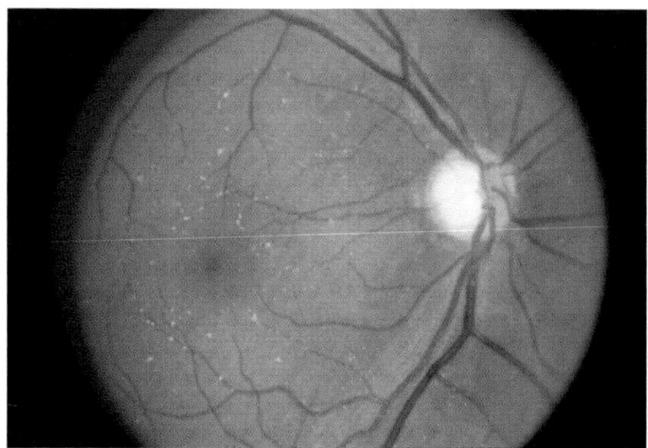

FIGURE 9.18.4 Talc retinopathy.

Presentation

- Talc particles lodged in the choriocapillaris and small retinal vessels are seen in chronic IV use of talc and cornstarch contained in illegal drugs. Neovascularization may occur.

- Tamoxifen (estrogen agent for breast cancer) causes crystalline retinal deposits and loss of vision due to maculopathy.
- Canthaxanthin (oral tanning agent) causes striking but asymptomatic retinal crystals.
- Oxalate crystals form in primary hyperoxaluria or due to methoxyflurane, an anesthetic.

Differential Diagnosis fundus albipunctatus, retinitis punctata albescens, familial drusen, Bietti's crystalline retinopathy, fundus albipunctatus.

Management if an acute episode of emboli, treatment includes the same maneuvers as for retinal artery occlusions.

9.19 Pattern Dystrophy

an autosomal dominant dystrophy of the RPE.

Presentation patients may have normal or mild decreased vision (about 20/30). Color vision is normal. Symmetric bilateral hy-

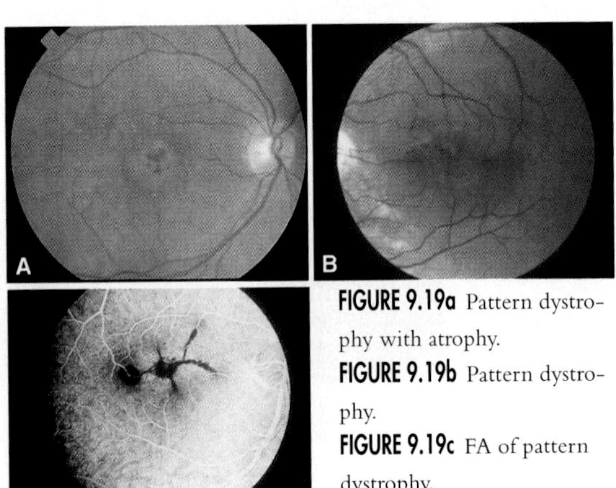

FIGURE 9.19a Pattern dystrophy with atrophy.
FIGURE 9.19b Pattern dystrophy.
FIGURE 9.19c FA of pattern dystrophy.

perpigmentation of the fovea often appears in a polymorphous or butterfly pattern.

Differential Diagnosis drug-induced degenerations, angioid streaks, rubella retinopathy, myotonic dystrophy.

Management EOG is subnormal. FA better demonstrates the blocking pattern of the RPE hyperpigmentation. No treatment is known.

9.20 Cone Dystrophies

cone dystrophies are less common than rod dystrophies and usually are autosomal dominantly inherited.

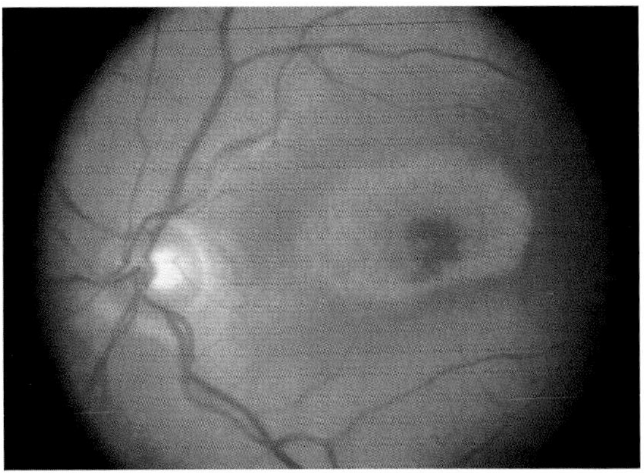

FIGURE 9.20 Bull's eye appearance of cone dystrophy.

Presentation this bull's eye maculopathy may present at birth with congenital nystagmus or in adults with low progressive bilateral visual loss, photophobia, and poor color vision. Vision is worse during the day than at night. Early, the fundus is essentially normal; later, nystagmus, temporal pallor of the optic disc, spotty pigment clumping in the macular area, and tapetal-like retinal sheen may appear.

Differential Diagnosis Stargardt's disease, chloroquine retinopathy, central areolar choroidal dystrophy, AMD, RP, optic neuropathy, non-physiologic visual loss.

Management FA may help detect the bull's eye pattern. ERG studies have a reduced single-flash photopic response and a reduced flicker response. Low-vision aids may be helpful in this incurable disease.

9.21 Idiopathic Parafoveal Telangiectasia

abnormal capillary vessels in the parafoveal region.

Presentation patients are usually age 50 to 60 years and present with minimal visual loss. Symmetric, bilateral temporal areas of perifoveal capillary telangiectatic vessels are seen clinically and on FA. The incompetent vessels hyperfluoresce. CME and mild exudate occur. Retinochoroidal anastomoses may be seen as temporal, right-angled vessels.

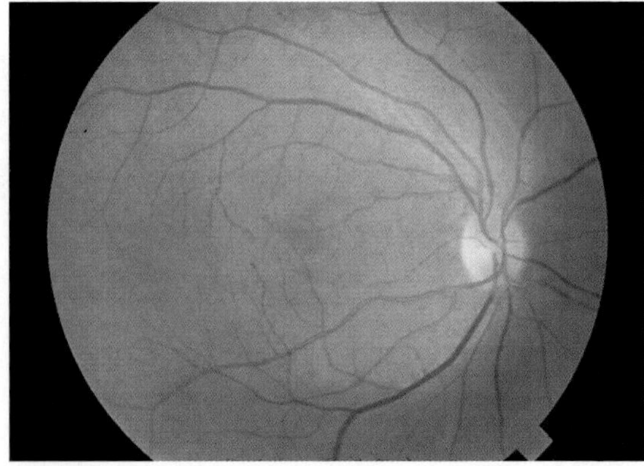

FIGURE 9.21 Idiopathic parafoveal telangiectasias with temporal capillary abnormalities.

Differential Diagnosis BRVO, radiation retinopathy, uveitis, CNV.

Management observation is necessary to detect CNV. Photocoagulation may be successful in preventing exudation and visual loss, although it is not generally recommended.

9.22 Sickle Cell Retinopathy

predominantly affects patients of African and Mediterranean heritage. Heterozygotes (sickle cell hemoglobin, sickle cell thalassemia) tend to have worse ocular disease than do homozygotes (SS), who have worse systemic disease.

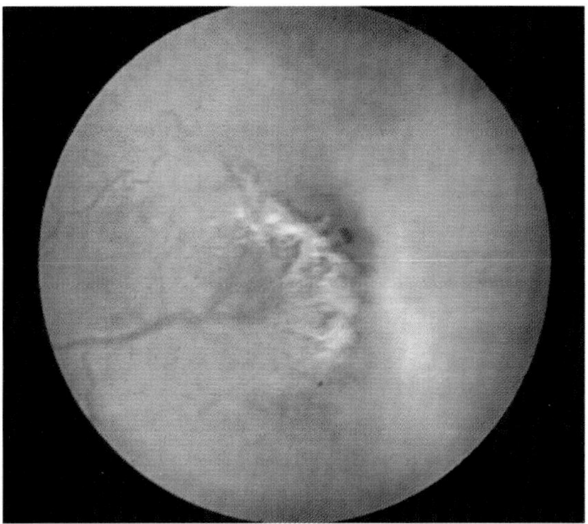

FIGURE 9.22 Sickle cell retinopathy—"sea-fan". (With permission from Yannuzzi L, Guyer D in The Retina Atlas, Mosby, 1995)

Presentation usually patients are asymptomatic. Flashes, floaters, and loss of vision occur with advanced disease.

- Nonproliferative: peripheral vascular occlusions (stage 1) cause tortuosity of retinal veins and hemorrhage. Hemorrhage causes black sunbursts (RPE reaction causing spiculated, midperipheral fundus lesions), salmon patches (intraretinal hemorrhage), and refractile deposits (hemosiderin). Chronic occlusion causes AV anastomosis formation (stage 2), which appears as dilated preexisting capillaries. Sclerosed peripheral retinal vessels or abnormal dull gray peripheral areas (result of ischemia) are seen in the fundus.

- Proliferative: due to ischemia, peripheral retinal neovascularization forms in the shape of a "sea fan" (stage 3). These frequently autoinfarct and regress. Complications from neovascularization include VH (stage 4), retinal breaks at the base of sea fans, and tractional retinal detachments (stage 5). Angioid streaks, comma-shaped capillaries of the inferior fornix conjunctiva, central retinal artery occlusion, and macular arteriolar occlusions may be seen.

Differential Diagnosis peripheral retinal neovascularization may be caused by sarcoidosis, diabetes, BRVO, embolic disease, Eales' disease, ROP, familial exudative vitreoretinopathy, chronic myelogenous leukemia, radiation retinopathy, pars planitis, carotid–cavernous fistula, ocular ischemic syndrome, talc retinopathy, and collagen vascular disease.

Management segmental scatter laser photocoagulation may be performed in ischemic areas to cause regression of active neovascularization. Retinal detachment and nonclearing VH require surgery.

9.23 Retinitis Pigmentosa

a group of inherited, degenerative pigmented retinopathies. May have varied inheritance.

Presentation symptoms include progressive loss of night and peripheral vision. Characteristic fundus findings are pigment deposits along arterioles (bone spiculing), narrowing of arterioles, vitreous cells, and "waxy" optic nerve pallor. ERG is diminished, and visual field loss is progressive.

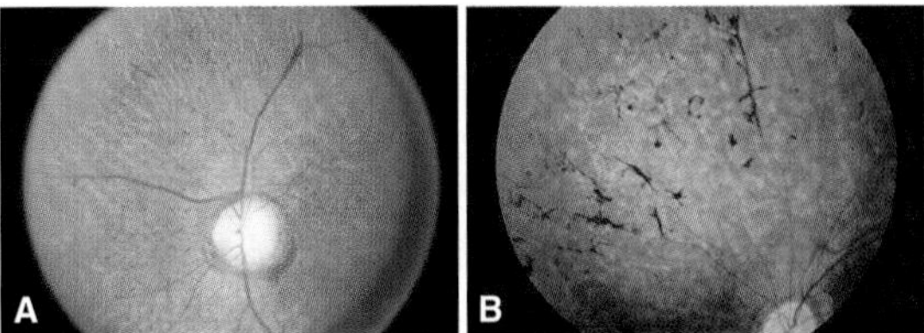

FIGURE 9.23a RP nerve head waxy pallor and attenuated vessels.
FIGURE 9.23b Bone spicules in the periphery of RP.

CME, epiretinal membrane, and posterior subcapsular cataract may ensue. RP syndromes include the following:

- Abetalipoproteinemia (Bassen-Kornzweig disease): celiac syndrome; fat malabsorption and secondary vitamin-A, D, E, K deficiency; diarrhea; chronic progressive ophthalmoplegia.
- Kearns-Sayre syndrome: chronic progressive ophthalmoplegia, ptosis, heart block.
- Lawrence-Moon or Bardet-Biedl syndrome: mild mental retardation, obesity, polydactyly, hypogonadism, nystagmus, optic nerve atrophy.
- Leber's congenital amaurosis: congenital poor vision, nystagmus, nonrecordable ERG.
- Refsum's disease: increased serum phytanic acid; cerebellar ataxia, polyneuropathy, anosmia, ichthyosis, partial deafness, enlarged cornea nerves.
- Usher's syndrome: congenital deafness, type I total deafness and no vestibular function, type II partial deafness and normal vestibular function.

Differential Diagnosis

night-blindness disorders include gyrate atrophy, choroideremia, vitamin-A deficiency, and congenital stationary night blindness. A pigmented retinopathy may be caused by phenothiazine toxicity, syphilis, congenital rubella, resolution of an exudative retinal detachment (toxemia of pregnancy or Harada's disease), pigmented paravenous retinochoroidal atrophy, myotonic dystrophy, Stickler's syndrome.

Management genetic counseling is recommended for all patients. Evaluate for legal blindness (patients frequently develop a visual field of <10° of arc). Systemic diseases must be detected and treated.

- Abetalipoproteinemia (Bassen-Kornzweig disease): check the serum lipoprotein electrophoreses. Treat with fat-soluble vitamin supplements and dietary fat restriction.
- Kearns-Sayre syndrome: obtain serial EKGs to rule out heart block.
- Refsum's disease: check serum phytanic acid. Treat with low-phytanic acid diet.

9.24 Choroideremia

rare, X-linked retinal dystrophy that affects males in the second decade and presents with night blindness.

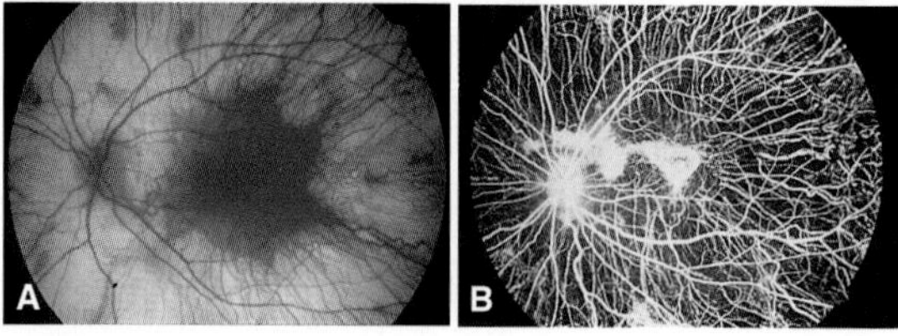

FIGURE 9.24a Choroideremia.
FIGURE 9.24b FA of choroideremia.

Presentation vision may remain fairly good until the fourth or fifth decade. Women may be asymptomatic carriers. Retinal findings include dispersed pigment granules throughout the fundus, accompanied by atrophy of the choroid, sparing the macula.

Differential Diagnosis RP, gyrate atrophy, albinism, thioridazine retinopathy.

Management no treatment is known. Patients may benefit from genetic counseling.

9.25 Gyrate Atrophy

recessively inherited retinal dystrophy caused by a defect in the enzyme ornithine transferase.

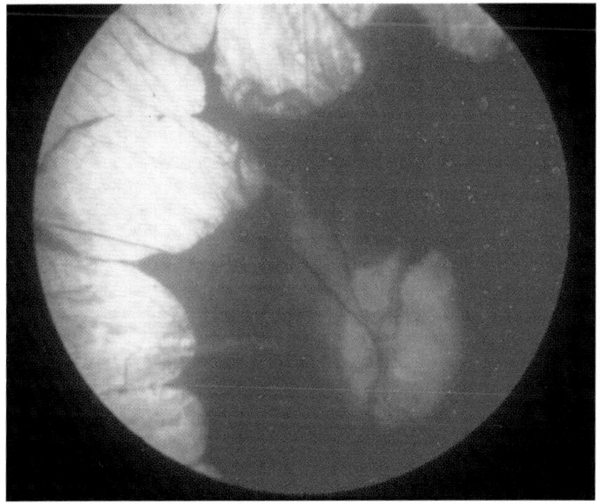

FIGURE 9.25 Gyrate atrophy.

Presentation patients present in their 20s and 30s with poor night vision. The fundus findings are scalloped and well-circumscribed areas of chorioretinal atrophy in areas of the equatorial retina. The atrophy expands centrally and peripherally. Retinal vessels and optic discs are normal.

Differential Diagnosis paving-stone degeneration, choroideremia, high myopia, thioridazine retinopathy.

Management visual prognosis may be improved by restricting arginine in the diet and adding pyridoxine.

9.26 RADIATION RETINOPATHY

patients with any irradiation of the head in total doses over 3000 rads are at risk for this slowly progressive occlusive vasculopathy.

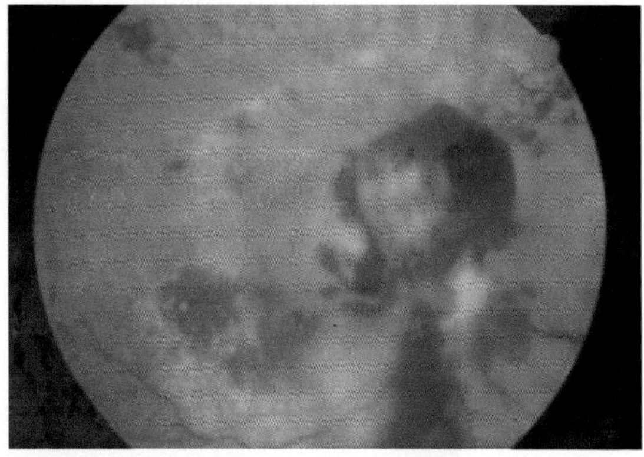

FIGURE 9.26 Radiation retinopathy. (With permission from Yannuzzi L, Guyer D in The Retina Atlas, Mosby, 1995)

Presentation visual loss is delayed 6 months to years after therapy. Findings include cotton-wool spots, vascular sheathing, vascular occlusions, microaneurysms and telangiectasias, neovascularization, and exudates. Visual loss results from foveal nonperfusion, macular edema, VH, retinal detachment, or neovascular glaucoma.

Differential Diagnosis diabetic retinopathy, BRAO, venous occlusive disease, retinal telangiectasia.

Management resultant macular nonperfusion is irreversible.

9.27 SOLAR RETINOPATHY

Presentation sun-gazing patients with visual loss (up to 20/200) present with yellow-white foveolar lesions that are replaced

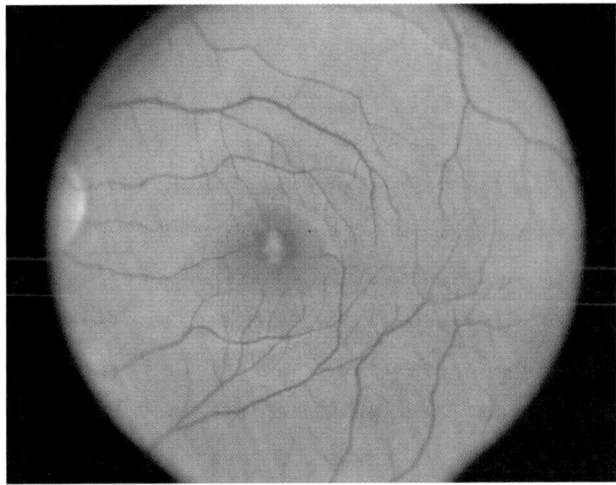

FIGURE 9.27 Solar retinopathy. (With permission from Yannuzzi L, Guyer D in The Retina Atlas, Mosby, 1995)

with a red foveolar depression surrounded by a pigmented halo. Vision improves in 3 to 6 months (usually to > 20/40).

Differential Diagnosis blunt ocular trauma, RP.

Management no treatment. Observation is warranted.

Chapter 10

SURGICAL RETINA

Naresh Mandava, Yale L. Fisher, Jason S. Slakter

10.1 Peripheral Retinal Degenerations

10.1.1 Lattice Degeneration—the most common peripheral vitreoretinal degeneration. Predisposes to retinal detachments.

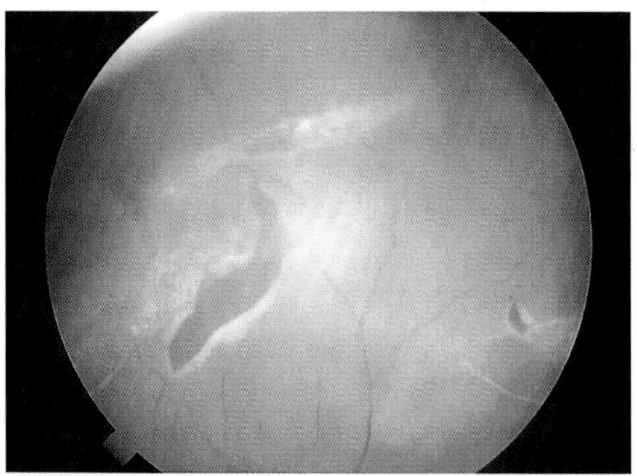

FIGURE 10.1.1 Retinal tear on edge of lattice degeneration.

Presentation common in high myopia. Occurs in all age groups. Incidence is 7 to 10% and occurs bilaterally 40 to 50% of the time. There is localized inner retinal atrophy (retinal thinning) with RPE hypertrophy in a round, oval, or linear shape. Location is usually anterior to the equator and parallel to the ora serrata, but radial perivascular lattice also occurs. White lines (lattice "wicker") represent sclerotic blood vessels. Atrophic holes occur within the lattice. Liquefied vitreous may overlie lattice, and there is increased vitreous adhesion at lattice margins, leading to risk of retinal tears.

Differential Diagnosis peripheral cystoid degeneration, chorioretinal scars (i.e., previous vasculitis).

Management

- Rarely needs treatment, and risk of retinal detachment is only 0.3%. Retinal tears usually occur adjacent to lattice but also may be found in remote locations. Consider treatment of lattice in the fellow eye of a retinal detachment or intraoperatively during retinal detachment repair. Treatment involves laser to surround the lattice lesion 360°.
- Follow-up: retinal detachment warnings (immediate follow-up for increase or change in the quality of flashes or floaters, onset of a dark curtain or shadow in peripheral vision, or loss of vision), yearly examination.

10.1.2 Peripheral Cystoid Degeneration—a common chorioretinal degeneration of peripheral retina.

Presentation occurs in nearly all eyes with advanced age. "Salt and pepper" peripheral chorioretinal degeneration may be associated with the cystic changes beginning in the outer plexi-

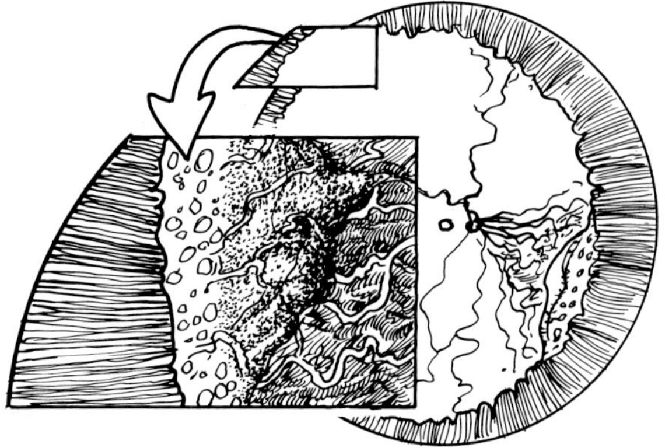

FIGURE 10.1.2 Peripheral cystoid degeneration.

form layer and sometimes enlarging into all layers of the retina. Advanced cystic changes lead to senile retinoschisis.

Management does not predispose to retinal detachment except rare instances when a full-thickness hole develops, or when there is retinoschisis.

10.1.3 Cobblestone Degeneration (or Paving-Stone Degeneration)—atrophy of outer retina, RPE, and choroid.

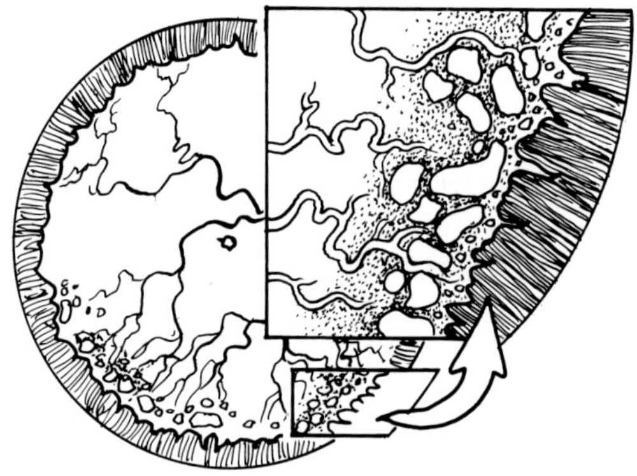

FIGURE 10.1.3 Cobblestone degeneration.

Presentation localized patches of 1 to 2 disc diameters of atrophied retina. White sclera and overlying traversing choroidal vessels are visible. Most common in the inferior periphery.

Management does not predispose to retinal detachment.

10.1.4 Ora Bays—pars plana tissue found posterior to ora serrata. Can be enclosed or partially enclosed by normal retinal tissue. Incidence is 4%.

Presentation brown islands or peninsulas of tissue surrounded by normal retina.

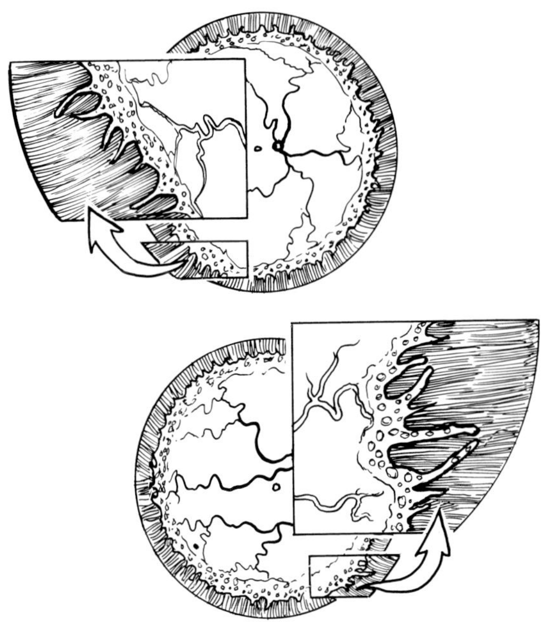

FIGURE 10.1.4 Ora bays.

Differential Diagnosis choroidal nevus, choroidal melanoma.

Management retinal detachment warnings; 16% associated with retinal tear posterior to lesion, only with concomitant posterior vitreous detachment.

10.1.5 Meridional Folds—radial, linear elevation of redundant peripheral retina aligned with ora bay, dentate process (an anterior extension of retinal tissue), or meridional complex (dentate process aligned with ciliary process in same meridian).

Presentation incidence is 25% with 50% bilaterality. Lesion is 0.6 to 6.0 mm long, usually nasal and above or below horizontal meridian.

Management none. There is no association with retinal breaks.

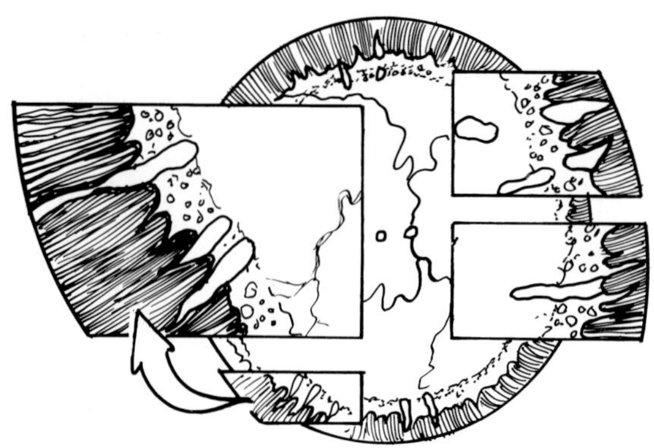

FIGURE 10.1.5 Meridional folds.

10.1.6 Retinal Tuft—a fingerlike projection of retinal tissue within the vitreous base.

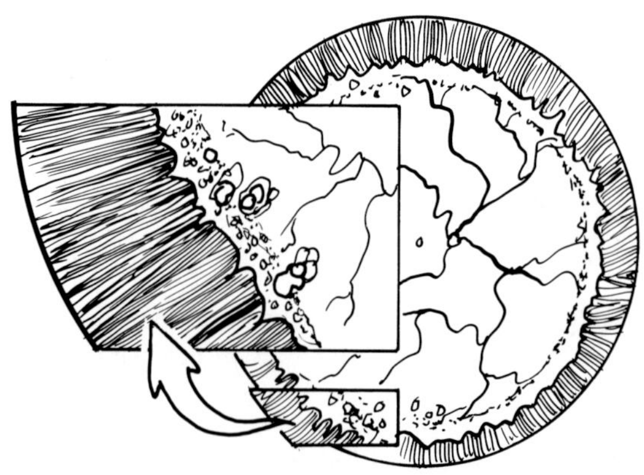

FIGURE 10.1.6 Cystic retinal tuft.

Presentation

- Noncystic retinal tuft: narrow base less than 0.1 mm, no associated cystic retinal degeneration, no association with retinal breaks.
- Cystic retinal tuft: base greater than 0.1 mm, cystic change in inner retina of tuft, 50 to 60% incidence.

About 6.5% of retinal detachments are caused by a break at the cystic retinal tuft.

- Zonular traction tuft: fibroglial strand extending from peripheral retina over pars plana, 10% incidence. 2 to 5% incidence of partial- or full-thickness retinal breaks.

Management symptomatic cystic retinal tufts are treated. Any lesion within the vitreous base need not be treated (the full extent of the vitreous base may be difficult to assess).

10.1.7 White without Pressure

10.1.7 White without Pressure—white peripheral retina due to a phenomenon related to the orientation of dense vitreous collagen in periphery.

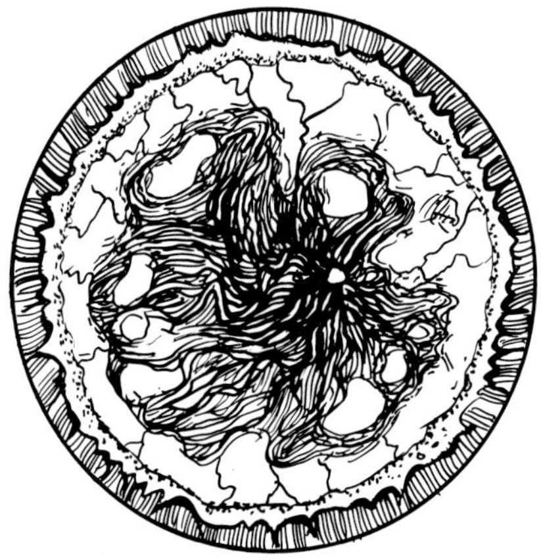

FIGURE 10.1.7 White without pressure.

Presentation well-demarcated zones of peripheral retinal whitening present without scleral depression. They simulate the white appearance of peripheral retinal tissue during scleral indentation.

Differential Diagnosis extraocular tumor, commotio retinae.

Management no association with retinal detachment. May be seen more frequently in fellow eye of patients with giant retinal tears.

10.1.8 Pars Plana Cysts—a normal finding in the pars plana.

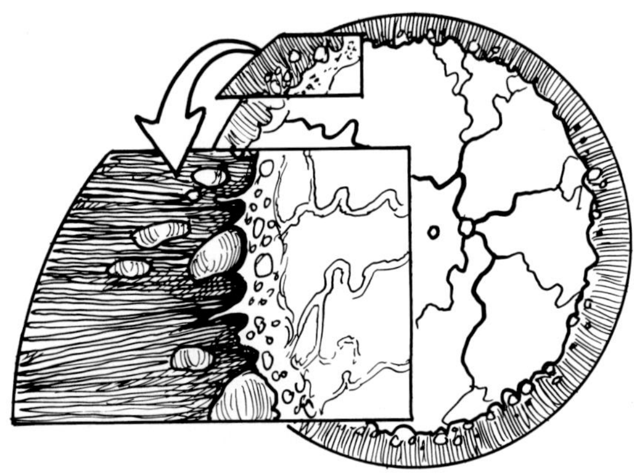

FIGURE 10.1.8 Pars plana cyst.

Presentation cysts in the posterior pars plana are visualized by scleral depression. Usually multiple, bilateral lesions, located temporally.

Management no clinical significance.

10.2 Posterior Vitreous Detachment

separation of the posterior hyaloid face from the retinal surface due to degeneration of the formed vitreous. The incidence of PVD increases with age (63% in patients over 70 years old) and after cataract surgery (more commonly with posterior capsular breaks) and trauma.

Presentation floaters (described as "cobwebs" or "flies") that move with eye movement; may have flashes that indicate vitreoretinal traction. Slit-lamp biomicroscopy with 78- or 90-diopter

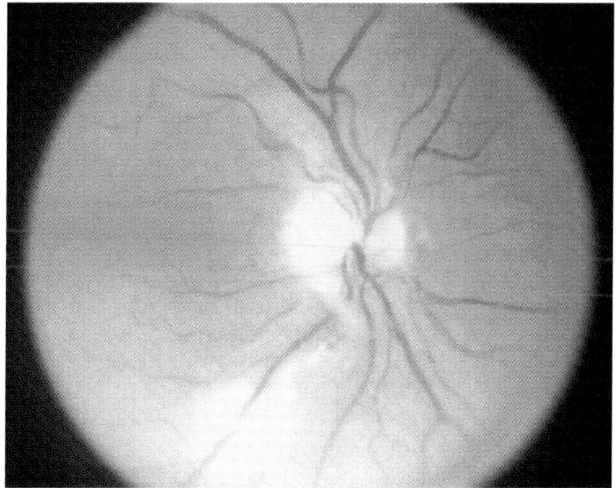

FIGURE 10.2 Posterior vitreous detachment with Weiss' ring.

lens may reveal a Weiss' ring (circular vitreous opacity floating in front of optic nerve representing previous adhesion of posterior hyaloid face to margins of the disc). B-scan confirms the diagnosis. PVD may be associated with vitreous hemorrhage or retinal tear. Of patients with a PVD and vitreous hemorrhage, 70% will have a retinal tear, whereas only 2 to 4% without hemorrhage have a retinal tear. Overall, 10 to 15% of patients with PVD have a retinal tear.

Differential Diagnosis

vitritis (does not have pigmented cells but may have associated manifestations of posterior uveitis), migraine (flashes in a zigzag, often C-shaped pattern, may have associated aura or headache, and may have scotomata but not moving floaters), retinal tear, retinal detachment, vitreous hemorrhage.

Management

- All patients require examination of the periphery to the ora (indirect ophthalmoscopy with scleral depression). A retinal tear or detachment requires immediate treatment. Pigment cells in the anterior vitreous or vitreous hemorrhage in an acute PVD increases suspicion of retinal tear or detachment.

- If vitreous hemorrhage obstructs view of the peripheral retina, B-scan is performed to rule out retinal break or detachment. Give patients retinal detachment warnings (immediate follow-up for increase or change in the quality of flashes or floaters, onset of a dark curtain or shadow in peripheral vision, or loss of vision).
- Follow-up: if there is no retinal tear, perform a scleral depression examination in 2 weeks, 2 to 3 months, and 6 months. If there is no visible retinal tear secondary to mild retinal or vitreous hemorrhage, examine daily for 1 to 3 days and then every 1 to 2 weeks to rule out retinal detachment.

10.3 Retinal Break

a tear or hole in the retina, which can lead to retinal detachment. Vitreous traction can produce an acute retinal tear. Degeneration or thinning of retinal tissue can lead to asymptomatic retinal holes.

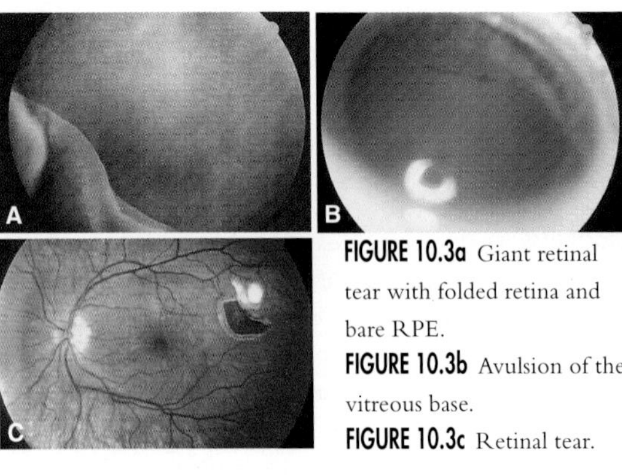

FIGURE 10.3a Giant retinal tear with folded retina and bare RPE.
FIGURE 10.3b Avulsion of the vitreous base.
FIGURE 10.3c Retinal tear.

Presentation flashes of light and floaters (described as "cobwebs" or "flies"), which move with eye movement. Retinal examination may reveal a full-thickness defect in the retina, often associated with pigment cells in the anterior vitreous ("tobacco dust"), posterior vitreous detachment, vitreous or preretinal hemorrhage, operculum of retinal tissue floating above the retinal hole, horseshoe flap tear. Adjacent retinal pathology or etiology of the break may be identified (i.e., lattice degeneration, cystic retinal tuft, retinal atrophy). A giant retinal tear is greater than 3 clock hours and is posterior to the ora serrata. A retinal dialysis is a retinal tear at the ora serrata.

Management all symptomatic retinal breaks should be treated. Asymptomatic retinal breaks should be treated if large or secondary to trauma or if the fellow eye has a history of retinal detachment. Consider treatment of asymptomatic horseshoe tears.

- Argon laser (see Section 17.11.5, Retinal Tears): use triple-mirror or wide-field contact lens.
- Indirect laser for anterior lesions too peripheral for contact lens.
- Cryotherapy if poor visualization or anterior break (i.e., retinal dialysis).
- Follow-up: give patients retinal detachment warnings (immediate follow-up for increase or change in the quality of flashes or floaters, onset of a dark curtain or shadow in peripheral vision, or loss of vision). Treated patients are examined with scleral depression in 1 week, 1 month, 2 to 3 months, and 6 months, and are encouraged to limit activity for 1 to 2 weeks until the retinal laser has the maximal effect. Untreated patients are examined at 6 months. Patients with large retinal tears above the horizontal meridian may benefit from positioning with the retinal break in the most dependent position to prevent retinal detachment.
- Complications: retinal detachment unrelated to treatment, macular pucker secondary to laser treatment or retinal break itself.

10.4 Retinal Detachment

detachment of the neurosensory retina related to rhegmatogenous (retinal break) or nonrhegmatogenous (exudative or tractional) etiology.

10.4.1 Rhegmatogenous Retinal Detachment—retinal break with subsequent passage of fluid into the subretinal space leading to detachment.

Presentation flashes of light, floaters, curtain or shadow starting from peripheral visual field, loss of central vision. Examination may reveal elevation of retina (transparent tissue with branching vessels) with corrugated folds, pigment cells in anterior vitreous, vitreous hemorrhage, relatively lower intraocular pressure than the fellow eye, afferent pupillary defect in larger detachments. Signs of chronicity include vitreous haze, preretinal or subretinal fibrous proliferation, fixed folds (see Section 10.4.4, Proliferative Vitreoretinopathy), pigmented demarcation line between attached and detached retina (indicates at least 3-month duration), and intraretinal macrocysts. Etiologic factors include myopia, lattice degeneration, trauma, aphakia, tractional retinal detachment, degenerative retinal diseases (Marfan, Ehlers-Danlos, Wagner's, Stickler's, Pierre Robin syndromes, familial exudative vitreoretinopathy, juvenile and senile retinoschisis, atopic dermatitis, acute retinal necrosis), macular hole (high myopia, trauma), CMV retinitis. Examination tips: Start by identifying the configuration of the detachment, which will identify the most likely location of the causative retinal breaks. Areas of lattice, hemorrhage, pigmentation, or other abnormalities should be examined carefully.

- Inferior detachments: retinal breaks are located on the higher side of the detachment. If the detachment is equal on both sides, the break is near the 6-o'clock position. If one sector or quadrant is detached, the break is near the upper edge. If the detachment is bullous, the break is above the horizontal meridian.

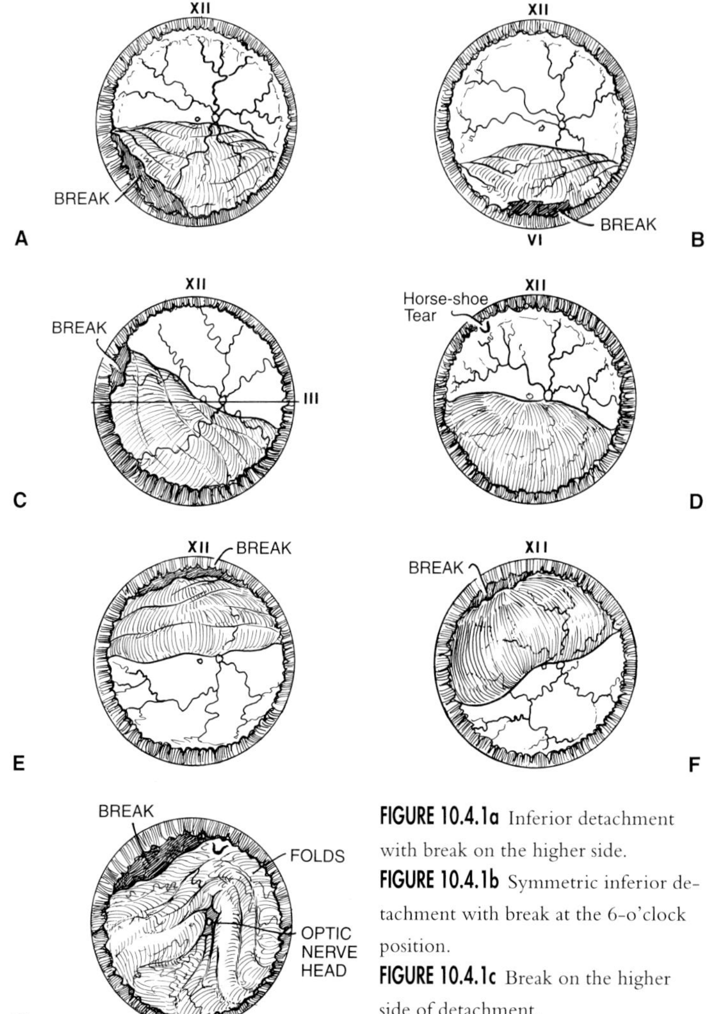

FIGURE 10.4.1a Inferior detachment with break on the higher side.

FIGURE 10.4.1b Symmetric inferior detachment with break at the 6-o'clock position.

FIGURE 10.4.1c Break on the higher side of detachment.

FIGURE 10.4.1d Peripheral sinus with bullous detachment.

FIGURE 10.4.1e Symmetric superior detachment with break between the 10- and 2-o'clock positions.

FIGURE 10.4.1f Bullous detachment with break between the 10- and 12-o'clock positions.

FIGURE 10.4.1g Total or subtotal retinal detachment with superior break and folds to the optic nerve head.

- Superior detachment: if detachment crosses the vertical midline, the retinal break is near the 12-o'clock position. If one sector or quadrant is detached, the break is near the upper edge.
- Total retinal detachment: the break is typically between the 10- and 2-o'clock positions.

Differential Diagnosis

"pseudo-retinal detachment" (similar funduscopic appearance to retinal detachment), juvenile retinoschisis, senile retinoschisis, branch retinal artery occlusion (severe nerve fiber layer edema can simulate a detachment), choroidal detachment (serous or hemorrhagic, epiretinal membrane), choroidal mass (uveal melanoma, metastatic carcinoma), exudative retinal detachment, tractional retinal detachment.

Management

- Indirect ophthalmoscopy with scleral depression of the affected eye and the fellow eye is necessary.
- Documentation and preoperative strategy are enhanced by detailed color fundus drawings.
- Contact lens biomicroscopy (triple mirror) provides increased resolution of retinal detail and may be helpful when a retinal break is not found.
- B-scan is used when media opacity is present and also to assess the current vitreoretinal dynamics or attachments.
- Rhegmatogenous retinal detachments require expedient treatment.
- Macula-off detachment: no benefit known for emergent surgery, recommend repair within 1 day to 1 week. Anecdotal benefit of early surgery if macula is off for less than 24 hours.
- Macula-on detachment: surgery immediately or within 24 hours with appropriate positioning of patient to prevent shift of subretinal fluid and detachment of macula.
- Small subclinical detachments can occasionally be treated with barrier laser surrounding the lesion to the ora serrata.

- Scleral buckle: silicone rubber (hard) or sponge (soft) elements that are sutured to the external sclera to indent the eye and reduce the retina to RPE distance, thereby allowing resorption of subretinal fluid by the RPE. External drainage of fluid is frequently done in addition to remove significant accumulation of fluid.
- Vitrectomy: vitreous is surgically excised, usually through trans–pars plana incisions. Further microsurgical techniques are used to flatten the retina, including retinotomy, internal fluid drainage, membrane peel, endolaser, air–fluid exchange, and silicone oil.
- Pneumatic retinopexy: intravitreous gas injection through the pars plana is used to tamponade the break. Preinjection cryotherapy or postinjection laser photocoagulation is used. Postoperative positioning is important.
- Superior break: pneumatic retinopexy (if between 8- and 4-o'clock positions and less than 1 clock hour) or scleral buckle.
- Posterior break: vitrectomy or possibly pneumatic retinopexy followed by laser.
- Inferior break: scleral buckle.
- Presence of PVR.
  - Early: scleral buckle, vitrectomy to remove pigment debris.
  - Grade C1 to C2: scleral buckle; if inadequate support of breaks, then a vitrectomy is needed.
  - Grade C3 or worse: vitrectomy with or without scleral buckle.
- Previous retinal procedure: revision of scleral buckle; vitrectomy if break is posterior to buckle or PVR is present.

10.4.2 Exudative Retinal Detachment—retinal detachment without a retinal break due to subretinal fluid caused by various conditions.

Presentation decreased vision, scotoma; transparent, elevated retina with a smooth surface. Detachment may be bullous with characteristic shifting fluid of varying turbidity. Etiologic

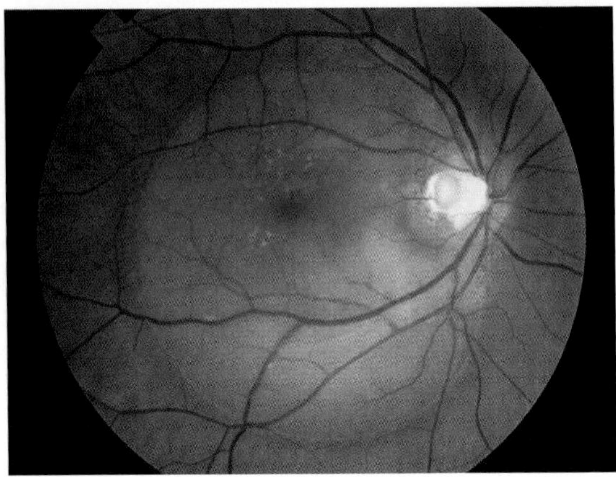

FIGURE 10.4.2 Optic pit with neurosensory detachment.

factors include tumors—primary choroidal (melanoma, hemangioma), metastatic (breast, lung); inflammation—scleritis, choroiditis (Harada's syndrome), retinitis (toxoplasmosis, ARN); vascular factors—Coats' disease, acquired peripheral angioma, retinal vein occlusion; macular diseases—central serous choroidopathy, age-related macular degeneration, or other diseases causing choroidal neovascularization (idiopathic disease, presumed ocular histoplasmosis syndrome, multifocal choroiditis); optic nerve diseases—morning glory, optic nerve pit; systemic diseases—toxemia of pregnancy, malignant hypertension, lupus choroidopathy, thrombotic thrombocytopenic purpura, bilateral diffuse uveal melanocytic proliferation; idiopathic uveal effusion; iatrogenic factor—cryotherapy.

Differential Diagnosis

rhegmatogenous or tractional retinal detachment, pseudo–retinal detachment (similar funduscopic appearance to retinal detachment), juvenile retinoschisis, senile retinoschisis, branch retinal artery occlusion (severe nerve fiber layer edema can simulate a detachment), choroidal detachment (serous or hemorrhagic, epiretinal membrane), choroidal mass (uveal melanoma, metastatic carcinoma, hemangioma) seen on B-scan or transillumination (all may have an exudative component of detachment as well as mass effect).

Management appropriate treatment of underlying cause of exudation.

- Laser photocoagulation or cryotherapy directly (i.e., Coats' disease, acquired hemangioma, choroidal neovascularization).
- Radiation (i.e., choroidal hemangioma, metastases).
- Medical treatment (i.e., steroids for lupus).
- See other specific treatments in corresponding sections.

10.4.3 Tractional Retinal Detachment

—vitreoretinal traction causing a retinal elevation, sometimes associated with a secondary retinal tear (combined detachment).

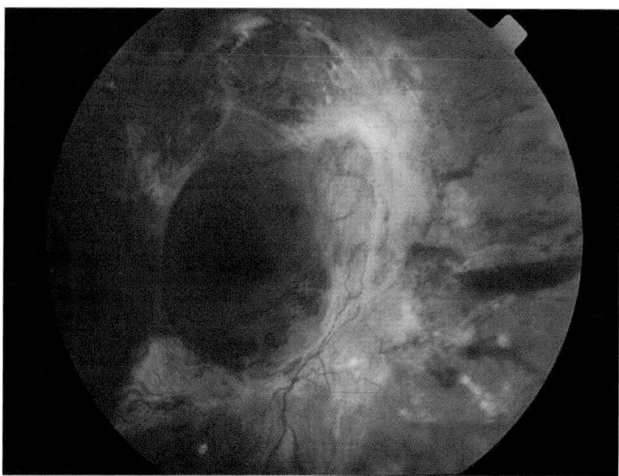

FIGURE 10.4.3 Proliferative diabetic retinopathy: extensive fibrovascular proliferation along the arcades, with a shallow superior tractional detachment of the macula.

Presentation white tractional bands on retina and in vitreous; high points of detachment correspond with traction sites. Detachments are concave and without folds. Secondary breaks may occur near sites of traction. Chronic detachments may develop a demarcation line. Etiologic factors include diabetic retinopathy, sickle cell retinopathy, toxocariasis, other diseases causing peripheral retinal neovascularization (sarcoidosis, branch retinal vein occlusion, embolic disease, Eales disease, retinopathy of prematurity, familial exudative vitreoretinopathy, chronic myelogenous leukemia, radiation retinopathy, pars planitis, carotid–cavernous fistula, ocular ischemic syndrome, and collagen–vascular disease).

Differential Diagnosis rhegmatogenous or exudative retinal detachment.

Management

- Indirect ophthalmoscopy with scleral depression of the affected eye and the fellow eye is necessary. B-scan is used to assess vitreoretinal dynamics or attachments.
- Indications for surgery include macula-off detachment or threatened macular detachment. Vitrectomy and membrane peeling of epiretinal fibrovascular membranes are the methods of treatment.

10.4.4 Proliferative Vitreoretinopathy—secondary complication of rhegmatogenous retinal detachment due to fibroglial proliferation on the retinal surface or subretinal in response to liberation of RPE cells. PVR can be present when the detachment is long-standing or can develop after surgery either from iatrogenic retinal breaks, further liberation of pigment cells and inflammation, or natural history.

Presentation grading system:

A Pigment clumping, vitreous haze

B Wrinkling of retinal surface, rolled edge of retinal break, vessel tortuosity

C-n Fixed folds in n quadrants (n = 1 to 3)

D-n Fixed folds in four quadrants

- D-1 Wide funnel detachment
- D-2 Narrow funnel detachment
- D-3 Closed funnel detachment

Management

- Primary detachment with PVR: high encircling buckle may be used for low-grade C-1. In the presence of

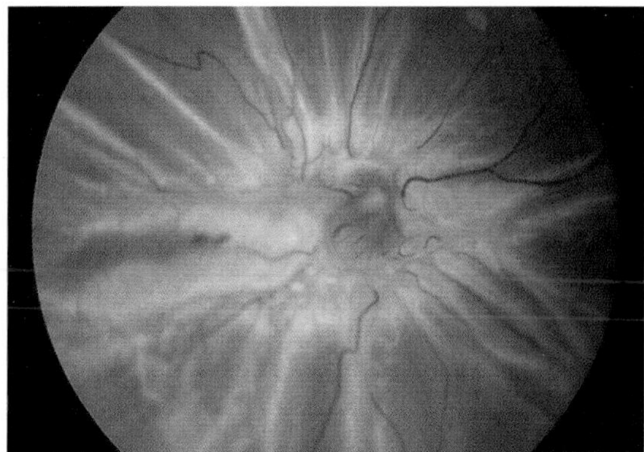

FIGURE 10.4.4 Grade-C proliferative vitreoretinopathy with fixed folds.

macular pucker or more fixed folds, consider vitrectomy.

- Redetachment secondary to PVR usually requires vitrectomy, membrane peeling, air–fluid exchange, gas tamponade, selective use of silicone oil, and occasionally retinotomy or retinectomy.
- Complications: chronic retinal detachment, hypotony, rubeosis, neovascular glaucoma, blind painful eye.

10.5 Retinoschisis

splitting at the level of the inner retina caused by degenerative (senile) form or hereditary (juvenile) form.

10.5.1 Senile Retinoschisis

10.5.1 Senile Retinoschisis—degeneration causing coalescence of cystoid spaces of peripheral cystoid degeneration forming schisis cavity in the inner retina.

Presentation

- Usually bilateral, inferotemporal location, dome-shaped schisis cavity evidenced by elevation of a very thin transparent layer of retina with retinal vessels. Sclerotic

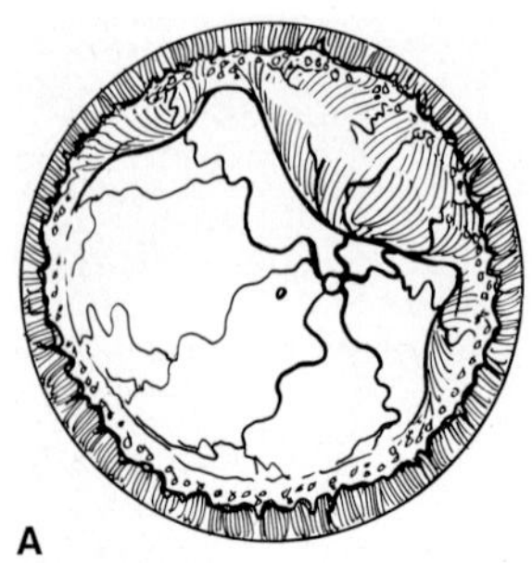

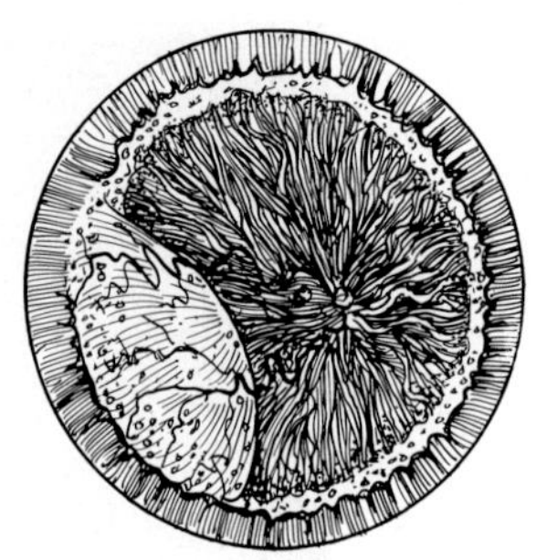

FIGURE 10.5.1a Superior retinal detachment.
FIGURE 10.5.1b Senile retinoschisis in inferotemporal quadrant.

white retinal vessels with "frosting" of inner wall of schisis cavity may be seen.

- Differentiation of retinoschisis and retinal detachment:

Retinal Detachment	Retinoschisis
Unilateral	Bilateral
Corrugated	Smooth
Undulation with movement	Stiff, no movement
Relative scotoma	Absolute scotoma
Demarcation line if chronic	No demarcation line
White spots subretinal if chronic	"Frosted" inner surface of schisis

Management

- Scleral depression to rule out outer lamellar breaks, which may lead to retinal detachment.
- Retinal detachment warnings.
- Follow-up: every 6 months to rule out retinal detachment.

10.5.2 Juvenile Retinoschisis—an X-linked recessive inherited disorder causing splitting of the retina in the nerve fiber layer.

Presentation visual loss, sometimes with family history; 100% have bilateral macular cystoid changes radiating from the fovea; vitreous hemorrhage (most common cause in children),

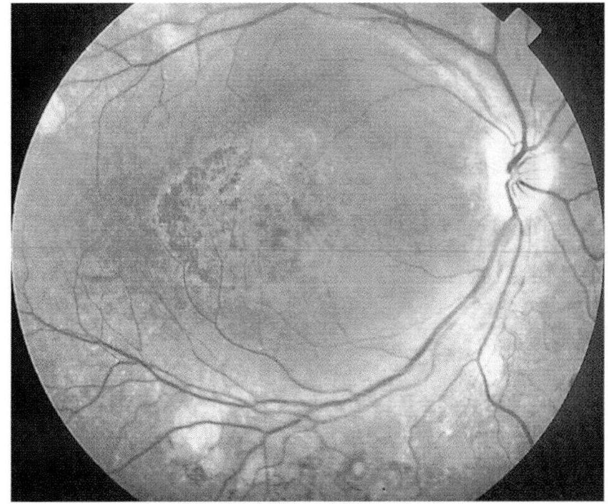

FIGURE 10.5.2 Juvenile retinoschisis with cystoid macular changes.

hemorrhage into schisis cavity, amblyopia, retinal detachment if outer and inner lamellar breaks are present.

Differential Diagnosis retinal detachment (especially exudative).

Management

- Retinal detachment requires surgical repair.
- Amblyopia requires patching of the better eye.
- Follow-up: every 4 to 6 months if no signs of retinal detachment. Amblyopia requires guidelines for occlusion therapy.

10.6 Choroidal Detachment

elevation of the retina and choroid secondary to transudate or hemorrhage into the suprachoroidal space.

10.6.1 Serous Choroidal Detachment—causes include hypotony (wound leak, overfiltration postfiltering procedure, cyclodialysis cleft, ruptured globe), scleritis or choroiditis (Harada's syndrome), idiopathic uveal effusion, tumors (primary choroidal, metastatic), and postsurgical (heavy laser photocoagulation, cryotherapy, scleral buckle).

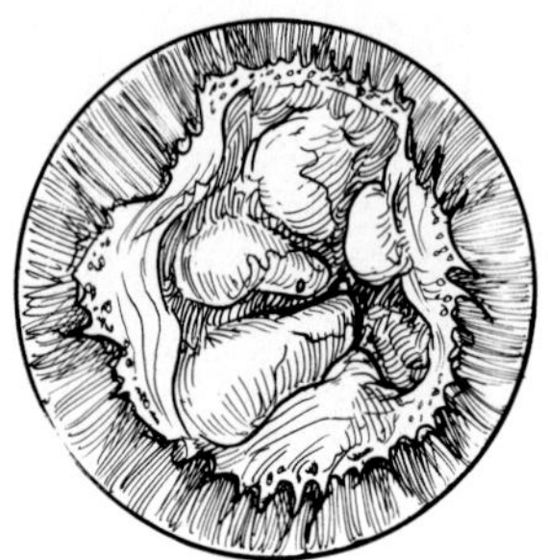

FIGURE 10.6.1 Serous choroidal detachment.

Presentation may be asymptomatic or cause decreased vision. Low IOP (<5 to 6 mm Hg), shallow anterior chamber. Quadrantic elevation of retina and choroid due to partitioning by the vortex veins distinguishes from retinal detachment.

Differential Diagnosis hemorrhagic choroidal, retinal detachment, retinoschisis, choroidal mass.

Management

- Cycloplegia (cyclopentolate 1% tid, homatropine 2% bid).
- Topical steroids (prednisolone acetate 1% q1 to 2 h).
- Consider oral steroids.
- Retina-to-retina contact ("kissing choroidals") requires surgical drainage.
- Manage or repair causative problem (see Sections 8.8.2, Wound or Bleb Leaks, and 8.8.3, Hypotony).
- Hypotony requires frequent IOP checks every 1 to 2 days.

10.6.2 Hemorrhagic or Expulsive Choroidal Detachment—bleeding into suprachoroidal space after intraocular surgery (due to rupture of posterior ciliary artery secondary to rapid globe decompression) or from choroidal neovascularization or trauma.

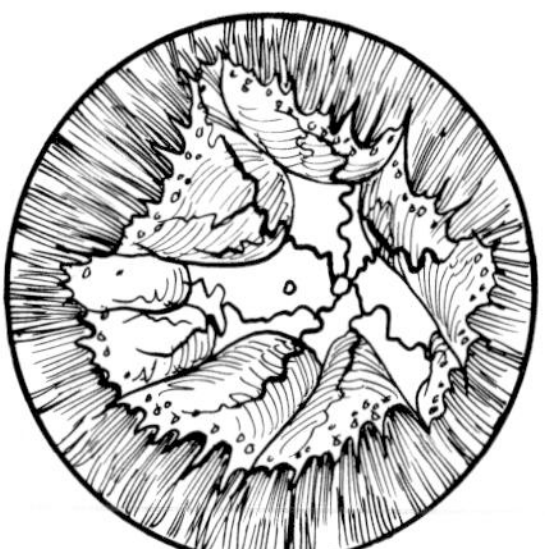

FIGURE 10.6.2 Hemorrhagic choroidal detachment.

Presentation more common in myopes, the elderly, diabetics, and hypertensives. Can present intraoperatively or immediately postoperatively with loss of red reflex, shallowing of anterior chamber, and rapid expulsion of intraocular contents from open surgical wounds. Postoperatively, patients present with pain, red eye, loss of vision, and high IOP. Can be distinguished from serous choroidal detachment by transillumination.

Differential Diagnosis serous choroidal detachment, retinal detachment, retinoschisis, choroidal mass.

Management

- Close wound as rapidly as possible. Surgical drainage is considered intraoperatively.
- For non-expulsive choroidal hemorrhage, consider surgical drainage after 7 to 10 days. Position to keep blood away from macula.
- Cycloplegia (cyclopentolate 1% tid, homatropine 2% bid).
- Topical steroids (prednisolone acetate 1% q1 to 2 h).

10.7 Diabetic Retinopathy (Proliferative)

the proliferative form of diabetic retinopathy may require surgical intervention. Angiogenic factors are released because of retinal ischemia, leading to neovascularization and fibrous proliferation. These two factors may progress to vitreous hemorrhage and tractional retinal detachment.

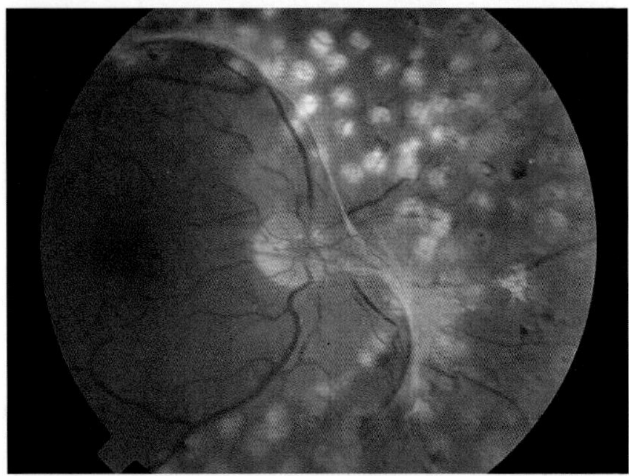

FIGURE 10.7 Proliferative diabetic retinopathy with PRP and moderate regression of neovascularization.

Presentation

decreased vision, metamorphopsia (if traction), floaters (if vitreous hemorrhage), pain (if neovascular glaucoma). Examination may reveal neovascularization of disc or retina with or without vitreous hemorrhage fibrovascular bands along arcades ("wolf jaw"), retinal elevation adjacent to tractional membranes, macular edema, ischemia, tractional retinal detachment (flashes, decreased vision if macula involved), rhegmatogenous retinal break or detachment (combined detachment), neovascularization of the iris or angle with or without neovascular glaucoma.

Management

- Aggressive panretinal photocoagulation to cause neovascular regression urgently.
- Indications for vitrectomy: vitreous hemorrhage that is nonclearing for 6 months, bilateral, in a monocular

eye, or recurrent; early vitrectomy for type I diabetics, premacular subhyaloid hemorrhage; hemolytic glaucoma in aphakic or pseudophakic eye; tractional retinal detachment, macula off (evaluate status of other eye, visual needs, potential for both visual recovery and visual loss); combined retinal detachment (tractional and rhegmatogenous); macular pucker or edema secondary to traction (same consideration as macula-off TRD).

- Follow-up: dependent on severity of disease: every 2 to 3 months if stable.

10.8 Macular Hole

a dehiscence of retinal tissue in the macula in the form of a round hole. May be related to age (idiopathic), trauma, epiretinal membrane traction, or cystoid macular edema with rupture of cyst. In idiopathic macular hole, contraction of the adherent prefoveolar vitreous cortex causes an early foveolar detachment. Continued traction leads to a retinal dehiscence and eventually a full-thickness macular hole.

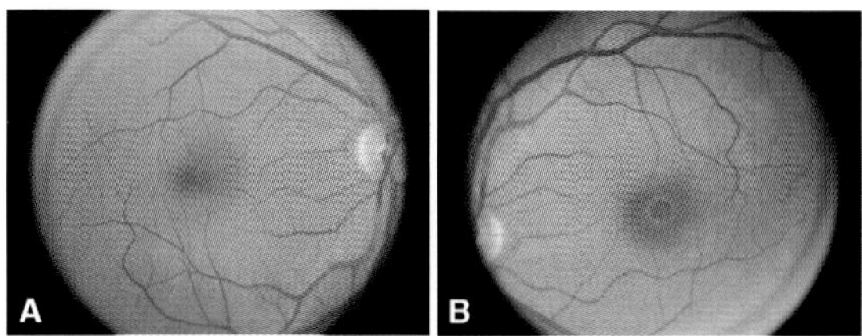

FIGURE 10.8a Stage 2 macular hole with 20/40 visual acuity.
FIGURE 10.8b Stage 3 macular hole after 2 months with visual acuity of 20/400.

Presentation

- Impending hole: metamorphopsia, normal vision.
- Full-thickness hole causes decreased vision to 20/50 to 20/800 (mean, 20/200).

- Stage 1A (impending macular hole): yellow spot (foveolar detachment), loss of foveal reflex and foveolar depression.
- Stage 1B (impending or occult hole): yellow ring, contracted prefoveolar vitreous still attached.
- Stage 2: pseudo-operculum (no retinal tissue) forms anterior to retinal plane; less than 400-μm retinal dehiscence present.
- Stage 3: full-thickness macular hole, 400 to 600 μm, surrounding gray rim of retinal detachment; positive Watzke's sign (a narrow slit beam is presented on the fovea, and the patient reports a broken line of light); yellow-white opacities in the hole at the level of RPE; epiretinal membrane on margins of the hole (10 to 20%); pseudo-operculum (75 to 85%).
- Stage 4: Same as stage 3 hole, but with posterior vitreous detachment (Weiss' ring or B-scan evidence of PVD).

Differential Diagnosis

- Of impending macular hole (yellow spot): drusen, solar maculopathy, central serous chorioretinopathy, epiretinal membrane with foveolar detachment.
- Of full-thickness hole: pseudohole (hole in epiretinal membrane—negative Watzke's sign, usually has PVD), large cyst with cystoid macular edema (negative Watzke's sign, fluorescein shows CME), geographic atrophy of RPE, central serous chorioretinopathy.

Management

vitrectomy with intraocular gas tamponade and strict facedown positioning for several weeks.

- Indications for treatment: stage 2 or worse (50% of stage 1 holes spontaneously resolve), functional visual deficit (worse than about 20/50), status of fellow eye, < 1 year of visual loss.
- Follow-up: Amsler's grid daily; examination every 4 to 6 months; 10 to 15% will develop a hole in the fellow eye (<5% if PVD is present); RD warnings for high myopes and post-traumatic macular holes.

10.9 Idiopathic Epiretinal Membrane

fibroglial membrane proliferation on premacular area causing distortion of normal retinal architecture. Caused by posterior vitreous detachment.

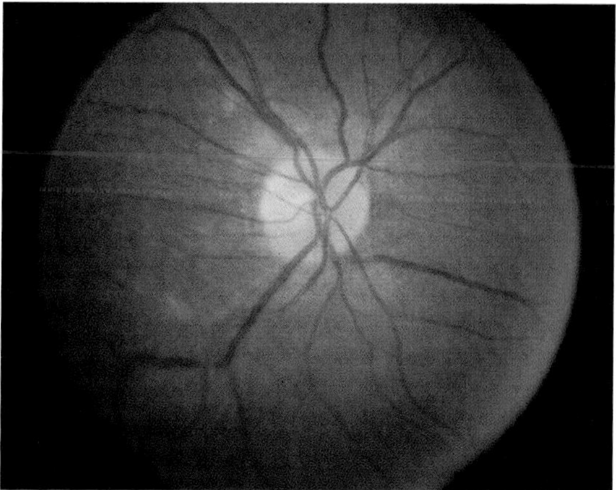

FIGURE 10.9 Epiretinal membrane extending from the disc toward the macula.

Presentation

- Early (cellophane maculopathy): glittery light reflex in macular area with normal vision and no symptoms.
- Mild: increased cellophane appearance with retinal wrinkling, distortion of retinal capillaries, vision typically better than 20/40 with mild metamorphopsia.
- Macular pucker: more significant distortion of retinal vessels and wrinkling; may have retinal edema by fluorescein; hemorrhages or cotton-wool spots; pseudohole may be present; visual loss may be 20/200 with metamorphopsia.

Differential Diagnosis

idiopathic macular hole, secondary causes of epiretinal membrane (retinal vascular disease [diabetes, vein occlusion], retinal tear or detachment, posterior uveitis).

Management no known treatment for secondary macular edema; vitrectomy and membrane peeling in select cases.

- Indications for surgery: functional visual deficit worse than 20/60, severe distortion of vision, less than 1 year of visual loss. Patients should understand that vision usually stabilizes after the acute growth of the membrane (period of weeks to a few months).
- Follow-up: Amsler's grid every 6 to 12 months (only 10% will have a decline in vision).

Chapter 11
OCULAR NEOPLASMS

Julia Hsu, René Rodriguez-Sains,
David H. Abramson

11.1 Iris Tumors and Nodules

11.1.1 Iris Nevus—a benign lesion of the iris composed of an accumulation of melanocytes that replaces a portion of the iris stroma. There is a very low chance of malignant transformation.

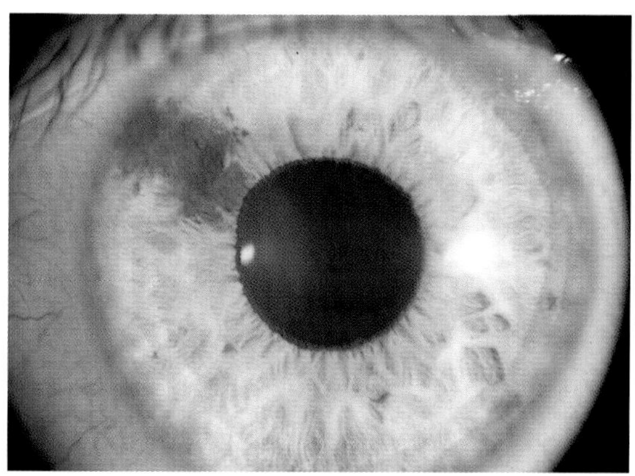

FIGURE 11.1.1 Iris nevus.

Presentation an incidental finding in light-skinned individuals with lightly pigmented irides. Patients with the atypical mole syndrome or dysplastic nevus syndrome have a higher incidence. The majority are located in the inferior quadrants of the iris. Lesions may be circumscribed or diffuse, pigmented or amelanotic. Light or amelanotic lesions may have a "tapioca appearance." There may be associated ectropion iridis, sector cortical cataract (in quadrant of the lesion), or an irregular pupil.

Differential Diagnosis iris freckle, iris melanoma, Lisch nodules, ocular melanocytosis (for diffuse nevus).

Management lesions should be photographed and followed to monitor for growth. If growth is documented, consider malignant transformation and sector iridectomy.

11.1.2 Iris Freckle

11.1.2 Iris Freckle—a flat area of pigmentation on the anterior surface of the iris that is composed of melanocytes with increased pigmentation. There is no malignant potential.

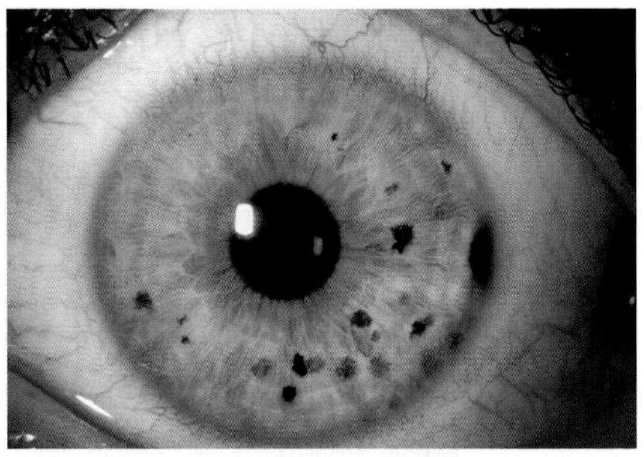

FIGURE 11.1.2 Iris freckle.

Presentation usually an incidental finding. There is a higher incidence in the atypical mole syndrome. In contrast to the iris nevus, the iris freckle does not affect the underlying iris architecture.

Differential Diagnosis iris nevus, iris melanoma, Lisch nodules.

Management clinical documentation. No treatment is necessary.

11.1.3 Iris Pigment Epithelial Cyst—a localized, smooth brown elevation of the iris stroma, secondary to a separation of the two epithelial layers. Cysts may be congenital or acquired (due to traumatic perforation, surgery).

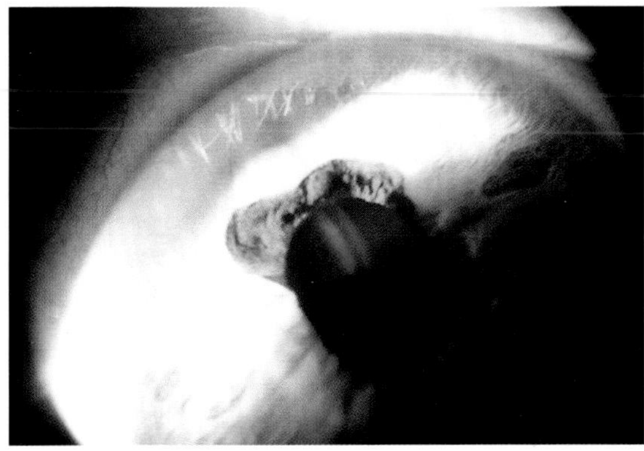

FIGURE 11.1.3 Iris pigment epithelial cyst.

Presentation usually an incidental finding. May be found anywhere between the pupillary margin and the ciliary body. Some lesions may break free and may be seen in the anterior or posterior chamber or in the vitreous. Lesions may transilluminate and may be better seen after dilation.

Differential Diagnosis iris and ciliary body melanomas.

Management ultrasound biomicroscopy may be useful in diagnosis. No treatment is necessary. If cysts enlarge and impinge on the visual axis, consider surgical excision.

11.1.4 Iris Melanoma—a malignant pigmented tumor of the iris stroma.

Presentation higher incidence in light-skinned individuals with blue irides. Patients may be asymptomatic. Lesions may be circumscribed or diffuse, nodular or flat, with variable pig-

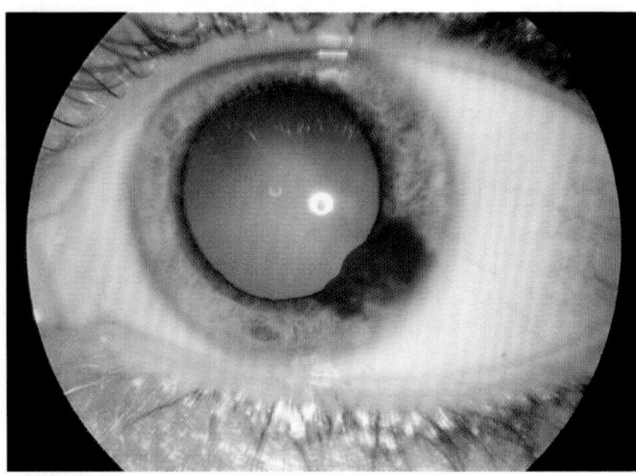

FIGURE 11.1.4 Iris melanoma.

mentation ranging from amelanotic to dark brown. A majority (80%) are located in inferior quadrants. A small circumscribed lesion may be difficult to differentiate from iris nevus. Other findings may include ectropion iridis, sector cataract, secondary glaucoma, and prominent vascularity. Large tumors may cause secondary visual loss, spontaneous hyphema, corneal edema, and band keratopathy (due to corneal compression). Patients with diffuse melanomas typically present with acquired hyperchromic heterochromia and secondary glaucoma.

Differential Diagnosis

- Circumscribed: iris nevus, primary iris cyst, iris atrophy, iris foreign body, metastatic carcinoma to iris, adenoma of pigment epithelium, iris hemangioma, pigment epithelial hyperplasia.
- Diffuse: iris nevus syndrome, siderosis, pigmentary glaucoma, congenital heterochromia.

Management

- Circumscribed: Periodic observation with photodocumentation every 6 months because only a small percentage (5%) of suspicious lesions demonstrate growth over the first 5 years. Potential for metastasis is very low if lesion is limited to the iris. In the past, excision was performed for growth. Many experts now recommend treatment for secondary glaucoma only.

- Diffuse: because overall biological behavior of these tumors is benign and slow growing, observe and treat any secondary glaucoma. In cases of severe glaucoma that have failed medical treatment, consider enucleation. Filtering surgery may promote metastasis.

11.1.5 Juvenile Xanthogranuloma—a benign inflammatory condition of childhood in which characteristic cutaneous papules appear but resolve spontaneously. Iris infiltration is the most common ocular manifestation. May also rarely involve orbit, eyelids, cornea, episclera, ciliary body, choroid, and optic disc.

Presentation orange cutaneous papules associated with yellow to gray, ill-defined nodular iris lesions. Diffuse infiltration may result in heterochromia. Spontaneous hyphema may occur as a result of vascularity of lesions. Secondary glaucoma may develop because of tumor infiltration of the angle.

Differential Diagnosis retinoblastoma, sarcoid, leukemia, foreign body, medulloepithelioma.

Management treatment options include local corticosteroids, irradiation, combined steroids and irradiation, or local excision.

11.1.6 Leiomyoma (Uveal)—a rare, benign smooth muscle tumor. May occur in the choroid, ciliary body, or iris.

Presentation typically a localized, flat to mildly elevated, light to nonpigmented, vascular lesion in the area of the iris sphincter muscle. May also occur peripherally and in the anterior chamber angle. Commonly associated with ectropion iridis in the same sector.

Differential Diagnosis iris lesions: amelanotic iris melanoma, metastatic carcinoma.

Management iris lesions may be diagnosed clinically and followed by periodic examination without treatment. Although fine-needle aspiration biopsy with electron microscopy and immunohistochemistry may help to distinguish the lesion from amelanotic melanoma, neither lesion requires treatment. There is no known metastatic potential.

11.1.7 Leukemic Iris Nodules

—the most common site of ocular manifestation of leukemia is the uveal tract. May also affect the vitreous, retina, optic disc, and orbit (see Sections 6.10.2 and 15.9).

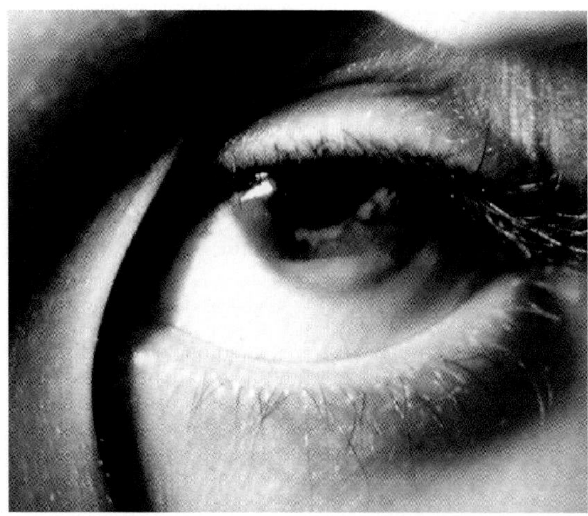

FIGURE 11.1.7 Iris involvement in leukemia with hypopyon.

Presentation iris involvement may be unilateral or bilateral and often appears as diffuse or nodular white lesions, with or without marked vascularity, with tumor cells in the anterior chamber. A pseudohypopyon is often present, secondary to collection of tumor cells in the anterior chamber. Secondary glaucoma may occur as a result of infiltration of the angle and obstruction to outflow. The iris stroma may become distorted or discolored secondary to diffuse thickening. Heterochromia may result.

Differential Diagnosis retinoblastoma, uveitis, trauma.

Management systemic workup if no prior diagnosis is made. Treatment consists of systemic chemotherapy with localized radiation therapy. Topical steroids cause quick but temporary resolution. This may occur with primary diagnosis, but if there is a recurrence in a previously treated patient, CNS involvement is common, and treatment should include the CNS.

11.1.8 Melanocytosis—there are two subcategories of congenital ocular melanocytosis: ocular melanocytosis and oculodermal melanocytosis. Both are associated with hyperpigmentation of the uveal tract and episclera, with a predisposition to ipsilateral melanoma of the uvea, meninges, orbit, and CNS. The oculodermal variant differs only in that it is associated with hyperpigmentation of the periorbital skin (nevus of Ota).

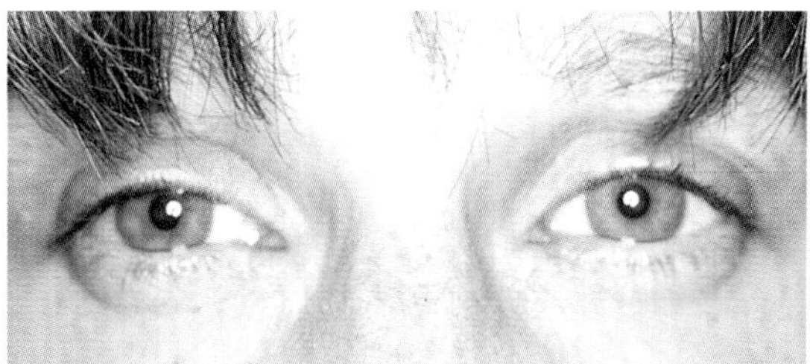

FIGURE 11.1.8 Iris melanocytosis.

Presentation usually unilateral lesions of blue to gray-brown patches of pigmentation of the episclera and sclera. Uveal tract pigmentation may be diffuse or sectoral. Heterochromia may be present secondary to diffuse iris involvement. In oculodermal melanocytosis, brow and lid pigmentation is also present.

Differential Diagnosis Sturge-Weber syndrome, racial pigmentation.

Management because hyperpigmented areas have a predisposition to develop malignant melanoma, regular close follow-up every 6 to 12 months is required. Any suspicious lesions should be worked up accordingly for malignant melanoma. Although oculodermal melanocytosis is more common in blacks and Asians, Caucasians are more likely to develop melanoma, both of the skin and of the eye.

11.1.9 Brushfield's Spots (Down's Syndrome)—elevated white to light yellow spots consisting of areas of iris stromal hyperplasia surrounded by a ring of relative hypoplasia.

Presentation lesions are found in the periphery of the iris and occur in groups of 10 to 20. They are usually found incidentally. Lesions occur in up to 90% of patients with Down syndrome and are more common in light irides. Similar lesions may be found in up to 24% of the normal population and are called Wolfflin nodules. Other associated findings in Down syndrome include epicanthal folds, ectropion, hypertelorism, and mongoloid slant. Keratoconus is present in 5 to 10% of cases (see Section 15.2, Down Syndrome).

Differential Diagnosis sarcoid nodules, iris nevus or freckle.

Management no treatment is necessary.

11.1.10 Lisch Nodules (Neurofibromatosis)—iris hamartomas consisting of collections of glial cells and melanocytes. These are the most common ocular manifestation of neurofibromatosis (see Section 15.19.1, Neurofibromatosis).

Presentation typically appears as multiple flat or slightly elevated, circular pigmented lesions over the iris. Lesions are almost always bilateral and are uncommon in patients under age 5 years.

Differential Diagnosis iris nevus.

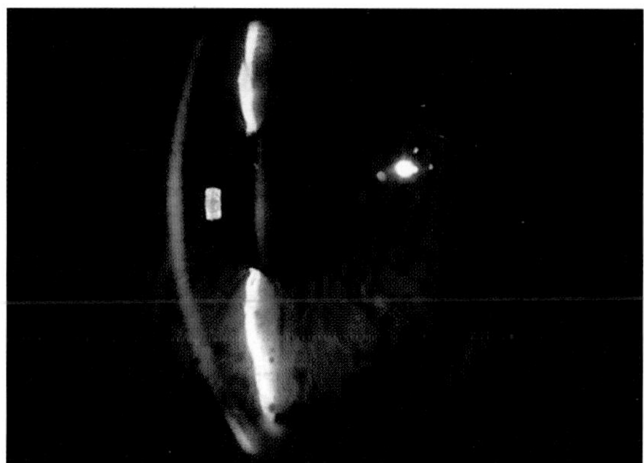

FIGURE 11.1.10 Lisch nodules.

Management clinical documentation and follow-up.

11.2 Ciliary Body Tumors

11.2.1 Ciliary Body Melanoma

11.2.1 Ciliary Body Melanoma—a melanocytic tumor of the ciliary body. Because of their location, small lesions usually are not detected.

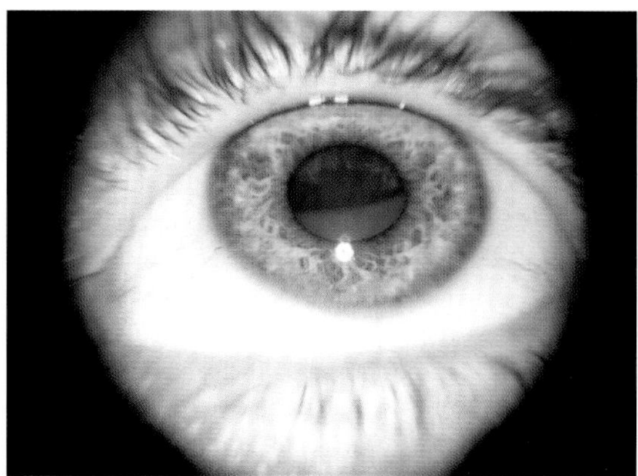

FIGURE 11.2.1 Ciliary body melanoma.

Presentation lesions may be nodular or diffuse and are located near the equator of the lens. Erosion may occur into the anterior chamber or through the sclera, which results in a pigmented epibulbar mass. Dilated episcleral vessels may be present over the quadrant of the tumor ("sentinel vessels"). In rare instances, lesions may extend 180° to 360° around the ciliary body and are referred to as "ring melanomas." Small lesions are typically asymptomatic. Patients with larger lesions may present with painless blurred vision secondary to astigmatism or lens subluxation. The intraocular pressure may be lower in the affected eye because of decreased aqueous production. However, patients may present with angle-closure glaucoma secondary to anterior displacement of the iris. Other findings may include cataract, hyphema, vitreous hemorrhage, and retinal detachment.

Differential Diagnosis ciliary body cysts, medulloepithelioma, leiomyoma.

Management treatment options include local excision (cyclectomy), brachytherapy, proton-beam irradiation, enucleation.

11.2.2 Medulloepithelioma (of the Ciliary Epithelium)

a congenital tumor of the nonpigmented ciliary epithelium that arises from the primitive medullary epithelium. May be benign or malignant. Also known as a diktyoma, amnonteratoid medulloepithelioma, or teratoneuroma.

Presentation patients typically present in childhood, with the majority between 2 and 4 years of age. Lesions may occasionally occur in adults. Typical appearance is that of a lightly pigmented ciliary body mass. Lesions may be visible at the iris root if the tumor erodes into the anterior chamber. Rare lesions may also develop in the optic nerve, with secondary disc swelling and proptosis. Common presenting signs and symptoms include pain, decreased visual acuity, and leukocoria. Other findings include lens subluxation, cataract formation, rubeosis iridis, and secondary glaucoma.

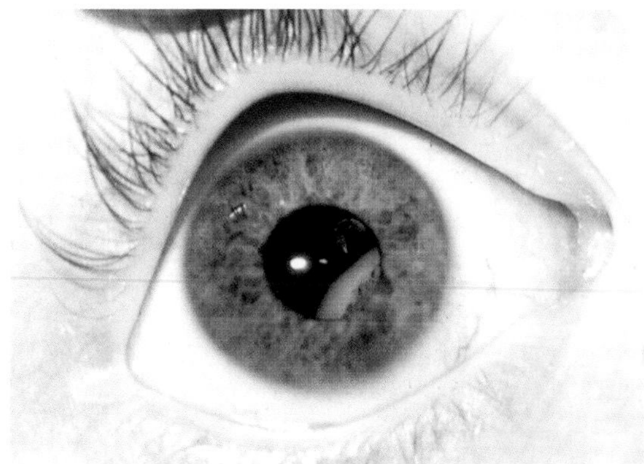

FIGURE 11.2.2 Medulloepithelioma.

Differential Diagnosis persistent hyperplastic primary vitreous, pars planitis, nematode endophthalmitis, congenital glaucoma, retinoblastoma, primary tumors of the pigmented ciliary epithelium, malignant melanoma.

Management clinical appearance is the most useful feature for diagnosis. There is no established role for other ancillary tests. Consider excisional biopsy for certain lesions localized to the iris. Treatment options include observation, local resection, or enucleation, depending on the size and location of the tumor. Most involved eyes are enucleated because of pain or blindness or because retinoblastoma cannot be definitely ruled out. Distant metastasis is rare, even in cases of frank malignancy.

11.3 Choroidal Tumors

11.3.1 Choroidal Nevus

11.3.1 Choroidal Nevus—a pigmented choroidal tumor of benign melanocytes, usually (90%) located posterior to the equator.

Presentation generally an incidental finding on routine examination. Typical appearance is that of a flat to mildly elevated

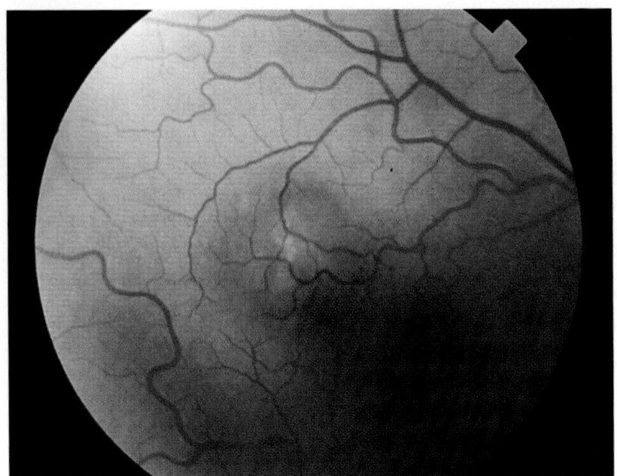

FIGURE 11.3.1 Choroidal nevus.

(<1.5 mm in height), gray to brown lesion. There may be associated overlying cystic degeneration of the retina, drusen, neovascular membranes, orange pigment, serous fluid, and visual field defects. Lesions close to the fovea may produce visual loss and/or field defects. Choroidal nevi are distinguished from malignant melanomas by basal size and thickness. Lesions thicker than 2.5 mm are almost always melanomas, whereas lesions thinner than 1 mm are virtually always nevi. Flat lesions of greater than 10 mm in basal size are at increased risk for malignancy. There is a higher incidence in patients with atypical mole syndrome.

Differential Diagnosis

- Choroidal melanoma, congenital hypertrophy of the retinal pigment epithelium, combined hamartoma, hyperplasia of the retinal pigment epithelium, subretinal hemorrhage.
- For amelanotic lesions: choroidal hemangioma, metastatic tumor, choroidal osteoma.

Management

for non-suspicious-appearing lesions, regular yearly examination and photodocumentation are sufficient. For lesions that are suspicious for malignancy, obtain baseline photos and ultrasound for accurate measurements of tumor size. Follow by close observation and photos approximately every 6 months to monitor for evidence of growth. If growth is documented, consider malignant transformation.

11.3.2 Choroidal Melanoma

11.3.2 Choroidal Melanoma—a malignant melanocytic tumor, usually affecting light-skinned individuals in the sixth to seventh decades of life. It is the most common primary intraocular cancer in adults.

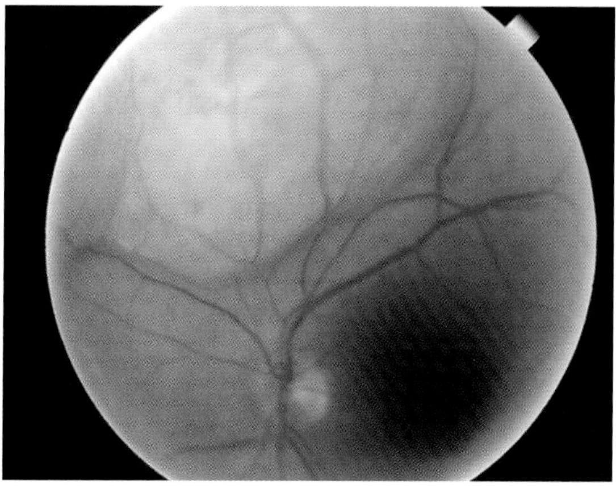

FIGURE 11.3.2 Choroidal malignant melanoma.

Presentation lesions typically appear as a nodular, well-defined, pigmented subretinal mass that may have varying degrees of overlying orange pigment and serous fluid. There may be variable pigmentation, with some lesions being amelanotic. Tumors may break through Bruch's membrane and take on a mushroom shape in cross section. Certain tumors may assume a diffuse rather than nodular growth pattern and cause choroidal thickening without obvious elevation. Patients may be asymptomatic or may present with blurred vision, visual field loss, floaters, photopsia, and, very rarely, pain. Other findings may include serous retinal detachment, angle-closure glaucoma, rubeosis iridis, vitreous and subretinal hemorrhages, and lens subluxation.

Differential Diagnosis choroidal nevus, circumscribed choroidal hemangioma, retinal pigment epithelium abnormalities (reactive hyperplasia, congenital hypertrophy, adenoma, combined hamartoma, adenocarcinoma), disciform scar, metastatic carcinoma, melanocytoma of the optic nerve, choroidal osteoma, retinal cavernous hemangioma, posterior scleritis, choroidal detachment, uveal effusion syndrome, hemorrhagic detachment of retina.

Management ultrasonography is useful in establishing the diagnosis and defining the extent of the lesion. Treatment options include radiation therapy (brachytherapy), proton-beam irradiation, and enucleation. Rarely, local excision is possible. A systemic workup for metastasis should include physical examination, liver function tests, chest radiograph, and abdominal CT scan in selected cases.

11.3.3 Choroidal Metastasis—the most common intraocular cancer in adults, with the posterior choroid being the most common site of involvement.

Presentation patients may be asymptomatic or complain of painless blurred vision or loss of vision. Tumors are usually bilat-

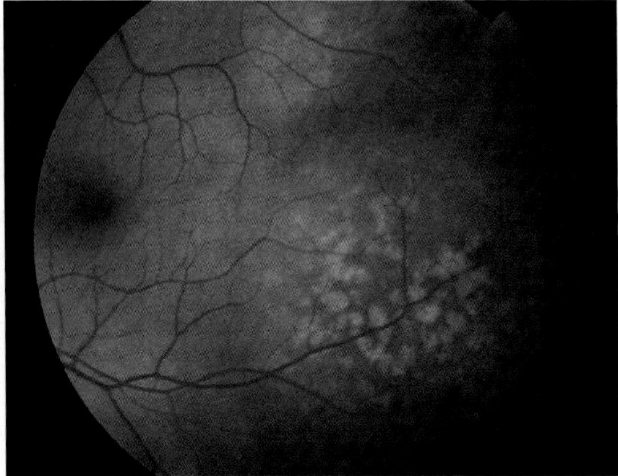

FIGURE 11.3.3 Choroidal metastatic lesion.

eral and multiple. Typical appearance is that of a yellowish, flat, ill-defined lesion with varying degrees of brown pigmentation on the surface, obscuring most choroidal markings. There may be associated serous retinal detachment.

Differential Diagnosis amelanotic nevus, amelanotic melanoma, choroidal osteoma, posterior scleritis, retinitis, choroiditis, choroidal hemangioma, rhegmatogenous retinal detachment, uveal effusion syndrome, central serous chorioretinopathy, Harada's disease.

Management because the overall patient prognosis is poor, treatment is targeted toward alleviation of pain, diplopia, and visual loss. Treatment approach depends on the type of primary tumor, and modalities include chemotherapy, hormonal therapy, radiation, and occasionally enucleation.

11.3.4 Cavernous Hemangioma of the Choroid—a benign and most common vascular tumor of the uveal tract. Lesions are divided into localized and diffuse forms.

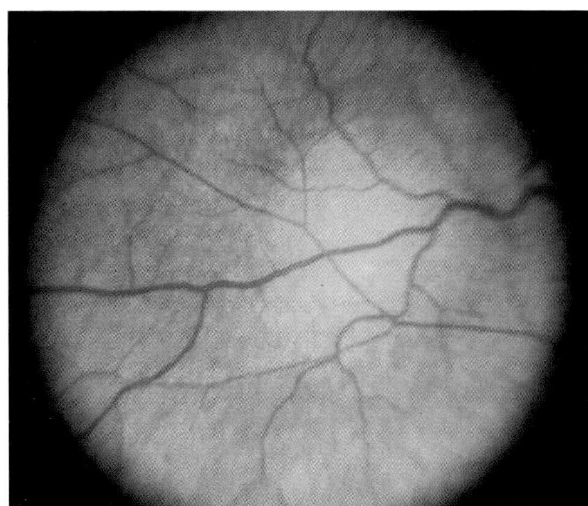

FIGURE 11.3.4 Choroidal hemangioma.

Presentation

- Localized: lesions are unilateral and unifocal, with no associated systemic disorders. Typical appearance is that of an orange-red lesion in the posterior pole, with frequent involvement of the macular area. There may be overlying yellow-white areas, as well as clumps of black pigment in the RPE. Subfoveal lesions tend to cause ipsilateral hyperopia (due to anterior displacement of retina). Patients present with visual loss at an early age and may develop secondary amblyopia. Patients with parafoveal lesions usually remain asymptomatic until age 20 to 40 years, when a serous retinal detachment develops, and they present with blurred vision and metamorphopsia.
- Diffuse: lesions are typically seen as a part of the Sturge-Weber syndrome and are ipsilateral to the facial hemangioma. Tumors have ill-defined borders, tend to be thickest over the macular area, and extend over a large area of the posterior choroid. The diffuse orange-red thickening of the posterior pole ("tomato catsup fundus") produces a bright red reflex. The majority of patients present at an early age (50% by age 8 years) with visual loss due to secondary hyperopia, amblyopia, or retinal detachment. Other complications include cataract and glaucoma.

Differential Diagnosis

for localized lesions: amelanotic choroidal melanoma, metastatic carcinoma, choroidal osteoma, central serous chorioretinopathy, granuloma, age-related macular degeneration, retinoblastoma, posterior scleritis.

Management

- Asymptomatic circumscribed lesions are typically stationary and do not require treatment.
- For secondary serous detachment, light argon-laser photocoagulation is used to create chorioretinal adhesions. Brachytherapy has been shown to be effective in shrinking tumors.
- Diffuse lesions are difficult to manage. Large tumors often produce hyperopic refractive error. The approach

consists of corrective lenses and prevention of amblyopia. Retinal detachment may require photocoagulation, posterior sclerotomy, and scleral buckle.

11.3.5 Choroidal Osteoma—an idiopathic, benign bony tumor of the choroid.

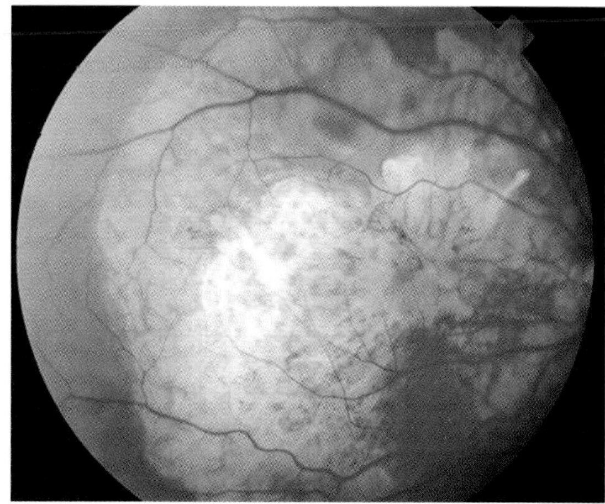

FIGURE 11.3.5 Choroidal osteoma.

Presentation the majority (70 to 80%) of lesions are unilateral. Lesions are typically yellow to orange, minimally elevated, with well-defined margins, which may have a scalloped appearance. Variable amounts of pigmentation may be seen on the surface of the tumors, and there may be associated serous subretinal fluid. Lesions may occur around or next to the disc, as well as in the macular area. Subretinal neovascularization is a common complication. Lesions are typically found in young females between 10 and 30 years of age. Patients may be asymptomatic or present with mild to severe visual impairment if there is macular involvement. Other findings on examination may include scotoma and metamorphopsia.

Differential Diagnosis amelanotic choroidal nevus, amelanotic choroidal melanoma, circumscribed choroidal hemangioma, metastatic carcinoma, organized subretinal hemorrhage, leiomyoma, age-related macular degeneration, posterior scleritis, neurilemmoma.

Management ultrasound and CT scan demonstrate characteristic calcification that aids in diagnosis. Fluorescein angiography may delineate overlying subretinal neovascular membranes. Lesions may show slow enlargement over long periods of time. Cases may be followed with simple observation alone but should be monitored closely for the development of any subretinal neovascular membranes. If present, these are treated with laser photocoagulation.

11.4 Retinal Pigment Epithelium Tumors

11.4.1 Congenital Hypertrophy of the Retinal Pigment Epithelium

11.4.1 Congenital Hypertrophy of the Retinal Pigment Epithelium—a flat, well-demarcated, darkly pigmented lesion consisting of hypertrophic retinal pigment epithelium that contains large pigment granules.

Presentation usually an incidental finding on routine examination. Lesions are typically unilateral, and a majority (70%) are located in temporal quadrants. Lesions may be either solitary or multifocal ("bear tracks"), consisting of a group of up to 30 lesions in a sectoral distribution. Some solitary lesions may contain lacunae or irregular borders secondary to foci of depigmentation, whereas others may also have surrounding halos. Lesions typically stop abruptly at the ora serrata and the optic disc (as opposed to melanocytomas). Multiple and bilateral lesions appear to be associated with Gardner's syndrome and familial adenomatous polyposis. On visual field testing, an absolute scotoma may be present because of degeneration of overlying retinal pigment epithelium.

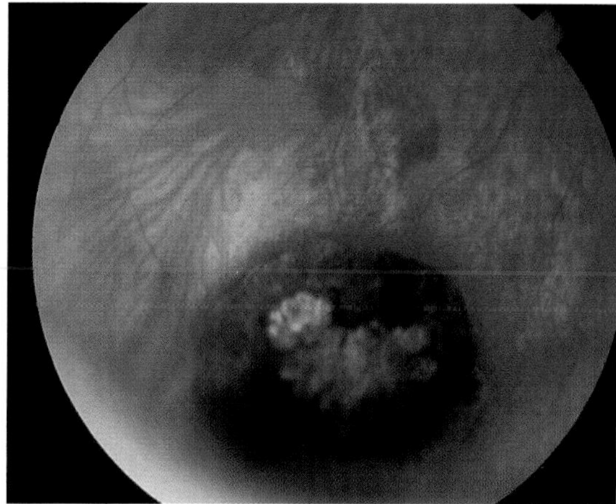

FIGURE 11.4.1 Congenital hypertrophy of the retinal pigment epithelium.

Differential Diagnosis

- Solitary: malignant melanoma, choroidal nevus, chorioretinal scar.
- Multifocal: malignant melanoma, choroidal nevi, reactive hyperplasia of retinal pigment epithelium, sector pigmentary dystrophy of the retina.

Management fluorescein angiogram demonstrates a stationary pattern throughout. Clinical documentation and periodic observation are sufficient. The majority of lesions are stationary, but in some instances there may be very slow and minimal enlargement. There is no tendency for malignant transformation. If Gardner's syndrome or familial adenomatous polyposis is suspected, regular screening and follow-up by an internist or gastroenterologist are indicated.

11.4.2 Combined Hamartoma of the Retinal Pigment Epithelium and the Retina—a tumor consisting of retinal pigment epithelial cells, retinal blood vessels, and glial cells.

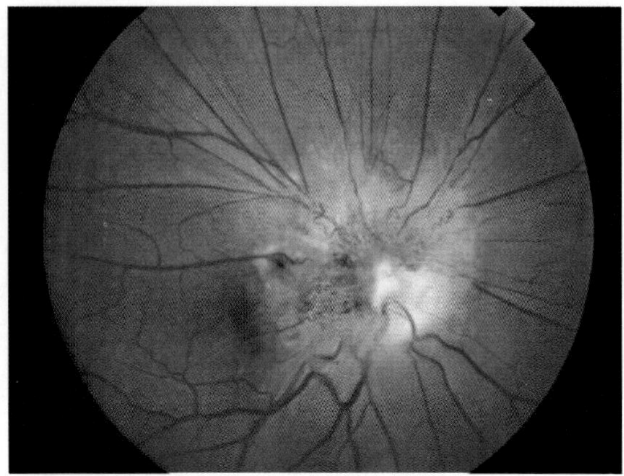

FIGURE 11.4.2 Combined hamartoma of the retina and the retinal pigment epithelium.

Presentation patients, 20 to 45 years of age, typically present with painless blurred vision; 20% may have normal visual acuity. The typical appearance is that of a unilateral, darkly pigmented, and slightly elevated lesion occurring adjacent to or over the optic disc, although in some cases it may be located in the periphery. Contraction of glial cells in the lesion produces traction on the surrounding retina and vessels toward the lesion, as well as accumulation of subretinal exudates.

Differential Diagnosis malignant melanoma, choroidal nevus, reactive retinal pigment epithelial hyperplasia, melanocytoma of the optic nerve, unifocal hypertrophy of the retinal pigment epithelium, adenomas of the retinal pigment epithelium. In children, consider retinoblastoma.

Management fluorescein angiography demonstrates the typical appearance. Although most lesions are stationary, in some cases there may be minimal enlargement. If there is marked retinal traction and secondary visual loss, vitrectomy and membrane peel may be attempted. There is no well-established treatment.

11.5 Retinal Tumors

11.5.1 Retinoblastoma—see Section 12.2.2.

11.5.2 Capillary Hemangioma—a vascular tumor that consists of a proliferation of retinal capillaries.

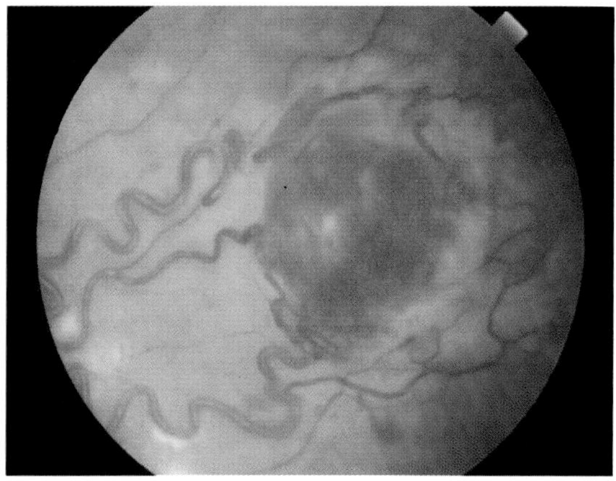

FIGURE 11.5.2 Capillary hemangioma.

Presentation typical appearance is that of an orange-red tumor supplied and drained by dilated, tortuous afferent and efferent vessels that extend back to the optic disc. Some lesions demonstrate exudation and vitreous contraction bands. Other lesions may arise from the disc. Lesions may be found incidentally, or patients may present with painless blurred vision. The usual presentation is in the second or third decade of life. Multiple and/or bilateral lesions are suggestive of von Hippel-Lindau syndrome. Retinal detachment commonly results from accumulation of subretinal fluid and exudate, as well as from traction.

Differential Diagnosis

- Peripheral: Coat's disease, racemose hemangioma, retinal cavernous hemangioma, nematode endophthalmitis, retinoblastoma, retinal astrocytoma, familial exudative vitreoretinopathy, peripheral hemorrhagic exudative chorioretinopathy, intraretinal macroaneurysm, sickle cell retinopathy.
- Of the optic disc: diffuse type resembles papilledema, papillitis.

Management fluorescein angiography demonstrates characteristic pattern. Small lesions that are asymptomatic may be followed by periodic examination every 3 to 4 months. Treatment is indicated for larger tumors and in cases where there is retinal detachment or accumulation of subretinal fluid or exudate. Treatment modalities include laser photocoagulation, cryotherapy, scleral buckling, and vitrectomy. Multiple lesions, a positive family history, or positive findings on review of symptoms indicate that a workup is necessary for von Hippel-Lindau syndrome (see Section 15.19.4).

11.5.3 Retinal Cavernous Hemangioma—a vascular malformation consisting of dilated, endothelial lined venous aneurysms which are connected by small orifices.

Presentation the typical appearance is that of a dark "cluster of grapes," without associated exudation or feeder vessel. Lesions may occur either in the retina or over the optic disc and may be associated with overlying fibroglial tissue as well as areas of hemorrhages. In some cases, there may be associated dermatologic and CNS vascular malformations. Patients are usually asymptomatic. Some cases may be complicated by vitreous hemorrhage or retinal traction from severe fibrogliosis.

Differential Diagnosis peripheral: Coat's disease, retinal astrocytoma, sickle cell retinopathy.

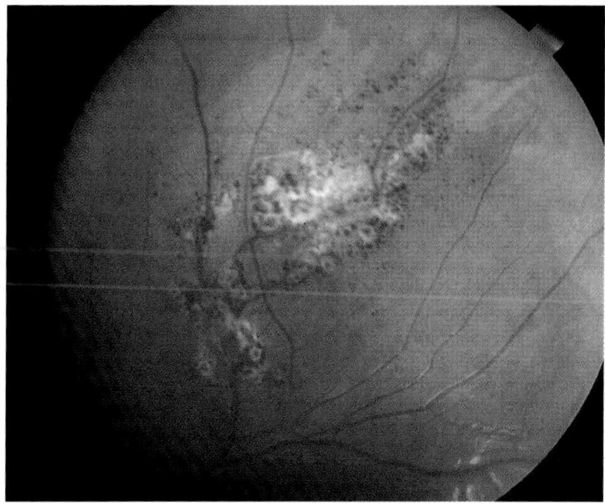

FIGURE 11.5.3 Retinal cavernous hemangioma.

Management fluorescein angiography reveals a typical diagnostic pattern. Periodic examination is sufficient because the majority are asymptomatic and stationary. A small number may demonstrate minimal enlargement. In cases of vitreous hemorrhage, consider treatment with either laser photocoagulation or cryotherapy.

11.5.4 Arteriovenous Malformation

—also known as racemose hemangioma. An aberrant anastomosis between a retinal artery and vein. If lesions are associated with a midbrain arteriovenous malformation, the condition is known as Wyburn-Mason syndrome. Other arteriovenous malformations may be present in the skin, orbit, mandible, and CNS.

Presentation lesions may range from a small, abnormal plexus to an extensive net of tortuous vessels. Symptoms vary with degree of optic nerve and retinal involvement. Patients may be asymptomatic or present with varying degrees of visual loss. Those with larger and more extensive lesions tend to have a higher incidence of other CNS vascular malformations.

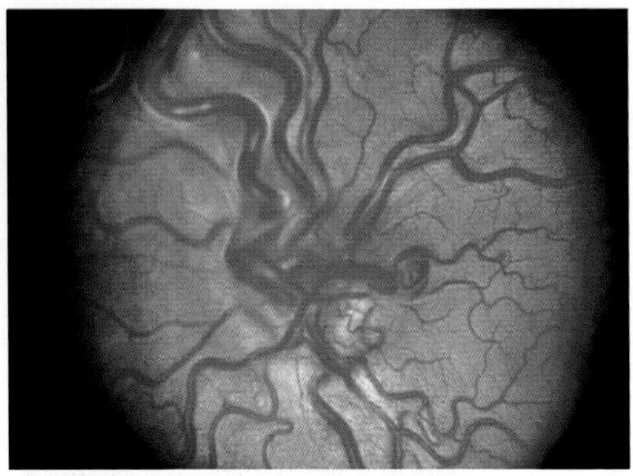

FIGURE 11.5.4 Arteriovenous malformation.

Differential Diagnosis congenital tortuosity of the retinal vessels, retinal capillary hemangioma.

Management fluorescein angiography is useful in diagnosis (distinguish from capillary hemangioma). Most lesions are stationary; therefore, no treatment is necessary. There is no consensus on the approach of destroying the lesion with cryotherapy or laser to prevent vitreous hemorrhage. MRI of the brain to rule out CNS arteriovenous malformation is indicated.

11.5.5 Astrocytoma

11.5.5 Astrocytoma—also known as astrocytic hamartoma. A benign tumor arising in the retina or optic disc. Lesions are rarely an isolated finding; they may be a manifestation of tuberous sclerosis (Section 15.19.2) or neurofibromatosis (Section 15.19.1).

Presentation tumors may be unilateral or bilateral, single or multiple. Retinal tumors range from small, smooth, translucent gray lesions in the nerve fiber layer to large, yellow, and calcified lesions that take on a "mulberry" appearance. Optic disc tumors are commonly referred to as giant drusen. Patients are usually asymptomatic. However, lesions in the posterior pole may produce painless blurred vision.

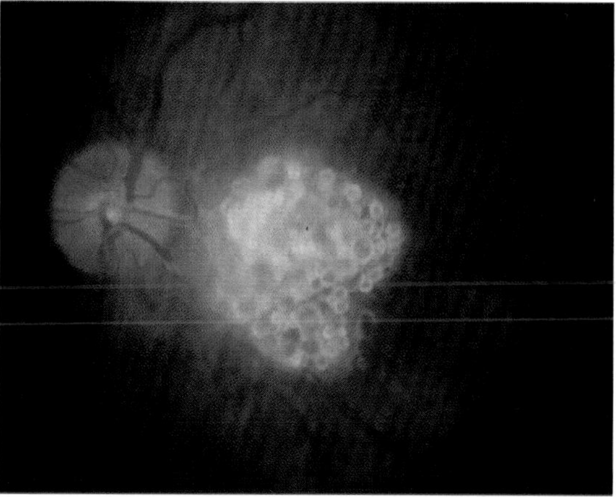

FIGURE 11.5.5 Astrocytoma.

Larger, calcified lesions may produce subretinal or vitreous hemorrhage.

Differential Diagnosis retinoblastoma, retinal capillary hemangioma, myelinated nerve fibers, optic disc drusen, massive gliosis of the retina, retinal granuloma.

Management fluorescein angiography and ultrasound are useful in diagnosis. Most lesions are asymptomatic and stationary; therefore, documentation and periodic follow-up are sufficient. There is no malignant or metastatic potential. Secondary retinal detachment and subretinal fluid collection may be treated with laser photocoagulation. Consider workup for tuberous sclerosis or neurofibromatosis.

11.6 Melanocytoma

a nevus variant that is located eccentrically over the optic disc.

Presentation usually an incidental finding. Lesions are typically unilateral, deeply pigmented (dark brown to jet black), and may

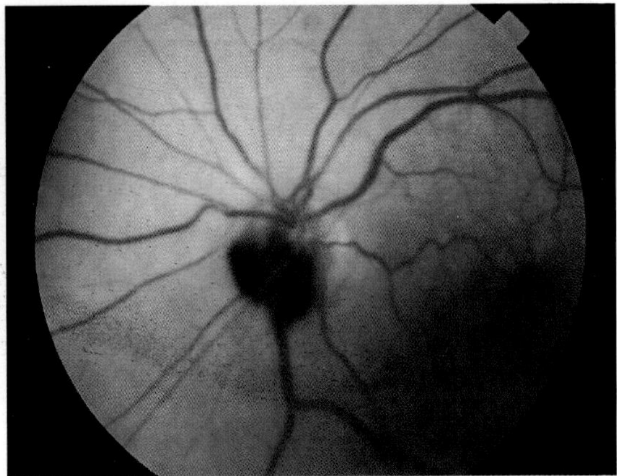

FIGURE 11.6 Melanocytoma.

be either flat or mildly elevated. Lesions commonly have fibrillated margins secondary to extension into the surrounding nerve fiber layer. Visual acuity is normal, although large lesions may cause blurred vision. There may be an associated afferent pupillary defect (30%), an enlarged blind spot (90%), or various nerve fiber layer visual field defects secondary to optic nerve compression.

Differential Diagnosis

malignant melanoma (melanocytoma equally common in blacks and whites versus <1% of melanoma in blacks), choroidal nevus, retinal pigment epithelium hypertrophy, juxtapapillary choroidal melanoma, retinal pigment epithelium hyperplasia, combined hamartoma of the retina and the retinal pigment epithelium.

Management

clinical diagnosis. Fluorescein angiography demonstrates hypofluorescence. Observation and regular follow-up with serial fundus photos are indicated. Approximately 10 to 15% may demonstrate slow growth but are benign. In cases of severe visual impairment and progressive growth, address the possibility of malignant transformation and consider enucleation.

Chapter 12

PEDIATRIC OPHTHALMOLOGY AND STRABISMUS

Tara Sweeney, Norman B. Medow, Renée Richards

12.1 Ophthalmia Neonatorum

12.1.1 Chemical Conjunctivitis—reaction of the newborn eye to instillation of prophylactic drops, commonly silver nitrate.

Presentation conjunctival injection and a watery discharge that lasts up to 48 hours after instillation of drops.

Differential Diagnosis chlamydial conjunctivitis, HSV, nasolacrimal dust obstruction.

Management this is a self-limited disorder. Warm compresses may be applied.

12.1.2 Bacterial Conjunctivitis—a conjunctival infection associated with mucoid discharge.

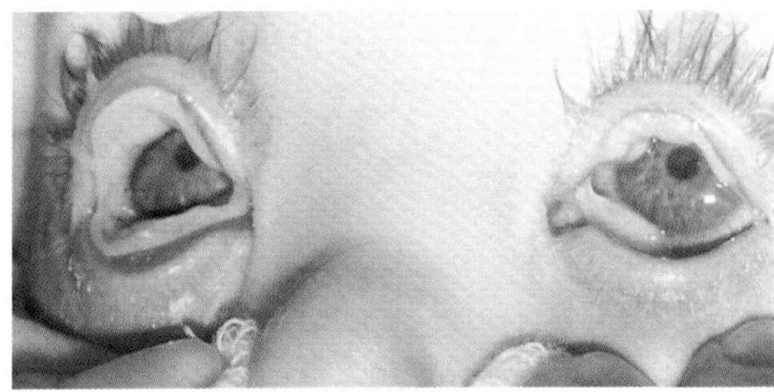

FIGURE 12.1.2 Bacterial conjunctivitis.

Presentation spectrum runs from itching, watery discharge, and low-grade conjunctival injection to eyelid edema, mucopurulent discharge, and severe injection. Corneal ulceration may occur.

Differential Diagnosis gonococcal, chlamydial, chemical conjunctivitis.

Management

- Gram's stain and cultures should be obtained prior to antibiotic therapy.
- Gram-positive organisms: treat with erythromycin–bacitracin ointment.
- Gram-negative organisms: treat with gentamicin ointment.
- Corneal ulcer: hospitalize and treat with rigorous, fortified therapy.

12.1.3 Gonococcal Conjunctivitis—a hyperacute bacterial conjunctivitis of the neonate.

Presentation typically presents as an aggressive conjunctivitis with copious mucopurulent discharge. Corneal ulceration may occur.

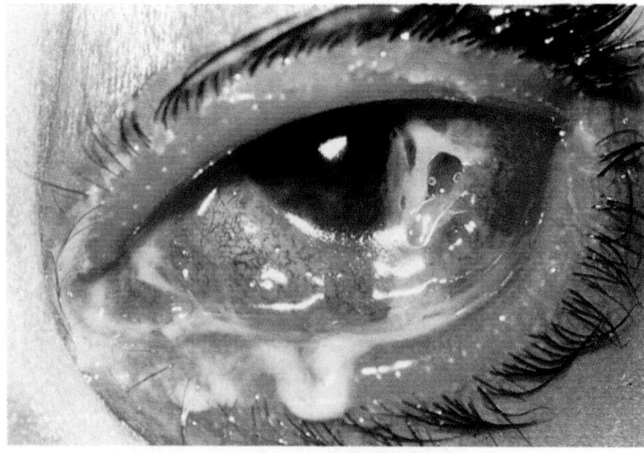

FIGURE 12.1.3 Hyperacute gonococcal conjunctivitis.

Differential Diagnosis streptococcal and other bacterial infections, chlamydial infection.

Management the suspicion or the diagnosis of gonococcal conjunctivitis is a pediatric emergency because of the virulence of the organism. Gram's stain (gram-negative diplococci and polymorphonuclear cells) and cultures, especially Thayer-Martin media, should be performed prior to antibiotic therapy. IV penicillin treatment (100,000 U/kg/day) should be started immediately. Topical bacitracin and saline lavage should be used daily. If cultures are positive, a systemic workup and infectious disease consultation are necessary. Concomitant chlamydial infection or syphilis may be present.

12.1.4 Chlamydial Conjunctivitis—a bacterial infection secondary to exposure to obligate intracellular parasites in the birth canal.

Presentation neonate usually develops red eye, eyelid edema, chemosis, and watery or mucopurulent discharge 3 to 5 days after birth. Conjunctival scarring and micropannus may result. Pneumonia and otitis media may present as later complications.

Differential Diagnosis gonococcal conjunctivitis, bacterial conjunctivitis, HSV, nasolacrimal duct obstruction, dacryocystitis.

Management take both bacterial and viral cultures. Check conjunctival scraping with Giemsa stain. If the diagnosis is suspected, treat the child with erythromycin suspension (50 mg/kg/day) for 3 weeks. The mother and her sexual partners should be treated with either oral tetracycline or erythromycin. Concomitant gonococcal infection may be present.

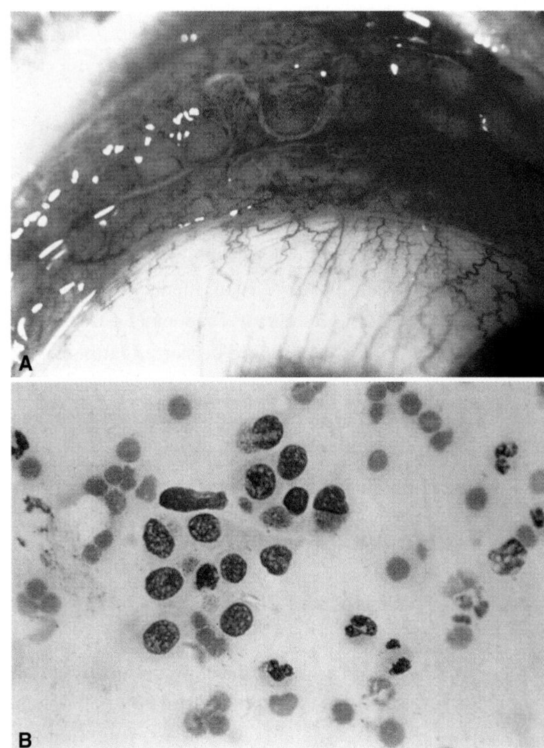

FIGURE 12.1.4a Chlamydial conjunctivitis.
FIGURE 12.1.4b Scraping of obligate intracellular parasites.

12.1.5 Herpes Simplex—special considerations in the neonate: represents primary herpetic disease. Call pediatric consultation to rule out systemic disease and consider use of acyclovir (see Section 5.1.1).

12.2 Leukocoria

12.2.1 Congenital and Developmental Lens Defects and Cataracts—see Chapter 7.

12.2.2 Retinoblastoma—a neuroblastic tumor that is the most common primary intraocular malignancy in children. It arises from either a heritable germline mutation or a somatic mutation in the long arm of chromosome 13.

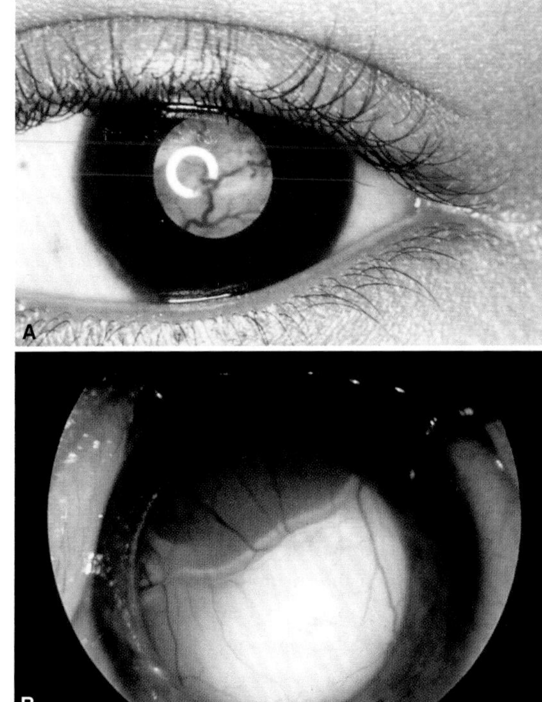

FIGURE 12.2.2a Retinoblastoma.
FIGURE 12.2.2b Retinoblastoma.

Presentation

The heritable form (autosomal dominant, 80 to 90% penetrance) is usually bilateral, whereas the nonheritable form is always unilateral. Retinoblastomas are typically detected when parents notice a "white reflex" in photographs of their children. Children also commonly present with strabismus. Often the diagnosis is made before the child is 2 years of age. Macular disease tends to be detected earlier than tumors of the midperiphery or anterior retina. Tumors may be detected as small subretinal masses, as larger, dome-shaped pearly pink elevations of the retina, or as preretinal masses with vitreous seeding. Iris neovascularization, pseudohypopyon, and VH may occur. Retinoblastoma may metastasize via the choroid to the bloodstream, via the optic nerve to the CNS, or via the sclera to the orbit. Metastases to the bone marrow are more common than to the liver and lung.

Differential Diagnosis congenital cataract, persistent hyperplastic primary vitreous, total retinal detachment, retinopathy of prematurity, Coat's disease, toxocariasis, astrocytic hamartoma, hemangioblastoma.

Management obtain family history (may be positive in up to 10% of children). Diagnosis is usually clinical; CT scan or ultrasound is helpful to detect calcification within the tumor and tumor extension. Biopsy is contraindicated because it will spread malignant tumor cells. Pediatric and radiation oncology consultation is recommended. Spontaneous regression has been reported; however, treatment options include irradiation and chemotherapy, brachytherapy, photocoagulation, cryotherapy, and enucleation. Relatives of children with retinoblastoma should be screened periodically.

12.2.3 Coat's Disease—a severe form of retinal telangiectasia and vascular anomalies occurring in both children and adults.

Presentation typically presents unilaterally, in a male, as an abnormal, white retinal reflex in the first decade of life. The vitreous is clear; there are no signs of turbidity with a very, almost diagnostic, yellow color to the retina. Because of vascular abnormalities, leaking vessels lead to intraretinal and subretinal exudation, especially in the macular area. This may further cause exudative retinal detachment, secondary cataract, and neovascular glaucoma.

Differential Diagnosis retinoblastoma, persistent hyperplastic primary vitreous, ROP, toxocariasis, sickle cell retinopathy, Eales' disease, fa-

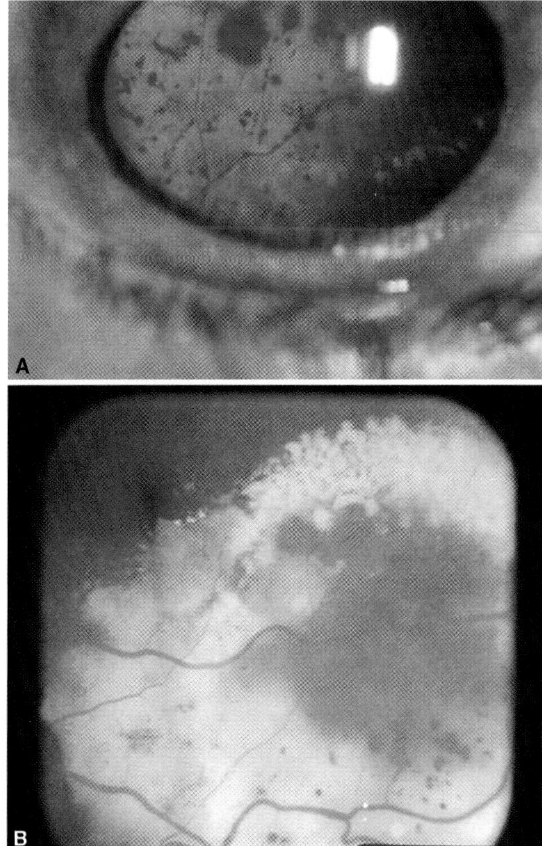

FIGURE 12.2.3a Coat's disease with subretinal exudate and serous retinal detachment.
FIGURE 12.2.3b Coat's disease with subretinal exudate and saccular aneurysms.

milial exudative vitreoretinopathy, cavernous hemangioma, leukemia, and anemia.

Management obtain family history; it should be normal. FA may demonstrate vascular anomalies and leakage from these vessels. The subretinal fluid of Coat's disease is brighter on MRI than is a retinoblastoma tumor mass. Laser photocoagulation and cryotherapy are used to destroy anomalous vessels to prevent further leakage. Patients may further require scleral buckle or filtering surgery.

12.2.4 Retinopathy of Prematurity (ROP)—a proliferative retinopathy of low birth weight infants subjected to oxygen therapy.

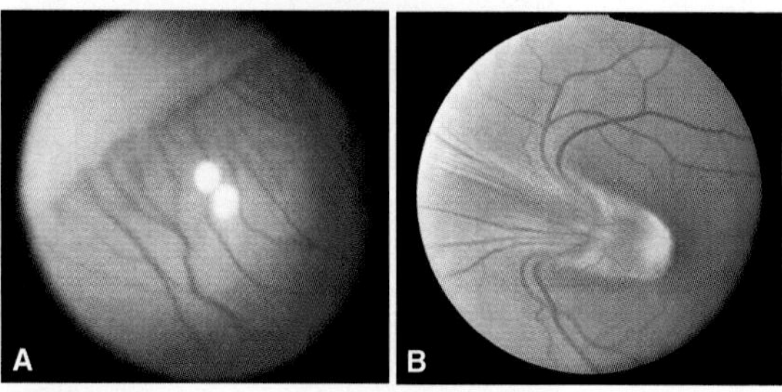

FIGURE 12.2.4a ROP: stage 2.
FIGURE 12.2.4b ROP: dragged macula.

Presentation infants in the neonatal intensive care unit are screened on weekly ROP rounds. Disease is classified according to three zones:

- Zone 1: a 60° circle (optic nerve to fovea is 30°) around the optic nerve.
- Zone 2: outside of zone 1 to the nasal ora serrata, and the same radius to the temporal periphery.
- Zone 3: the remaining anterior, temporal crescent.

Stages of disease range from a flat or ridged demarcation line separating vascular and avascular retina (stages 1 and 2), to a ridge with extraretinal fibrovascular proliferation (stage 3), to subtotal or total retinal detachment (stages 4 and 5). The presence of dilated and tortuous retinal or iris vessels is called "plus" disease and indicates risk of progression. Undiagnosed children may present with strabismic amblyopia, myopia, cataracts, glaucoma, a dragged macula, or retinal detachment.

Differential Diagnosis persistent hyperplastic primary vitreous, retinoblastoma, Coat's disease, toxocariasis, sickle cell retinopathy, familial exudative vitreoretinopathy, incontinentia pigmentosa.

Management obtain a prenatal and birth history. Infants of less than 36 weeks' gestation or less than 2000-g birth weight who have received oxygen are screened at discharge and at 7 to 9 weeks of age. Follow stage 1 and stage 2 disease every 2 weeks, or more often in presence of plus disease. When stage 3 "plus" disease occurs in either zone 1 or 2 for 5 contiguous or 8 total clock hours, laser photocoagulation or cryotherapy is used. Vitrectomy or scleral buckle surgery may be necessary for stages 4 and 5.

12.2.5 Toxocariasis

12.2.5 Toxocariasis—a systemic disease with ocular inflammation resulting from ingestion of *Toxocara canis,* a dog parasite.

Presentation typically presents as unilateral ocular inflammation in children with a history of playing with dirt in a sandbox. The larvae migrate to the retina and then die and cause inflammation and destruction. Inflammation may present as a posterior pole or peripheral, eosinophilic granuloma (a white domelike lesion, with overlying vitreous cells) or as a chronic endophthalmitis. Later sequelae include cataract, hypotony, a dragged macula and pseudoexotropia, or retinal detachment. Systemic disease may affect the liver and lungs.

Differential Diagnosis retinoblastoma, retinoma, ROP, other causes of posterior uveitis (toxoplasmosis, syphilis), trauma with intraocular foreign body, cataract.

Management obtain a careful social (pets) and family history. Check a blood *Toxocara* titer via ELISA and peripheral eosinophil count. Ultrasound the retinal lesion; a *Toxocara* granuloma rarely is calcified. Periocular or systemic steroids are the mainstays of treatment for ocular inflammation.

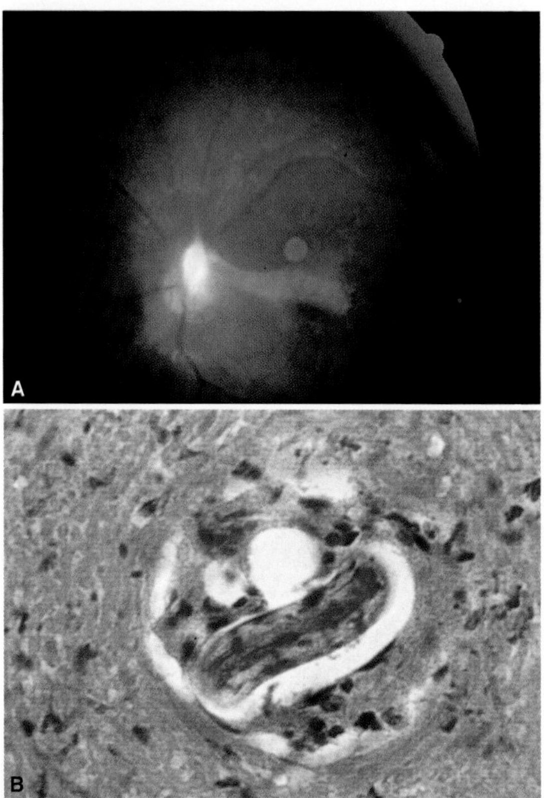

FIGURE 12.2.5a *Toxocara canis.*
FIGURE 12.2.5b *Toxocara canis* nematode.

12.3 Congenital Nasolacrimal Duct Obstruction

blockage of the tear outflow system usually due to a thin membrane below the nasolacrimal sac. Obstruction may also occur anywhere within the nasolacrimal system.

Presentation epiphora, full tear lakes, sticky eyelashes with a watery or mucoid discharge in the absence of either conjunctivitis or blepharitis, recurrent bacterial conjunctivitis.

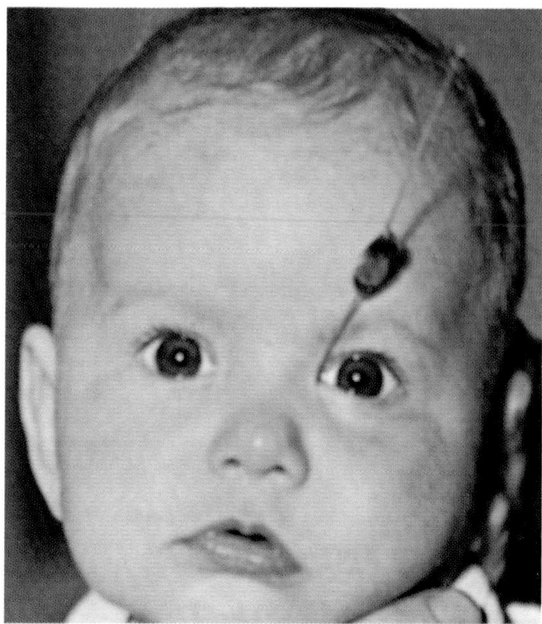

FIGURE 12.3 Probing of congenital nasolacrimal duct obstruction.

Differential Diagnosis punctal atresia and other congenital anomalies of the upper lacrimal system, congenital glaucoma, conjunctivitis, and blepharitis.

Management place fluorescein in the eye; if blocked, the yellow dye will roll down the child's face and cannot be recovered from the nose with a cotton-tip applicator after 10 minutes. Conservative therapy consists of gentle massage, warm compresses, and erythromycin ointment prn. Up to 90% of obstructions may resolve within the first year of life. We prefer to probe at about 1 year. Success rates are about 90% from 9 months to 15 months and then decrease precipitously for older children. If obstruction persists, patients may then require a second trial of probing with tube placement or a dacryocystorhinostomy.

12.4 Dacryocystocele

a cystic swelling of the lacrimal sac causing obstruction both above and below the sac.

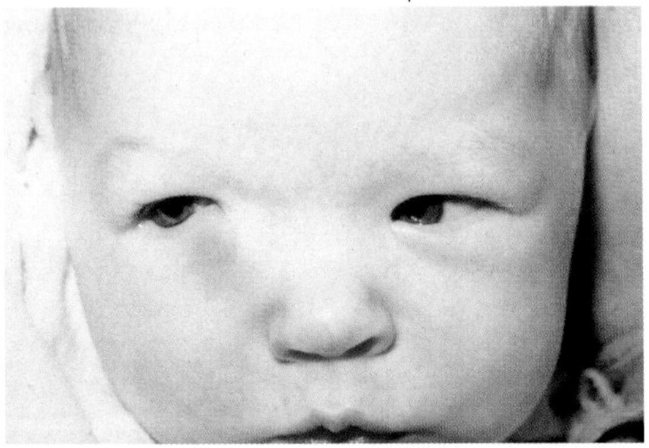

FIGURE 12.4 Dacryocystocele.

Presentation typically presents at birth as a bluish swelling below the medial canthus.

Differential Diagnosis encephalocele, hemangioma, nasolacrimal duct obstruction with dacryocystitis.

Management may resolve with massage and erythromycin ointment. If it persists beyond 1 month of age, patients should be probed. If dacryocystitis is present, systemic antibiotics and surgical drainage of the sac may be necessary.

12.5 Congenital Glaucoma

an anomalous chamber angle leading to high IOP and ocular damage.

Presentation may present as a primary or secondary disease. Photophobia is the most important presenting symptom. Infants may also present with tearing, myopia, amblyopia, and

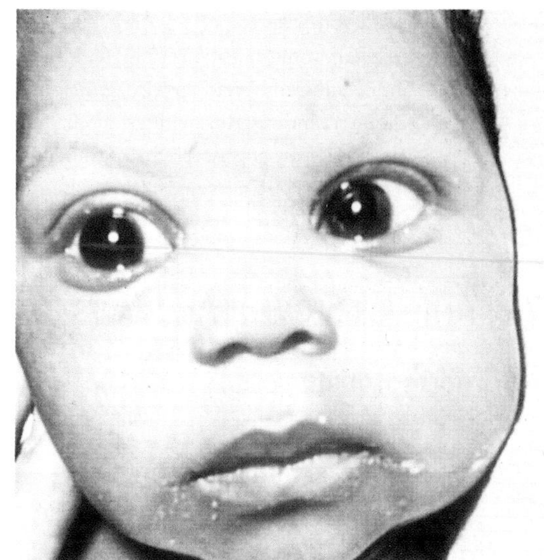

FIGURE 12.5 A two-month-old with congenital glaucoma.

corneal edema. Horizontal breaks in Descemet's membrane are known as Haab's striae. Buphthalmos may occur if high pressures are untreated. Older children with more subtle disease may present with mild corneal enlargement and optic nerve head cupping.

Differential Diagnosis

nasolacrimal duct obstruction (tearing); congenital hereditary stromal or endothelial dystrophy, metabolic disorders, birth trauma (corneal edema and striae). Associations include systemic syndromes such as Sturge-Weber syndrome or neurofibromatosis, congenital cataract, intrauterine rubella, aphakia, aniridia, trauma.

Management

check the family history, measure the corneal diameter and IOP, and try to perform gonioscopy and optic nerve visualization. Once diagnosis is made, there is a role for both temporary medical treatment and more definitive, surgical intervention. Oral Diamox (acetazolamide) may be used in a dosage of 5 to 10 mg/kg/day. Goniotomy, trabeculotomy, trabeculectomy with mitomycin, implant procedures, and cyclophotocoagulation are possible surgical interventions. Although glaucoma present at birth carries a poor prognosis, careful assessment for amblyopia is necessary. Optic nerve head cupping is reversible in children with careful pressure control.

12.6 Anterior Segment Anomalies

12.6.1 Birth Trauma—damage to the cornea secondary to passage through the birth canal or secondary to a forceps delivery.

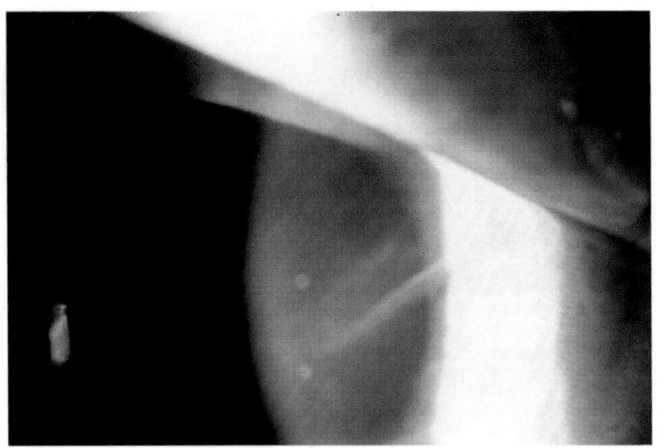

FIGURE 12.6.1 Traumatic forceps delivery.

Presentation vertical breaks in Descemet's membrane. May also have central corneal opacity.

Differential Diagnosis breaks may be confused with Haab's striae in congenital glaucoma.

Management
- Clear cornea: observation.
- Opacified cornea: antiamblyopia therapy and consideration of PK.

12.6.2 Megalocornea—horizontal corneal diameter greater than 12 mm in the newborn (normally, 9.5 to 10.5 mm).

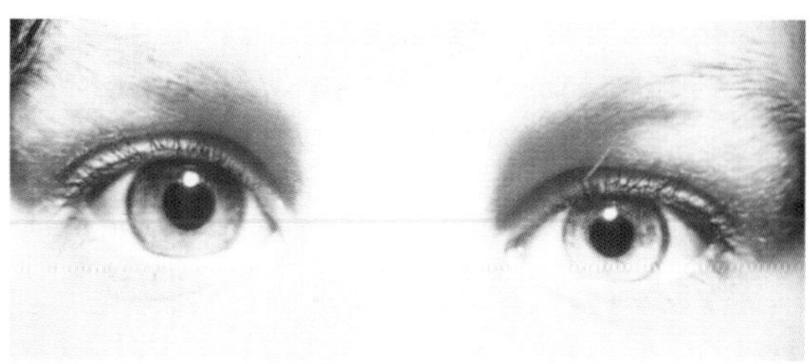

FIGURE 12.6.2 Megalocornea.

Presentation unilaterally or bilaterally enlarged corneas that may present with corectopia, iris hypoplasia, lens subluxation, and glaucoma.

Differential Diagnosis congenital glaucoma, anterior cleavage syndromes.

Management congenital glaucoma must be ruled out; then, follow the case for refractive changes and development of increased intraocular pressure.

12.6.3 Microcornea—horizontal corneal diameter less than 9 mm in the newborn (normally, 9.5 to 10.5 mm).

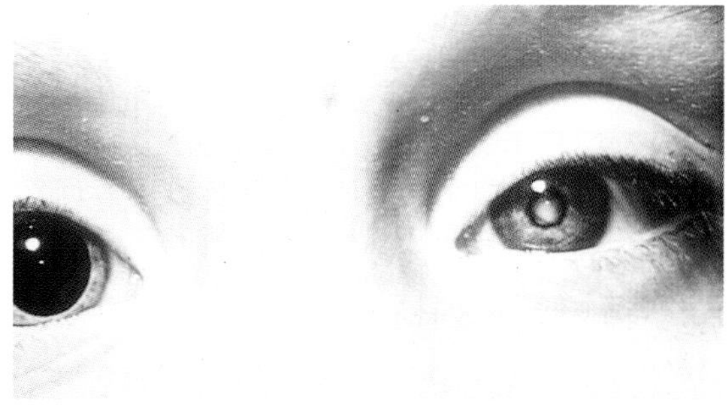

FIGURE 12.6.3 Microcornea with cataract.

Presentation may be an isolated finding or in conjunction with congenital cataracts and persistent hyperplastic primary vitreous.

Differential Diagnosis nanophthalmos, sclerocornea, congenital cataract, persistent hyperplastic primary vitreous.

Management if an isolated finding, no treatment. Otherwise treat other ocular abnormalities.

12.6.4 Posterior Embryotoxon—an anteriorly displaced Schwalbe's line (the junction of Descemet's membrane and the trabecular meshwork).

Presentation often referred to as a white corneal ring near the limbus on slit-lamp examination. May be present in about 25% of normal eyes. The abnormal line may be seen on gonioscopy.

Differential Diagnosis arcus juvenilis, Axenfeld-Rieger syndrome, Alagille syndrome, aniridia.

Management follow the case.

12.6.5 Axenfeld-Rieger Syndrome—a spectrum of anterior segment disorders previously separated into Axenfeld's and Reiger's anomalies and syndromes.

Presentation posterior embryotoxon is always present with iris strands or iris atrophy or hypoplasia. Other findings may include corectopia, iris–corneal touch, ectropion, and anterior chamber dysgenesis with glaucoma (50% incidence, may present in adulthood). Also associated with skeletal (craniofacial, shoulder) and dental abnormalities, and sometimes mental retardation.

Differential Diagnosis posterior embryotoxon, trauma, anterior uveitis.

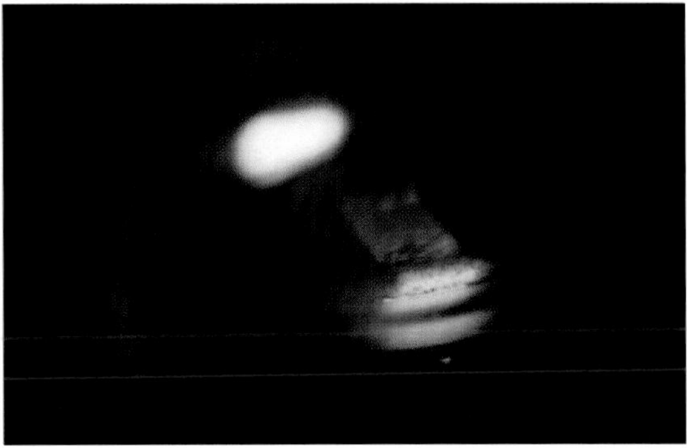

FIGURE 12.6.5 Prominent iris processes of Axenfeld's anomaly.

Management check and treat IOP, if elevated. Look for skeletal anomalies.

12.6.6 Peter's Anomaly—a group of disorders including a central corneal leukoma and abnormalities of the stroma, Descemet's membrane, and the corneal endothelium.

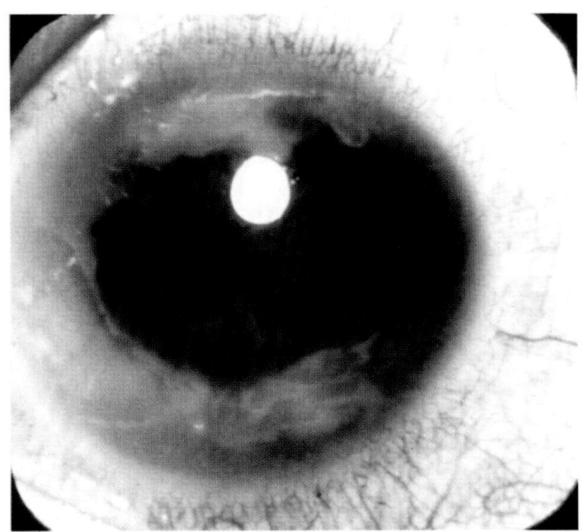

FIGURE 12.6.6a Rieger's anomaly.

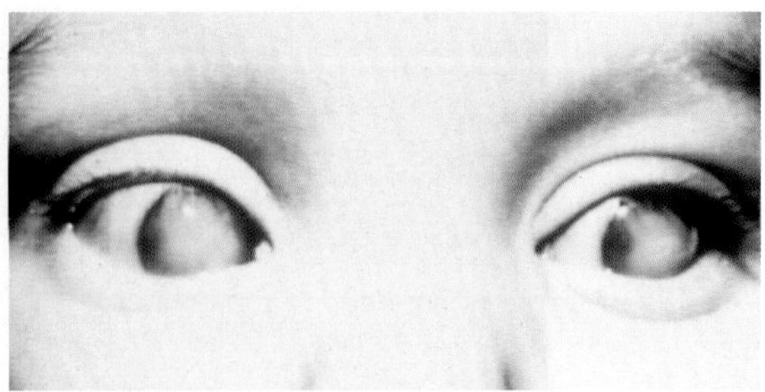

FIGURE 12.6.6b Bilateral Peter's Anomaly.

Presentation central corneal leukoma with iris adhesions to the edge of the leukoma; frequently with cataract and glaucoma. Systemic disorders such as craniofacial and skeletal disorders and cardiac defects may occur.

Differential Diagnosis trauma, dermoid cyst, sequelae of intraocular inflammation.

Management treat IOP. Corneal transplant and anterior segment reconstruction may be performed if the patient does not suffer from irreversible amblyopia.

12.7 Esodeviations

12.7.1 Pseudoesotropia—prominent epicanthal folds or a wide nasal bridge simulating an esotropic appearance.

Presentation parents often complain that the child's eye appears to turn inward. The child may also be referred in by the pediatrician for esotropia. However, there is no movement on cover–uncover testing (see Section 17.1.1).

Differential Diagnosis congenital esotropia, accommodative esotropia, disorders of epicanthal area such as the blepharophimosis syndrome.

Management follow the case closely. Check photographs for central corneal reflexes. Congenital and accommodative esotropias can occur in the setting of prominent epicanthal folds.

12.7.2 Congenital Esotropia—inward deviation of one or both eyes within the first six months of life.

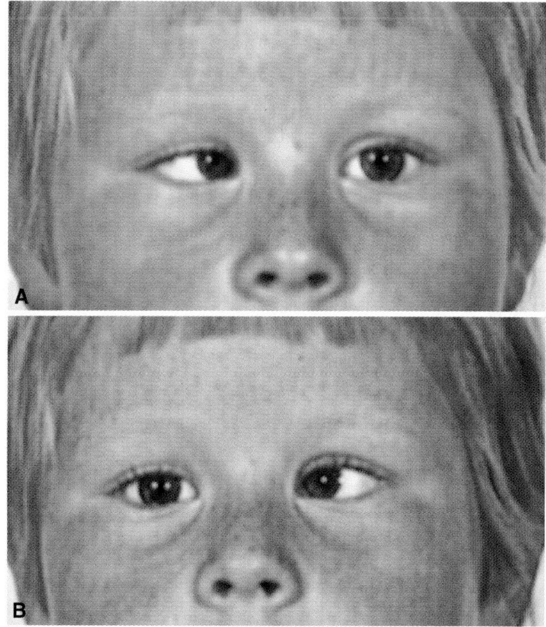

FIGURE 12.7.2a Congenital esotropia with left eye fixation.
FIGURE 12.7.2b Alternating esotropia with right eye fixation.

Presentation parents often notice that one or both eyes are looking inward. Children usually cross-fixate and have a large-angle comitant esotropia. Nystagmus and overaction of the inferior obliques or dissociated vertical deviation may be present. There is usually no accommodative component. Amblyopia may be present.

Differential Diagnosis accommodative esotropia, bilateral sixth nerve palsies, sensory deprivation, nystagmus blockage syndrome.

Management obtain a family history—it is often abnormal. Measure the deviation at distance and near and be sure that it is comitant; determine whether an "A" or a "V" pattern is present. Perform careful slit-lamp and fundus examinations to determine whether causes of sensory deviation are present. Correct any refractive errors that exist (cycloplegic refraction). If the child cries when one eye is covered, evaluate the fixation pattern and begin amblyopia therapy (patching). Once the vision appears equal in both eyes, surgical correction is performed, preferably before the age of 2 years. A bilateral medial rectus recession is commonly done. Surgery may also include the inferior obliques if there is significant overaction and a "V" pattern.

12.7.3 Accommodative Esotropia—a turning in of one or both eyes due to activation of the accommodative reflex.

Presentation patients usually present from 2 to 5 years of age with one eye turned in the majority of the time. Amblyopia is common. Cycloplegic refraction usually reveals greater than 2 D of hyperopia; however, the deviation may occur with low hyperopia and be secondary to a high AC/A ratio (the deviation is greater at near than at distance).

Differential Diagnosis congenital esotropia, sensory deprivation, sixth nerve palsy, nystagmus blockage syndrome, spasm of near reflex, Duane's syndrome type I, pseudostrabismus.

Management obtain a family history. Perform careful slit-lamp and fundus examinations to determine whether causes of sensory deprivation are present. Measure the deviation at distance and near and prescribe the full cycloplegic refraction. Determine whether there is an "A" or a "V" pattern. If a

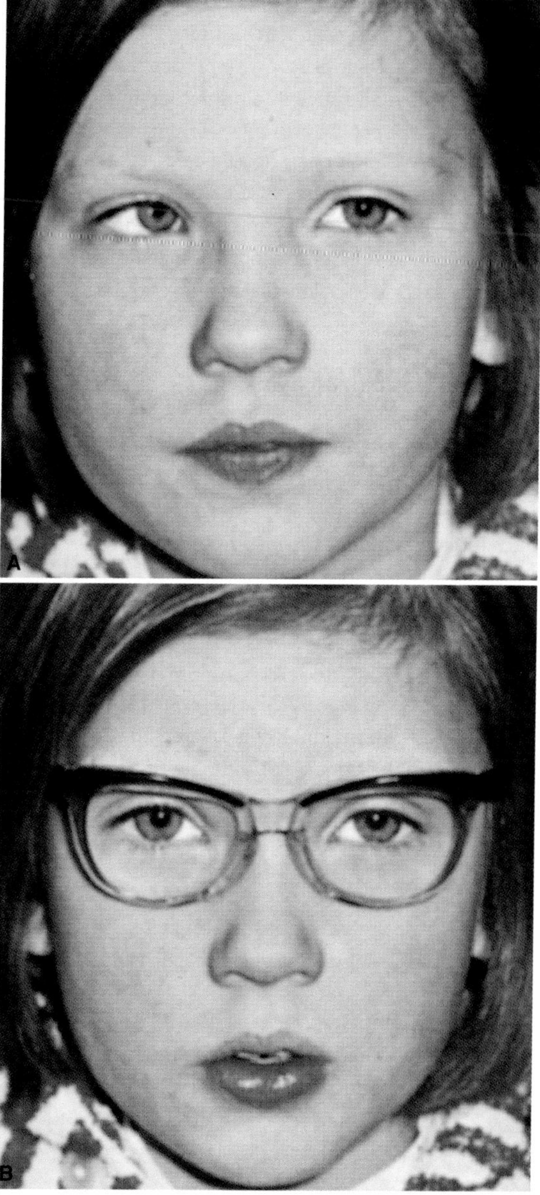

FIGURE 12.7.3a Accommodative esotropia.
FIGURE 12.7.3b With spectacle correction.

high AC/A ratio exists, consider bifocal therapy. If amblyopia is present, institute patching or atropine therapy. Once glasses are prescribed, see the child after 1 month of full-time wear. If the child improves with spectacle correction, orthoptic examination and cycloplegic refraction should be performed every 6 months in an effort to decrease the power of the spectacles and the bifocal. If the child's condition does not improve with spectacle correction, surgical options include a recession–resection or a bilateral medial rectus recession.

12.8 Exodeviations

12.8.1 Intermittent Exotropia—either eye may be turned outward.

Presentation frequently presents before 5 years of age. Parents often complain that in sunlight, after a nap, or toward the end of a day, the child may squint or their eye may turn toward the wall. On cover–uncover testing, there is refixation of the affected eye inward. The deviation is usually greater at distance than at near. There may be an "A" or a "V" pattern. Amblyopia is rare, and stereopsis and fusion are usually intact. May progress to a constant exotropia in older children and adults.

Differential Diagnosis convergence insufficiency, sensory exotropia, third nerve palsy, Duane's syndrome type II, constant exotropia, pseudoexotropia (large-angle kappa).

Management cycloplegic refraction to detect myopia. Therapeutic myopic spectacles may stimulate accommodative convergence. Institute antisuppression patching therapy. If deviation deteriorates, a recession–resection or a bilateral lateral rectus recession may be performed.

12.8.2 Convergence Insufficiency—decreased ability to focus on a near target.

Presentation children often present after 10 years of age complaining of headaches, blurred vision, and difficulty when reading for prolonged periods of time. The child has poor convergence amplitudes and the near point of convergence is remote. Accommodation amplitudes and near point of accommodation are usually normal. An exophoria may be present at near.

Differential Diagnosis intermittent exotropia, head trauma, or intracranial lesions causing convergence paralysis.

Management orthoptic exercises are the treatment of choice. Of all childhood strabismus, convergence insufficiency is the most treatable by orthoptic therapy. "Pencil push-ups" and other near-point exercises are prescribed. The child may be forced to exercise with base-out prisms to increase convergence amplitudes. If convergence paralysis is present, rule out an intracranial lesion. If accommodation amplitude is also affected, consider systemic disease.

12.9 Strabismus Syndromes

12.9.1 Nystagmus Blockage Syndrome—a manifest nystagmus that dampens on adduction.

Presentation the child usually presents with an eye turning inward and nystagmus. The nystagmus is dampened on adduction of the fixing eye and increases on abduction. A face turn is present.

Differential Diagnosis congenital esotropia, Ciancia syndrome, Duane's syndrome.

Management perform careful slit-lamp and fundus examinations. Prescribe hyperopic spectacles if indicated by cycloplegic refraction. Surgery may be performed to move the esotropic eye in the direction of the face turn.

12.9.2 Dissociated Vertical Deviation—a central disorder in which an eye may spontaneously and slowly drift upward.

Presentation commonly presents as part of the congenital esotropia syndrome. When the hypertropic eye fixates on a target, there is no corresponding hypotropia of the other eye. The eye under cover is always up.

Differential Diagnosis inferior oblique overaction, hypertropia.

Management a dissociated vertical deviation is often difficult to measure; base-down prism is often used over the deviating eye. If the deviation is cosmetically intolerable, unilateral or bilateral superior rectus muscle recession may be performed, with or without a Faden procedure. Anteriorization of the inferior oblique is performed for inferior oblique overaction.

12.9.3 Duane's Syndrome—an incomitant strabismus characterized by retraction of the globe on attempted adduction. Hypoplasia of the sixth nerve nucleus with paradoxical innervation of the lateral rectus from the third nerve is the cause.

Presentation limited abduction (type I), adduction (type II), or both (type III). Narrowing of the palpebral fissures on adduction is seen secondary to cocontraction of the medial and lateral recti. Eyes may be straight in the primary position in types I and III; mild esotropia may be present in type I, and exotropia is present in type II. Upshoot and downshoot phenomena have been described as an anomalous vertical deviation secondary to a tight lateral rectus. Abduction is usually severely limited, and a face turn for fusion is common.

Differential Diagnosis sixth nerve palsy, Goldenhar's syndrome, congenital esotropia.

Management treat any refractive error and amblyopia. Surgery is usually reserved for a face turn. A large medial rectus recession is usually performed but not resection of the lateral rectus.

12.9.4 Brown's Syndrome—a motility disorder of elevation in adduction due to an abnormal superior oblique tendon and trochlea.

Presentation may present as unilateral or bilateral inability to elevate the eye in adduction. There may be a hypotropia on primary gaze. Forced ductions show restriction of elevation in adduction. The patient may have an abnormal head posture: chin up, tilt to the affected side, and face turn away from affected side.

Differential Diagnosis inferior oblique palsy, trauma, tenosynovitis of the superior oblique tendon.

Management surgery may be performed for an abnormal hypotropia or an abnormal head posture. Weakening of the superior oblique tendon has variable results.

12.10 Complications of Strabismus Surgery

12.10.1 Residual and Secondary Deviations—a residual deviation is an undercorrected deviation. A secondary deviation may result from surgical overcorrection.

Presentation these deviations may present immediately after surgery or occur over time. For example, a congenital esotropia may be surgically corrected to a small-angle residual esotropia. Over time, the child may develop a secondary exotropia.

Differential Diagnosis lost or slipped muscle, accommodative component.

Management in adults only, adjustable suture techniques may help prevent large residual or overcorrected deviations. Prisms may be used or, if the deviation is large enough, a surgical correction may be recommended.

12.10.2 Conjunctival and Corneal Abnormalities—a surface abnormality resulting from surgical injury.

Presentation conjunctival scarring, inclusion cysts, allergic reactions, and foreign-body granulomas may all result in the postoperative period; keratitis or corneal abrasion may occur. Dellen may form quite rapidly and if surgery is performed on multiple recti. Anterior segment ischemia may result in corneal edema.

Differential Diagnosis infection, allergic reaction, trauma.

Management meticulous surgical technique is recommended to avoid inadvertent trauma to Tenon's capsule and the plica semilunaris. Topical corticosteroids may be used for granuloma formation, allergic reactions, and uveitis secondary to ischemia. Lubrication is the treatment of choice for dellen formation.

12.10.3 Lost or Slipped Muscle—an unexpected large change in position of the eye after surgery.

Presentation a lost muscle generally retracts into Tenon's capsule along the orbital wall during the surgical procedure, while a slipped muscle may be generally discovered postoperatively within its sheath. There is loss of rotation into the involved field of action.

Differential Diagnosis operation on the wrong muscles.

Management a lost muscle may be retrieved by careful exploration, often with great difficulty! If a lost or slipped muscle is suspected in the postoperative period, immediate surgery should be performed to avoid scarring and contracture.

12.11 Shaken-Baby Syndrome

a syndrome of child abuse with important retinal findings.

Presentation children are under 3 years of age with a history of having been violently shaken or abused. Ocular findings include extensive intraretinal and preretinal hemorrhages. Retinal folds and hemorrhagic schisis may be seen. Systemic findings may include developmental delay, intracranial hemorrhage, bone fractures, bruises, and other evidence of trauma.

Differential Diagnosis coagulation disorder, X-linked juvenile retinoschisis, birth trauma (retinal hemorrhages generally disappear by 1 month), trauma unrelated to child abuse (very rarely causes retinal heme, never extensively). Has not been documented with cardiopulmonary resuscitation.

Management social history and appropriate social services, CT of the head to rule out intracranial hemorrhage and skull fractures, careful examination for bruises, burn, cuts, and so on, radiography of ribs and long bones to rule out fracture. Retinal hemorrhages spontaneously resolve over several months. In severe cases, treatment is vitrectomy for VH, if the ERG has a normal b wave.

Chapter 13
NEURO-OPHTHALMOLOGY

Steven Rosenberg, Carolyn Lederman, Jeffrey Odel

13.1 Cranial Nerve Palsies

13.1.1 Isolated Oculomotor (III) Nerve Palsy—limitation of ocular motility with or without pupillary dilation associated with damage to the third cranial nerve.

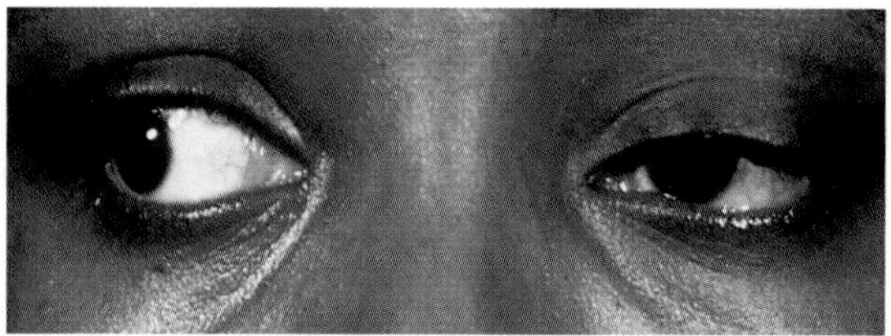

FIGURE 13.1.1 Right CN III palsy with ptosis and limited adduction.

Etiology aneurysm (20%) (classically of the posterior communicating artery); microvascular disease (20–40%), including diabetes and hypertension; trauma (including during birth and surgery); tumor (especially brainstem); congenital; Paget's disease; cavernous sinus syndrome; ophthalmoplegic migraine; numerous neurologic and systemic diseases, including collagen vascular disease, lymphoma, temporal arteritis, herpes zoster, meningitis (cryptococcal, carcinomatous, TB, sarcoid), sinusitis, encephalitis.

Presentation

- Symptoms: binocular double vision, drooping eyelid. Aneurysm can cause severe headache. Microvascular disease may cause a retroorbital burning pain.

- Findings

  Complete: limitation of eye movements in all directions except abduction (CN VI), intorsion, mild depression (CN IV); the affected eye may appear in the "down and out" position; ptosis is complete and may prevent diplopia.

  Partial: incomplete involvement of the extraocular muscles, with or without ptosis.

  Pupil involved: dilated, fixed pupil *or* definite pupillary dilation in the setting of a partial palsy.

  Pupil spared: normal pupil size and response *or* a slightly larger pupil in the setting of a complete palsy.

  Aberrant regeneration may be present: lid retraction in downgaze, lid elevation with or without pupillary constriction on adduction, globe retraction with vertical gaze.

- Associated findings

  Fascicular lesions: contralateral ataxia (Benedik's syndrome), contralateral hemiparesis (Weber's syndrome), alteration of consciousness (transtentorial uncal herniation).

  Nuclear lesion: may have bilateral ptosis, contralateral superior rectus palsy.

Differential Diagnosis

chronic progressive external ophthalmoplegia, Kearns-Sayre syndrome, Graves' orbitopathy, myasthenia gravis, orbital pseudotumor, gaze palsies, cavernous sinus thrombosis, pituitary apoplexy.

Management

- Age less than 40 years: emergent CT and MRI (rule out infarct, cavernous sinus mass, pituitary apoplexy), lumbar puncture and CSF studies, followed by angiogram to rule out aneurysm. Some centers have had success with MR angiography.
- Age more than 40 years: pupil involved. Emergent CT and MRI (rule out infarct, cavernous sinus mass, pituitary apoplexy), lumbar puncture and CSF studies, fol-

lowed by angiogram to rule out aneurysm; about 15% will still have a microvascular cause.

Pupil spared: check blood pressure, blood glucose, ESR in the elderly if temporal arteritis suspected and consider temporal artery biopsy.

Incomplete: observe daily for 5 to 7 days and then weekly for 1 month and monthly for 6 months. If not resolved in 3 to 4 months or pupil becomes involved, perform MRI; if normal, perform cerebral angiogram and CSF studies.

Complete: most likely microvascular; medical workup as above. Pursue imaging studies if palsy persists over 3 months, history of cancer, or evidence of aberrant regeneration.

13.1.2 Isolated Trochlear (IV) Nerve Palsy—limitation of eye movement isolatable to action of the superior oblique muscle.

Etiology trauma (most common, often bilateral); congenital or decompensated congenital palsy; microvascular disease, including diabetes and hypertension; tumor; rarely aneurysm.

Presentation

- Symptoms: binocular vertical double vision. Environment may appear slanted.
- Findings: hypertropia on the affected side, head tilt away from the hypertropic eye, inability to move the hypertropic eye inferonasally. Hypertropia worsens on gaze contralateral to the hypertropic eye and with head tilt to side of the hypertropic eye.

Differential Diagnosis comitant hypertropia, thyroid orbitopathy, myasthenia gravis, orbital pseudotumor, entrapment of contralateral inferior rectus, skew deviation, Brown's tendon sheath syndrome, superior oblique myokymia (recurring diplopia and tremulous sensation in one eye, benign).

Management

- Workup: history of duration (compare with old photographs), stability of degree of deficit, trauma, microvascular risk factors (measure blood pressure, serum glucose levels).

Conduct a three-step test: (1) determine which eye is hypertropic (should be the affected side), (2) determine whether hypertropia is worse on contralateral or ipsilateral gaze (should be worse on contralateral gaze), and (3) determine whether hypertropia worse on contralateral or ipsilateral head tilt (should be worse on ipsilateral head tilt).

Congenital: measure vertical fusional amplitudes: if greater than 3 PD, the lesion is overwhelmingly likely to be congenital or a decompensated congenital palsy and no further evaluation is necessary. Consider the tensilon test to rule out myasthenia if presentation is not classic (Section 13.7) and the double Maddox rod test if bilateral palsy is suspected (left hypertropia on right gaze, right hypertropia on left gaze) (Section 17.2.2). If progression or other neurologic signs or symptoms present, consider MRI and CT scan.

- Treatment: treat any underlying condition found. Acquired palsies tend to resolve in 2 to 6 months. As comitance spreads with chronicity, consider prisms or strabismus surgery.

13.1.3 Abducens (VI) Nerve Palsy—limited action of the lateral rectus secondary to damage to the fourth cranial nerve.

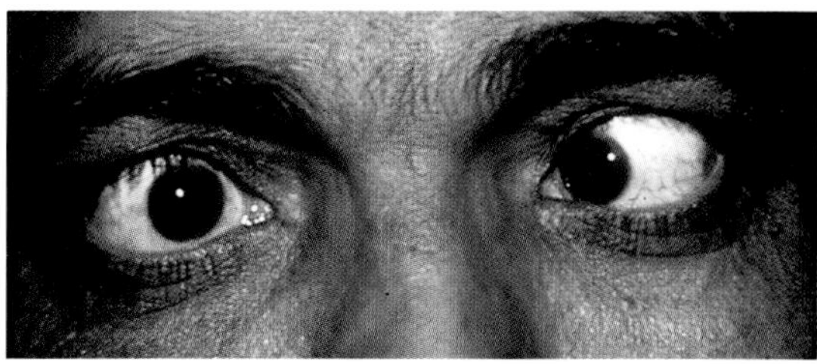

FIGURE 13.1.3 Bilateral CN IV palsy.

Etiology

microvascular disease, trauma (including shaken-baby syndrome), raised intracranial pressure (including pseudotumor cerebri), temporal arteritis, tumor (glioma, nasopharyngeal carcinoma, meningioma), aneurysm (especially in cavernous sinus), multiple sclerosis, vasculitis, syphilis, benign postviral, Mobius' syndrome (congenital CN VI and VII palsy). Bilateral: trauma, mass lesion, meningitis, aneurysm, trauma, multiple sclerosis, Wernicke's encephalopathy.

Presentation

- Symptoms: binocular, horizontal double vision.
- Findings: incomitant esotropia; diplopia worse on gaze in the direction of the eye affected, less or nonexistent on contralateral gaze; no restriction of forced duction.

Differential Diagnosis

thyroid orbitopathy, myasthenia gravis, orbital pseudotumor, Duane's retraction syndrome, convergence spasm (pupillary constriction on attempted abduction).

Management

- Workup: history of trauma, vasculopathic risk factors (evaluate for hypertension and diabetes).

  Age less than 14 years: MRI may not be necessary in patients younger than age 14 without other signs (especially if preceding viral illness), but follow such cases every 1 to 2 weeks for about 2 months. Alternatively, initially obtain an MRI (though glioma is a nonemergent diagnosis).

  Age 15 to 40 years: neurologic evaluation. Measure CBC, glucose, blood pressure. Consider the tensilon test.

  Age over 40 years: most likely vascular. If over age 55 and temporal arteritis suspected, obtain ESR, consider temporal artery biopsy. If not resolved in 6 months, reevaluate.

Obtain an MRI and lumbar-puncture results especially if other neurologic symptoms are present; if bilateral, and no history of heavy trauma; or if there is no resolution in 3 to 6 months.

- Treatment: treat any underlying condition found. Resolution should occur in 3 to 6 months. Consider prisms if double vision is intolerable during this time.

13.1.4 Facial (VII) Nerve Palsy—weakness of facial muscles on one side supplied by the seventh cranial nerve.

Etiology

stroke or central or brainstem tumor, multiple sclerosis, peripheral tumor including parotid and cerebellopontine angle, trauma, otitis media, herpes zoster (Ramsay Hunt syndrome), Guillain-Barré syndrome, Lyme disease, sarcoidosis, metastasis, microvascular disease (diabetes), syphilis, collagen vascular disease, Bell's palsy, (idiopathic).

Presentation

- Symptoms: drooping side of face, tearing or dryness of eye with poor closure of eye, change in taste or hearing (hyperacusis).
- Findings: weakness, paralysis of facial muscles; ectropion or poor closure of eye, exposure keratitis or other signs of dryness; if chronic, may have synkinesis—different branches of nerve are stimulated at the same time (similar to aberrant regeneration).

Differential Diagnosis

parkinsonism, basal ganglia lesion.

Management

- Workup: complete neurologic, ophthalmic, and otolaryngologic examination; history of hearing loss, ear pain. Determine whether the upper eyelid and forehead are involved—indicates peripheral lesion; if spared, indicates central lesion. If there is a history of trauma, obtain CT scan to rule out fracture. If there are other neurologic signs, obtain MRI of the head and brain (check the cerebellopontine angle especially if CN VIII is involved). Consider chest radiography, CBC with differential, ACE levels, Lyme disease and EBV titers, RPR, HIV, RF, ESR, and ANA. Bell's palsy is a diagnosis of exclusion.

- Treatment: as per etiology.

  Bell's palsy: observation is indicated. Consider steroids (oral prednisone 60 mg/day for 4 days, followed by taper). Surgical decompression may be performed by an ENT specialist.

  Ramsay Hunt syndrome: Consider acyclovir (800 mg) 5 times a day for 10 days.

  Poor lid closure: For mild exposure, artificial tears up to 6 times a day, with bed-time ointment lubricants; for more severe exposure, nonpreserved tears up to every hour or viscous lubricants every 3 to 4 hours. Consider lateral or complete tarsorrhaphy, or a gold weight implant in the upper lid.

13.1.5 Multiple Cranial Nerve Palsies (Cavernous Sinus Syndrome and Orbital Apex Syndrome)

—any combination of ipsilateral III, IV, V, or VI nerve palsies, or Horner's syndrome secondary to lesion of cavernous sinus or orbital apex.

Etiology

AV fistula, cavernous sinus thrombosis, metastatic or local spread of malignancy, intracavernous granulomatous process (e.g., sarcoid, TB), aneurysm, mucormycosis (especially in diabetic, can cause death), herpes zoster, Tolosa-Hunt syndrome (idiopathic inflammation of the orbital apex or anterior cavernous sinus associated with pain, possible mild proptosis), pituitary tumor or apoplexy, meningioma, mucocele.

Presentation

- Symptoms: double vision, drooping lids or inability to hold the eye open, pain or numbness of the face.
- Findings: any combination of findings of III, IV, V, or VI nerve palsies or Horner's syndrome, with all findings on same side of face. The pupil may be dilated, constricted or uninvolved. May have ocular bruit if secondary to AV fistula.

Differential Diagnosis

myasthenia gravis, chronic progressive external ophthalmoplegia, orbital lesions, brainstem disease, infectious or neoplastic meningitis, nasopharyngeal carcinoma, dorsal midbrain syndrome (Parinaud's), progressive supranuclear palsy, sarcoidosis, myotonic dystrophy, Guillain-Barré syndrome (Miller-Fisher variant, postviral, progressive), trauma affecting the subarachnoid space, thyroid orbitopathy.

Management

- workup: history of infection, neoplasm, anorexia, headache, increase in symptoms with fatigue, diabetes. Check for ocular bruit, examine the pupil, ocular motility, resistance to retropulsion, Hertel's exophthalmometry, full medical and nasopharyngeal examination (mucosal black crusts in mucor). Obtain CT scan or MRI of brain, orbit, and sinuses. Doppler may help to identify fistulas. Consider the tensilon test, lumbar puncture (up to 3 times to rule out neoplastic meningitis). Obtain CBC with differential, ESR, ANA, and RF.
- Treatment: as per etiology.

  Arteriovenous fistula: may follow if symptoms mild. Treat any elevated IOP (due to elevated episcleral venous pressure). Consider neuroradiology or neurosurgical referral.

  Infectious cavernous sinus syndrome, mucormycosis: Hospitalize and obtain infectious disease consultation.

  Tolosa-Hunt syndrome: treat with steroids as for orbital pseudotumor.

13.2 Pupillary Abnormalities

13.2.1 Anisocoria—relative difference in pupillary size; may be physiologic or pathologic.

Etiology

- More anisocoria in dim light: Horner's syndrome, uveitis, pharmacologic (miotics), aberrant regeneration of CN III, old Adie's tonic pupil.
- More anisocoria in bright light: CN III palsy, iris trauma (surgical, sphincter tear), pharmacologic (atropinics, adrenergics), Adie's tonic pupil.

- Physiologic anisocoria: usually equal in dim and bright light and less than 1 mm in difference.

Presentation unequal pupillary size.

Management depends on etiology.

13.2.2 (Relative) Afferent Pupillary Defect (APD)—

decreased or absent pupillary constriction of both eyes in response to light stimulus to the affected eye when compared with response to light stimulus to the contralateral eye.

Etiology any unbalanced damage to the anterior visual system to level of the pretectal nucleus (i.e., affecting pathways from one eye more than from the other) including but not limited to optic nerve disease (including glaucoma, neuropathy, compressive lesion such as a tumor), central retinal artery occlusion, central retinal vein occlusion, optic tract or chiasmal lesion.

Vitreous hemorrhage, macular degeneration, branch retinal vascular occlusions, retinal detachment, other retinal disease, or long-standing amblyopia may cause a milder relative APD. Cataract on the contralateral side is occasionally associated with APD. Postchiasmal lesions rarely cause an APD when there is asymmetric visual field loss.

Presentation

- Symptoms: usually decreased vision on the affected side.
- Findings: swinging flashlight test, in which pupillary responses are compared as a light is swung rhythmically from one eye to the other. Both pupils constrict when the normal eye is illuminated. When the light is swung to the affected eye, both pupils become relatively larger by dilating, sometimes after an initial constriction. If the affected pupil has an immobile pupil, a "reverse" APD is elicited by observing the contralateral reactive pupil with a second dim light during the swinging flashlight test. The normal pupil will dilate when the light is swung to the affected eye.

Management

- Workup: complete neuro-ophthalmic evaluation, including visual field examination, color vision, and Hertel's exophthalmometry. APD can be quantified with varying neutral-density filters over the normal eye until results of the swinging flashlight test are normal. Consider MRI of brain and orbits.

13.2.3 Horner's Syndrome—damage to sympathetic innervation resulting in miosis and ptosis on the affected side.

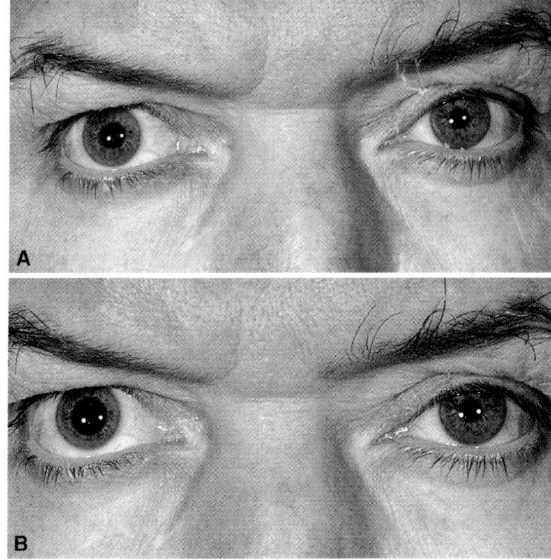

FIGURE 13.2.3a Horner's syndrome left eye.
FIGURE 13.2.3b After cocaine test.

Etiology

- First-order neuron: brainstem stroke, spinal cord tumors, cervical disc disease.
- Second-order neuron: apical lung lesion (Pancoast's tumor), thoracic artery aneurysm, trauma to brachial plexus, thoracic surgery.

- Third-order neuron (postganglionic): neck tumor, neck surgery, dissecting carotid aneurysm, cavernous sinus lesion.
- Congenital: birth trauma, selected causes from the above list.

Presentation

- Symptoms: eyelid droop; may notice relative pupillary difference.
- Findings: ptosis on the affected side, miosis on the affected side, anisocoria greater in dim than in bright illumination, increase in accommodative amplitude, apparent enophthalmos, decreased tear production on the affected side, facial anhidrosis (if first-order or second-neuron affected), heterochromia iridis (with lighted iris on the affected side) in congenital Horner's syndrome.

Management

- Workup (see also Section 13.2.1): determine onset of Horner's syndrome from history and photographs.

  Cocaine test: if positive, confirms Horner's syndrome. Instill one drop of cocaine 10% (or two drops of cocaine 5%) in each eye and wait 30 minutes. The affected pupil will dilate less than will the normal side. Note: Cocaine works by inhibiting re-uptake of norepinephrine by postganglionic nerve fibers.

  Hydroxyamphetamine 1% (Paredrine) is used to distinguish between preganglionic and postganglionic abnormalities. Instill one drop in each eye and wait 30 minutes. If the abnormal pupil dilates, then there is a preganglionic defect. If there is no dilation of the abnormal pupil, then there is a postganglionic defect. Note: Hydroxyamphetamine works by causing release of norepinephrine from preganglionic nerve fiber. Therefore, the third-order neuron must be intact for dilation to occur.

  After determining preganglionic or postganglionic etiology, target workup dependent on suspected site of damage to the sympathetic chain, after recording a careful history of trauma, surgery, and chest, neck, or CNS symptoms.

Preganglionic lesion: neurology referral. With chest or neck symptoms or history, consider chest radiograph (apical lordotic views), cervical spine CT. With CNS symptoms, consider MRI of the brain and cervical cord down to the second thoracic vertebra.

Postganglionic lesion: if old (check old photographs) and isolated, no workup is necessary. If associated with cluster headache, this is a benign condition, and no workup is necessary. If associated with severe head or neck pain, consider workup for carotid dissection (MRI or MRA, angiography).

- Treatment: dependent on the cause of Horner's syndrome. Ptosis surgery may be performed for cosmesis.

13.2.4 Argyll-Robertson Pupil—small, irregular pupils caused by tertiary syphilis.

Presentation

- Symptoms: usually asymptomatic.
- Findings: small (usually <2 mm), irregular pupils, usually bilateral and asymmetric; light-near dissociation (pupils react poorly to light, but do react with convergence); poor pharmacologic dilation; iris atrophy.

Differential Diagnosis

- Of small pupils: posterior synechiae due to anterior uveitis, miotics, old Adie's tonic pupil.
- Of light-near dissociation: pinealoma, midbrain stroke, Adie's tonic pupil, aberrant regeneration.

Management

- Workup: test pupillary responses to light and to near. Perform a full eye examination to look for other signs of syphilis; VDRL/FTA, lumbar puncture.
- Treatment: for tertiary syphilis, use penicillin IV.

13.2.5 Adie's Tonic Pupil—an idiopathic, benign interruption of parasympathetic supply causing a dilated pupil with light-near dissociation; usually unilateral.

Presentation

- Symptoms: pupillary inequality; may have blurred vision or light sensitivity.
- Findings: females 70%, irregularly dilated pupil on the affected side, minimal or no reaction to light, segmental constriction of sphincter (vermiform contractions: streaming of iris crypts), near response greater than light response, slow redilation after constriction, supersensitivity to pilocarpine, diminished deep-tendon reflexes. Note: Old Adie's pupil may constrict over time and dilate poorly in the dark.

Differential Diagnosis

herpes zoster, varicella, temporal arteritis, syphilis, orbital trauma, pharmacologic dilation. Of light-near dissociation: pinealoma, midbrain stroke, Adie's tonic pupil, aberrant regeneration.

Management

- Workup: examine the pupillary response in bright and dim illumination and at near. Look for vermiform contractions. Pilocarpine test: Adie's pupil is hypersensitive to dilute (⅛) pilocarpine. Instill one drop in each eye. The normal eye will constrict minimally or not at all. Adie's pupil will constrict. Note: Painful ciliary spasm may result from instillation of regular-strength pilocarpine.
- Treatment: none, but dilute pilocarpine may be given for cosmesis.

13.3 Developmental Optic Nerve Anomalies

13.3.1 Prepapillary Vascular Loop—blood vessels that project from the optic disc into the vitreous and return to the optic disc to continue their usual course; 80 to 90% are arterial in origin.

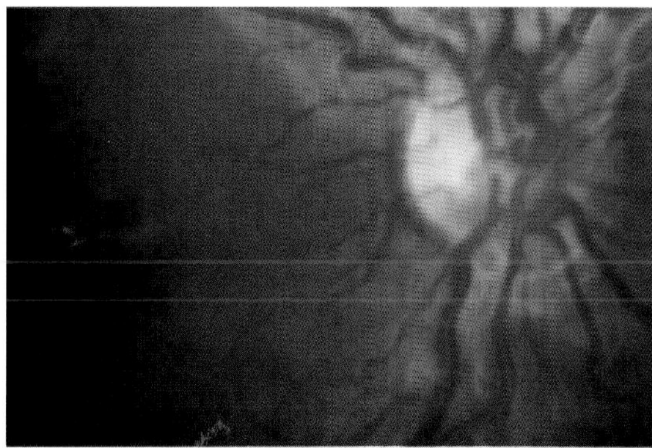

FIGURE 13.3.1 Peripapillary vascular loop.

Presentation incidental finding.

13.3.2 Optic Nerve Hypoplasia (and Aplasia)

—congenital disorder resulting in small optic nerves (or, extremely rarely, lack of optic nerve tissue in optic nerve aplasia); unilateral or bilateral, marked or minimal.

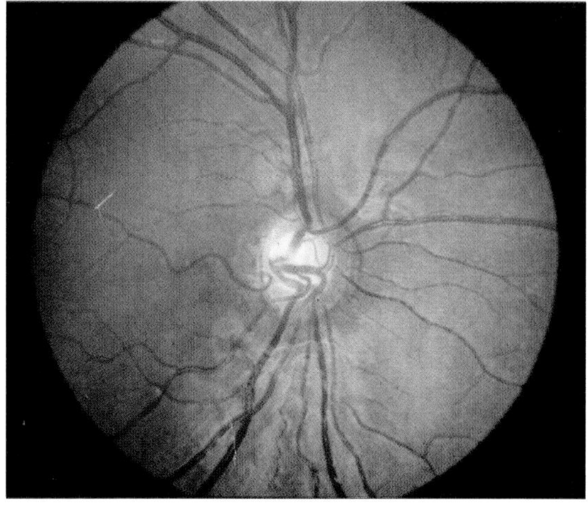

FIGURE 13.3.2 Optic nerve hypoplasia.

Etiology associated with maternal diabetes or maternal ingestion of quinine, LSD, anticonvulsants; congenital optic nerve glioma or craniopharyngioma.

Presentation

- Symptoms: may be asymptomatic, decreased visual acuity, nystagmus.
- Findings: visual acuity can vary from normal to very poor. Severe cases may result in APD, nystagmus, or strabismus (especially esotropic deviation in unilateral cases). May be isolated or accompany other ocular or brain malformations; small optic disc with peripapillary atrophy. Most commonly, the deficiency is on the nasal aspect of nerve. "Double ring sign" results from pigment changes at the junction of sclera and lamina cribrosa (outer ring) and termination of retinal pigment epithelium (inner ring).

Differential Diagnosis coloboma, staphyloma in myopia.

Management

- Workup: neuroimaging to rule out septo-optic dysplasia, or de Morsier's syndrome (absent septum pellucidum), with classic triad of short stature, nystagmus, and optic disc hypoplasia. Consider endocrinologic evaluation.
- Treatment: if unilateral, occlusion therapy of normal eye to treat possible overlying amblyopia.

13.3.3 Optic Nerve Pit—congenital malformation resulting in defect in optic nerve tissue.

Presentation

- Symptoms: asymptomatic and often found on routine examination. May have visual distortion or decreased acuity if associated with serous macular detachment.
- Findings: grayish appearing pit within the nerve substance, usually on the inferotemporal disc. May have associated serous macular detachment and schisis cavity. FA shows late leakage from the pit.

Differential Diagnosis glaucoma, optic nerve coloboma. Of serous detachment of the macula: central serous chorioretinopathy, AMD,

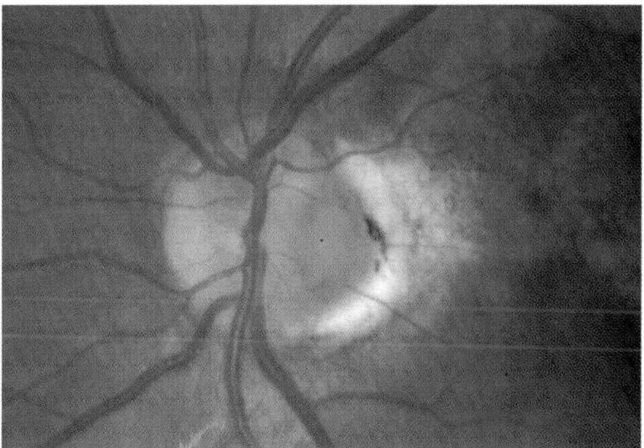

FIGURE 13.3.3 Optic nerve pit.

retinal detachment with macular involvement, pigment epithelial detachment.

Management

- Workup: close inspection of the disc, examination of the macula to rule out serous macular detachment, consider FA and baseline visual field.
- Treatment: sometimes helpful is laser photocoagulation to the peripapillary retina adjacent to the pit if serous macular detachment.

13.3.4 Optic Nerve Coloboma and Morning Glory Syndrome

13.3.4 Optic Nerve Coloboma and Morning Glory Syndrome—congenital defect of the optic nerve resulting from faulty closure of the embryonic optic cup.

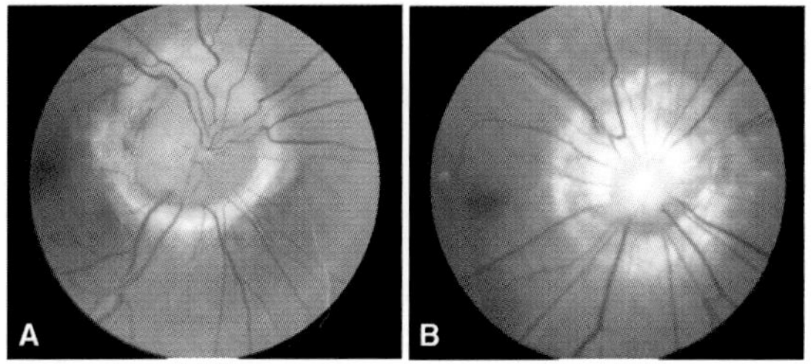

FIGURE 13.3.4a Optic nerve head coloboma.
FIGURE 13.3.4b Morning glory syndrome.

Presentation

- Symptoms: decreased visual acuity if macular fibers are involved. May be a nerve fiber layer visual field defect corresponding to the location of coloboma (therefore, usually superiorly).
- Findings: defect in optic nerve tissue; usually inferiorly. May be associated colobomas of retina, choroid, lens, or iris. "Morning glory" disc is a coloboma with blood vessels radiating radially from the center of disc, white central connective tissue, and surrounding pigmented chorioretinal tissue with female prediction.

Management

- Workup: close examination of the disc, visual field testing.
- Treatment: observation. Serous detachment is possible.

13.3.5 Tilted Disc—congenital anomaly associated with visual field defect.

Presentation

oval optic disc usually tilted so that the superior disc is elevated with a crescent inferonasally on the depressed side; irregular radiation of vessels; usually bilateral and associated with nasal visual field defects.

Differential Diagnosis

oblique insertion of the optic nerve in myopia, myopic crescent.

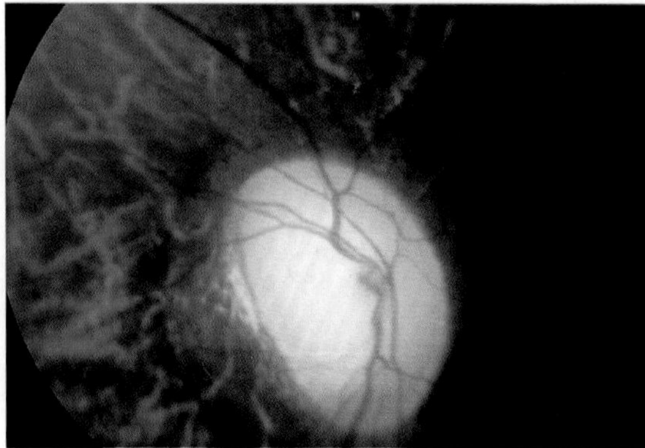

FIGURE 13.3.5 Tilted optic nerve head.

Management consider baseline visual field. Evaluation.

13.4 Optic Disc Pathology

13.4.1 Optic Neuritis—inflammation of the optic nerve.

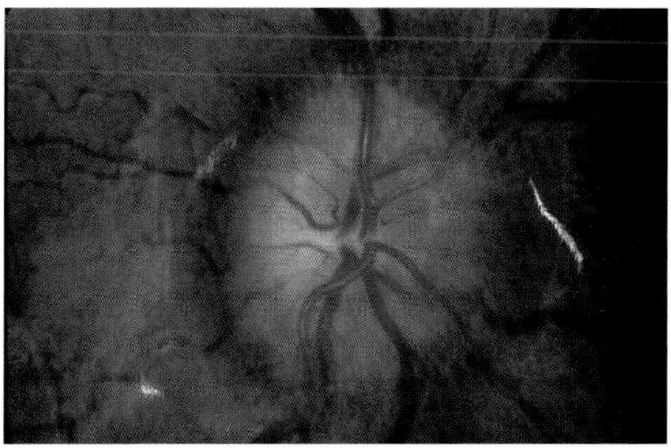

FIGURE 13.4.1 Optic neuritis with anterior swelling.

Etiology idiopathic, multiple sclerosis, postviral, granulomatous inflammation, syphilis, spread from contiguous sites of inflammation (meninges, sinus, orbit).

Presentation

- Symptoms: decreased vision; decreased color vision; ocular pain (90%), especially with eye movements; usually unilateral, but may be bilateral; flashes of light.
- Findings: most common under age 45 years; decreased visual acuity; afferent pupillary defect, if unilateral or asymmetric; decreased color vision; central or cecocentral field defect; swollen disc, or normal disc if retrobulbar optic neuritis. May have vitreous cells or sheathing of retinal venous sheathing. Visual acuity decreases until days 7 to 10 and then partially returns over months.

Differential Diagnosis AION (arteritic or nonarteritic), optic nerve infiltration (lymphoma, granulomatous, metastatic), papilledema, malignant hypertension, optic nerve compression from orbital tumor (optic nerve glioma), acute Leber's optic neuropathy, toxic or nutritional amblyopia.

Management

- Workup: perform complete ophthalmologic and neurologic examinations, including pupillary response and color testing. Check blood pressure. Check VDRL/FTA, ESR, CBC. Perform MRI to determine the presence and number of plaques and to rule out tumors. In children, etiology is usually postviral, and bilaterality is more common. Workup for meningitis if the patient is febrile, lethargic.
- Treatment: if a specific cause is found, treat the underlying disorder. If idiopathic or suspected multiple sclerosis, consider observation (see below). If no improvement, rule out tumor with MRI or CT. Consider diagnosis of anterior ischemic optic neuropathy. We recommend treatment for optic neuritis suspected to be caused by multiple sclerosis, which will be the case in over 60% of patients. IV corticosteroids lead to faster visual recovery and delayed onset of multiple sclerosis. Strongly consider treatment for plaques on MRI, previous episodes of neurologic symptoms, visual acuity of less than 20/200, bilateral affliction, and the occupational need for a quick recovery (e.g., a pilot). Consider IV methyl prednisolone (250 mg) over 30 minutes q6h for 12 doses, followed by oral prednisone (1 mg/kg/day) for 11 days and then tapered. (Do not treat initially with oral prednisone.)

13.4.2 Band Optic Atrophy

—atrophy of the optic nerve restricted to or approximating the horizontal meridian.

Etiology

pituitary adenoma, meningioma, craniopharyngioma, aneurysm, glioma, pituitary apoplexy.

Presentation

- Symptoms: none or a history of frequent accidents, falling down the stairs, bumping into doorways, and so on; may be associated with headache.

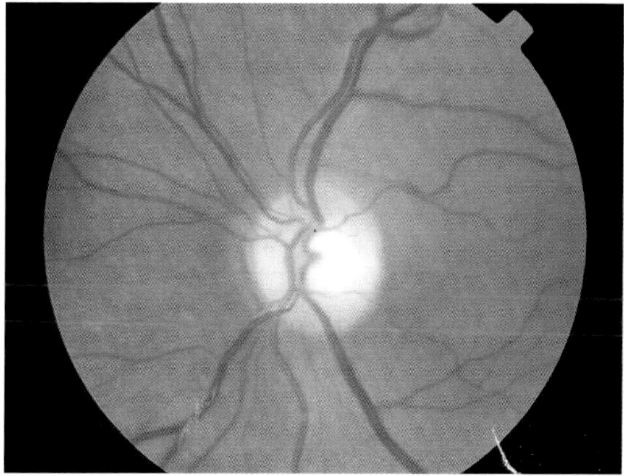

FIGURE 13.4.2 Band optic atrophy.

- Findings: usually associated with bitemporal hemianopsia from a chiasmal lesion.

Management

- Workup: full ophthalmic examination, including confrontational visual field testing; Humphrey, Goldmann, or other visual field test; MRI for evaluation of pituitary fossa; consider LP to rule out hemorrhage from tumor if headache is present.
- Treatment: as per etiology, referral to neurosurgery.

13.4.3 Papilledema—disc swelling specifically produced by elevated intracranial pressure.

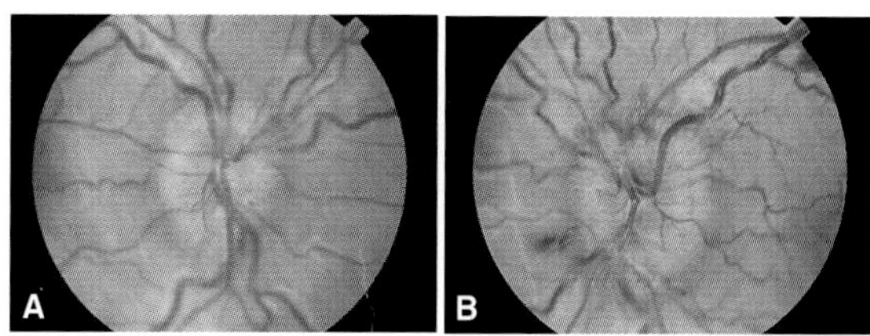

FIGURE 13.4.3a Papilledema: right eye.
FIGURE 13.4.3b Papilledema: left eye.

Etiology intracranial tumors, pseudotumor cerebri, subdural and epidural hematomas, subarachnoid hemorrhage, brain abscess, sagittal sinus thrombosis. Children: posterior fossa tumors.

Presentation

- Symptoms: headache, transient visual obscurations especially on bending over, nausea and/or vomiting, double vision, decreased vision (occasionally).
- Findings:

  Acute: bilateral asymmetric swelling of discs (takes 6 to 18 hours to develop), disc hyperemia with dilated capillaries, dilated veins, loss of spontaneous venous pulsations (though 20% of normals may have no spontaneous venous pulsations), flame-shaped hemorrhages at disc margin, enlarged blind spot, obscuration of blood vessels entering and leaving disc due to nerve fiber layer edema, soft exudates, concentric retinal folds (Paton's lines).

  Chronic: elevation of discs without hemorrhages ("champagne cork discs") (takes 6 weeks or more to develop), decrease of venous dilation, eventual atrophy of discs (pallor) with decrease of disc elevation.

Differential Diagnosis pseudopapilledema (see below), malignant hypertension, central retinal vein occlusion, ischemic optic neuropathy, optic neuritis, infiltration of optic nerve (lymphoma, granulomatous), orbital tumors (though rare to be bilateral).

Management

- Workup: check blood pressure. Consider emergent CT or MRI to rule out intracranial mass. Consider lumbar puncture and check opening pressure if CT or MRI is negative.
- Treatment: varied depending on cause of papilledema.

13.4.4. Pseudopapilledema—elevation of the optic disc not caused by elevated intracranial pressure.

Etiology optic nerve head drusen, hyperopia.

Presentation

- Symptoms: usually asymptomatic; may have associated nerve fiber layer visual field defect; visual loss only if secondary to optic nerve or macular insult (e.g., CRVO, disc infarction).
- Findings: absent central cup, anomalous vascular pattern (increased vessels, tortuosity, vascular loops, or vessels emanating from the center of disc), irregular disc margin; may have subretinal, intraretinal, or vitreous hemorrhages due to choroidal neovascularization; absence of hyperemia, exudates, cotton-wool spots, nerve fiber layer edema; presence of spontaneous venous pulsations (though 20% of normals do not have venous pulsations); may have visual field defects.

Differential Diagnosis see causes of papilledema, Section 13.4.3.

Management careful determination that this is not true papilledema. Ultrasound may detect buried drusen. FA (without injection) may show autofluorescence on drusen. Evaluate for pseudoxanthoma elasticum if optic nerve drusen.

13.4.5 Pseudotumor Cerebri—increased intracranial pressure with normal neuroimaging and normal CSF composition.

Etiology idiopathic, vitamin-A intoxication, tetracycline therapy, steroid withdrawal, naladixic acid, impairment of central venous drainage (i.e., intracranial venous sinus thrombosis), SLE.

Presentation

- Symptoms: headache, transient visual obscurations, blurred vision, nausea and/or vomiting, double vision.
- Findings: see Section 13.4.3; most common in obese, young females; may have sixth nerve palsy (unilateral or bilateral), intracranial pressure greater than 250 mm H_2O.

Differential Diagnosis see Section 13.4.3, Papilledema.

Management
- Workup: neuro-ophthalmologic examination, including motility and color plates. Quantify APD with neutral-density filters. Check blood pressure. Consider CT or MRI to rule out intracranial lesion, LP to check intracranial pressure, visual fields.
- Treatment: neurologist comanagement; weight loss.

  If asymptomatic: consider 6-month follow-ups or PRN. Treat for visual field loss, decreased acuity, or headache. Consider diuretics (acetazolamide, at least 1 g daily; sometimes furosemide). Discontinue any causative medications. Consider systemic steroids.

  If progressive visual field loss: consider surgery (optic nerve decompression or lumboperitoneal shunt).

13.4.6 Arteritic Ischemic Optic Neuropathy (Giant Cell Arteritis)—infarction of the optic disc, or rarely of the retrobulbar portion of the optic nerve; nearly always associated with GCA.

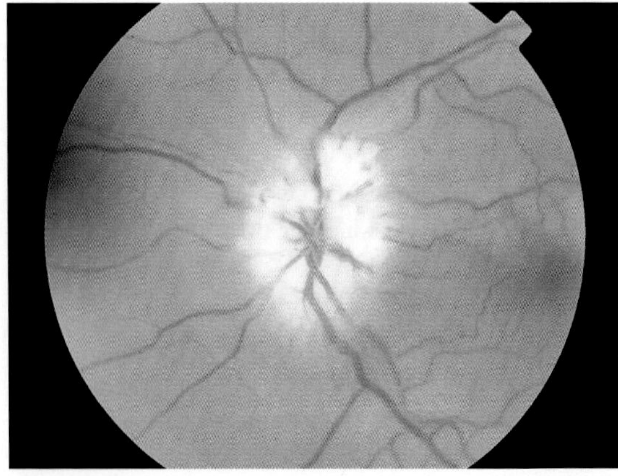

FIGURE 13.4.6 AION secondary to GCA.

Presentation

- Symptoms: acute, usually painless visual loss with altitudinal field defect. May be preceded by transient visual obscurations. Visual deficit is usually maximal at onset, but may progress for few days to several weeks. Associated headache, neck pain, jaw pain with chewing or talking (claudication), scalp tenderness, fevers, weight loss, and myalgias (shoulders, hips) may be present.
- Findings: age more than 55 years: optic disc edema. Visual field defect is usually in a nerve fiber bundle distribution. May have elevated ESR (90%) and palpable, tender temporal artery; usually coexistent anemia of chronic disease.

Differential Diagnosis

nonarteritic ischemic optic neuropathy, optic neuritis, orbital compressive lesion, CRVO, optic nerve infiltration (carcinomatous, granulomatous, lymphoreticular).

Management

- Workup: complete examination, including palpation of temporal arteries, ESR, CBC, ANA, FTA/VDRL. Check blood pressure and blood glucose. Consider temporal artery biopsy if GCA is suspected. If biopsy negative but a strong suspicion, biopsy the other side or treat empirically. FA may help distinguish the condition from a nonarteritic cause (choroidal ischemia present in arteritic AION).
- Treatment: systemic steroids (prednisone, 60 to 100 mg; or methylprednisolone, 250 mg IV q6h if within 48 hours, especially if visual loss is bilateral). Begin therapy as soon as the diagnosis is considered, because risk of contralateral involvement is 65%, usually within days. Taper steroids over months, following ESR, C-reactive protein, and symptoms.

13.4.7 Nonarteritic Ischemic Optic Neuropathy

—infarction of the optic disc, or rarely of the retrobulbar portion of the optic nerve, not related to GCA.

Etiology usually associated with hypertension. Other risk factors include small optic nerve and cup, smoking, hyperopia, diabetes, migraine, recent ophthalmic surgery.

Presentation

- Symptoms: acute, always painless, visual loss with frequently an altitudinal field defect. The visual deficit is usually maximal at onset, but may progress for few days to several weeks.
- Findings: age usually 45 to 65 years; small optic disc and cup; optic disc and nerve fiber layer edema may be sectoral; visual field defect usually in a nerve fiber bundle distribution; normal ESR. Later, optic atrophy and nerve fiber layer dropout develop rapidly. The second eye is at risk in 15 to 40% of cases. "Pseudo–Foster–Kennedy" is optic nerve atrophy on one side from previous AION and optic disc swelling on the currently affected side.

Differential Diagnosis arteritic ION, optic neuritis, orbital compressive lesion, CRVO, optic nerve infiltration (carcinomatous, granulomatous, lymphoreticular), hypotensive shock (bilateral, better prognosis).

Management

- Workup: rule out arteritic AION and examine ESR, CBC, ANA, FTA/VDRL, blood pressure, blood sugar. Carotid studies are not specifically indicated. FA shows delayed disc filling but normal choroidal filling, unlike in arteritic AION.
- Treatment: none. Optic nerve sheath fenestration has not been proven beneficial.

13.4.8 Toxic or Nutritional Optic Neuropathy

—optic neuropathy associated with poor nutrition, alcohol, and/or tobacco use; unknown if toxic effect of substances or associated vitamin deficiency.

Etiology tobacco and/or alcohol abuse; nutritional deficiency, specifically thiamine and vitamin B_{12}; toxic (methanol, ethambutol, chloramphenicol, isoniazid, rifampin, lead, digitalis).

Presentation

- Symptoms: slowly progressive, bilateral visual loss.
- Findings: mild to severe decreased visual acuity; always bilateral, though may be asymmetric; decreased color vision; bilateral central or centrocecal scotoma; optic disc normal early, but may become atrophic; splinter hemorrhages and tortuosity of small retinal vessels.

Differential Diagnosis

bilateral AION, hypotensive shock, radiation, infiltrative optic neuropathy, Leber's optic neuropathy, thyroid or other bilateral compressive optic neuropathy.

Management

- Workup: complete neuro-ophthalmologic examination, including color plates; visual field; detailed history of nutritional status, tobacco and/or alcohol abuse, medication and toxin exposure; CBC, serum vitamin B_{12} and folate levels;VDRL/FTA. Consider heavy-metal screen (lead levels).
- Treatment: cessation of alcohol and tobacco products; cessation of other possible toxic agents, as just listed; thiamine (100 mg PO bid), folate (1 mg PO qd), multivitamin daily (especially B complex). Refer to an internist for B_{12} deficiency.

13.4.9 Leber's Optic Neuropathy—hereditary optic neuropathy, transmitted by mitochondrial (maternal) DNA.

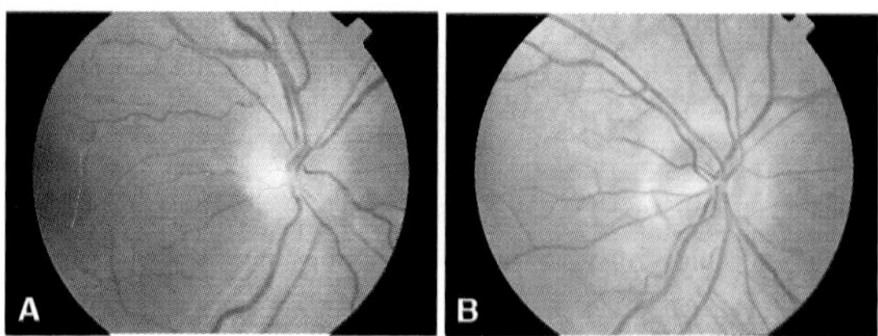

FIGURE 13.4.9a Leber's hereditary optic neuropathy.
FIGURE 13.4.9b Asymptomatic brother of patient; visual loss to count figures 2 months after the photograph.

Presentation

- Symptoms: usually young males (age 15 to 25 years); sudden, painless visual loss; may progress for weeks to months; bilateral, though onset may be delayed in the second eye.
- Findings: severe visual loss (20/200 to finger count); dense central or cecocentral scotoma; optic disc is normal or hyperemic and mildly swollen; abnormal telangiectatic vessels in the peripapillary nerve fiber level.

Differential Diagnosis

bilateral AION, hypotensive shock, radiation, infiltrative optic neuropathy, toxic or nutritional optic neuropathy, thyroid or other bilateral compressive optic neuropathy, optic neuritis.

Management

- Workup: rule out other causes of optic neuropathy (social history, family history). Consider CT or MRI to rule out compressive lesion. Consider a blood test (or muscle biopsy) to detect mitochondrial chromosomal mutations.
- Treatment: none is effective. Recommend genetic counseling.

13.4.10 Compressive Optic Neuropathy—optic neuropathy resulting from compression of the pregeniculate portion of the optic nerve.

Etiology

- Intraorbital: optic nerve meningioma, optic nerve glioma (age <20 years), thyroid orbitopathy, pseudotumor.
- Intracranial: meningioma, craniopharyngioma, pituitary tumors.

Presentation

- Symptoms: slowly progressive visual loss.
- Findings: decreased visual acuity, APD on the affected side, loss of color vision, possible proptosis and resistance to retropulsion if intraorbital lesion, normal or diffusely pale optic nerve, swollen optic nerve, optociliary shunt vessels (associated with meningiomas).

Differential Diagnosis AION, optic neuritis, infiltrative optic neuropathy, Leber's optic neuropathy, thyroid or other bilateral compressive optic neuropathy, optic neuritis.

Management

- Workup: CT or MRI of the orbit and brain. Any presumed optic neuritis that does not improve or AION that atypically progresses should be imaged to rule out compression.
- Treatment: see specific section by etiology.

13.4.11 Infiltrative Optic Neuropathy—optic neuropathy resulting from an infiltrative process of the optic nerve.

Etiology inflammatory (sarcoid), infectious (TB, cryptococcus, toxoplasmosis, toxocariasis, coccidiomycosis), leukemia, lymphoma, metastatic carcinoma.

Presentation

- Symptoms: slowly progressive visual loss.
- Findings: decreased visual acuity, from none to severe; characteristic grayish-white and swollen disc appearance; frequently bilateral.

Differential Diagnosis bilateral AION, hypotensive shock, radiation, infiltrative optic neuropathy, Leber's optic neuropathy, papilledema, pseudopapilledema, optic neuritis.

Management

- Workup: CT or MRI to evaluate optic nerves, systemic evaluation for the aforementioned processes.
- Treatment: depends on the underlying process.

13.4.12 Radiation Optic Neuropathy—optic neuropathy caused by radiation. The neuropathy is usually delayed by 2 years after standard doses of radiation but may be seen many years after treatment. The optic nerve may be affected by radiation to eye, orbit, sinus, nasopharynx, or brain.

Presentation Symptoms: decreased visual acuity, may be bilateral.

Differential Diagnosis bilateral AION, hypotensive shock, infiltrative optic neuropathy, Leber's optic neuropathy, thyroid or other bilateral compressive optic neuropathy, optic neuritis.

Management Workup: history of radiation to orbits or head, CT or MRI to evaluate the optic nerve, workup for other causes of optic neuropathy. No treatment available.

13.5 Tumors of Neural Origin

13.5.1 Optic Nerve Glioma—histologically benign, relatively circumscribed tumor of optic nerves and chiasm thought to be derived from mature, pilocytic astrocytes.

Presentation

- Symptoms: decreased visual acuity. Strabismus or nystagmus may be noted.
- Findings: age usually 2 to 6 years at presentation; relative afferent pupillary defect; optic atrophy or optic nerve swelling; mild proptosis if intraorbital (usually <3 mm, axial, nonpulsatile, not reducible); may have limited motility or nasal, downward global displacement. If a chiasmal lesion is present, nystagmus, hypothalmic and pituitary function disturbance, and symptoms of increased intracranial pressure (vomiting, lethargy, headache) may be present. Among children, 25 to 50% have neurofibromatosis with associated findings. Optic glioma in adults is extremely rare and is usually aggressive and fatal.

Differential Diagnosis other neoplasms (meningioma, lymphangioma, hemangioma, other neural tumors, rhabdomyosarcoma), acute ethmoiditis, hyperthyroidism, craniostenosis, retro-orbital hemorrhage secondary to trauma.

Management

- Workup: complete ophthalmic examination, including visual acuity, pupillary assessment, color plates, tonome-

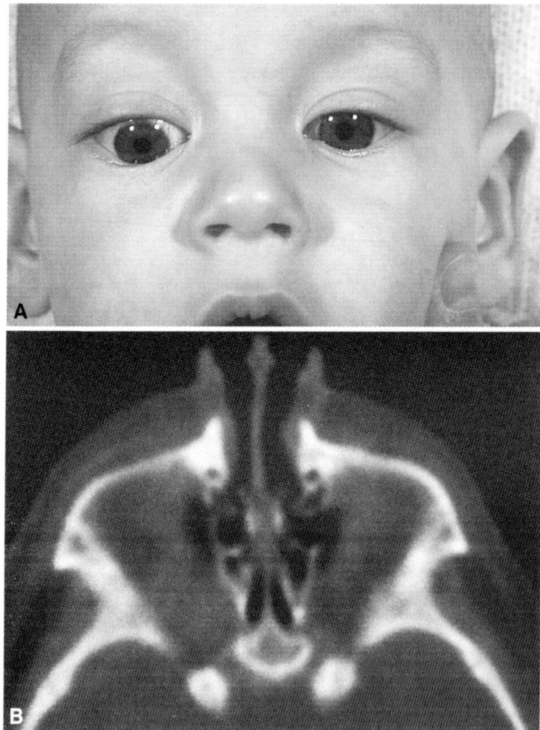

FIGURE 13.5.1a Inferior displacement of the globe in optic nerve glioma.
FIGURE 13.5.1b Enlarged optic nerve secondary to optic nerve glioma.

try, optic nerve evaluation. CT scan will show fusiform enlargement of optic nerve. Consider orbital ultrasound or MRI to define the lesion better.

- Treatment: observation—lesion may show spontaneous stabilization or regression. Consider radiation therapy or surgery for more aggressive tumors, but intervention has a high risk of visual loss or blindness.

13.5.2 Neurofibroma and Schwannoma—benign tumors derived from glial cells of peripheral nerves. Endoneural cells and axons may also be involved with neurofibromas. Schwannomas tend to be singular and encapsulated, whereas neurofibromas are more likely to be multiple, unencapsulated, and more likely to undergo malignant transformation.

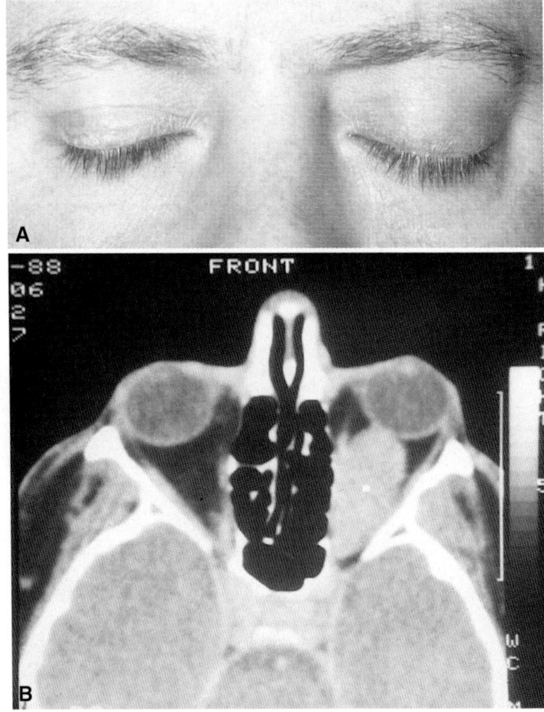

FIGURE 13.5.2a Proptosis due to a schwannoma.
FIGURE 13.5.2b Orbital space-occupying schwannoma.

Presentation

- Symptoms: "lump" around the eye if subcutaneous; if localized to the orbit, prominent eye or double or decreased vision.
- Findings: proptosis if orbital, but nodule if subcutaneous; wide age range but peak occurrence in fifth and sixth decades if not associated with neurofibromatosis.

  If associated with neurofibromatosis I (von Recklinghausen's disease): café au lait spots, pigmented skin lesions, multiple neurofibromas, Lisch nodules of iris, bone involvement and/or malformations.

If associated with neurofibromatosis II: bilateral acoustic neurofibromas. Café au lait spots and/or skin lesions are less common.

Differential Diagnosis lymphoma, other orbital tumors (including but not limited to meningioma, fibrous histiocytoma, hemangiopericytoma, hemangioma), metastatic disease, mucocele.

Management

- Workup: complete medical history (cancer, trauma); assessment of visual acuity, ocular movements, displacement; Hertel's exophthalmetry, tonometry, dilated examination, CT scan, MRI, or ultrasound (if an orbital lesion, usually a well-defined mass in superior orbit).
- Treatment: observation; surgical excision for cosmesis or for enlarging tumor with increasing visual signs or symptoms.

13.5.3 Meningioma

13.5.3 Meningioma—tumor arising from the arachnoid mater covering the CNS (including brain, spinal cord, optic nerve). May involve the optic nerve sheath primarily or, more commonly, extends secondarily into the orbit or optic nerve sheath from an intracranial lesion.

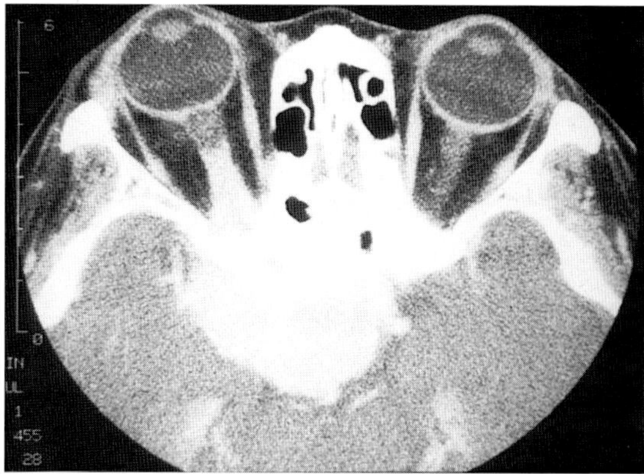

FIGURE 13.5.3 Optic nerve meningioma.

Presentation

- Symptoms:
  If optic nerve sheath involved: prominent eye, slow progressive loss of vision.
  If intracranial: may be asymptomatic until tumor very large.
- Findings: overall, 60% female; over 80% female with optic nerve sheath meningiomas. Patients are usually middle aged, but primary orbital meningiomas have a younger onset. Visual loss is painless and slow. Relative afferent pupillary defect and centrocecal scotoma may exist, as well as unilateral exophthalmos, optic atrophy, papilledema, optociliary shunt vessels. Tumor may be seen eroding into choroid if advanced. Strabismus or lid edema may be associated.

Differential Diagnosis

other intraorbital tumors, metastatic disease, mucocele, lymphoma.

Management

- Workup: complete ophthalmic examination including visual acuity, Hertel's exophthalmetry, pupillary response, confrontational fields, dilated examination, CT scan or MRI of head and orbits (tumor mass may be seen intracranially or enlargement of optic nerve often with "railroad track" appearance).
- Treatment:
  If primary intraorbital: usually observed every 3 to 6 months.
  If visual field progresses or there is visual loss: surgical excision is possible but leads to further visual loss.
  If intracranial involvement: refer to neurosurgeon.

13.6 Blepharospasm

13.6.1 Benign (Essential) Blepharospasm—bilateral, involuntary, intermittent or constant blinking caused by contraction of orbicularis oculi muscles.

Presentation

- Symptoms: excessive blinking, twitching, or closing of eyes.
- Findings: bilateral involvement (necessary for diagnosis but may begin as unilateral transiently); age 40 to 70 years at presentation; females more than males by 2 : 1; brows low, lower lids high. Other muscles (e.g., jaw, neck) may be involved in 75% of patients, but no other neurologic signs should be present. There is altered affect, and spasms disappear while asleep or during concentration.

Differential Diagnosis

hemifacial spasm, facial myokymia, trigeminal neuralgia, prior Bell's palsy (postparalytic spasm), Parkinson's disease, progressive supranuclear palsy, Huntington's disease, multiple sclerosis, stroke (bihemispheric), Tourette's syndrome, tardive dyskinesia.

Management

- Workup: assessment for other muscular involvement, presence of ocular irritation, other neurologic signs. Ensure that spasms are bilateral and disappear during sleep or activity, such as singing. Consider CT or MRI for any atypical presentation (for cerebellopontine angle tumor).
- Treatment: haloperidol, clonazepam, and other medications usually elicit a poor response. Botulinum toxin injection is usually successful. Rarely, consider selective facial nerve section or orbicularis myectomy.

13.6.2 Hemifacial Spasm—unilateral episodic spasm of muscles supplied by facial nerve (VII) caused by irritation of the nerve.

Presentation

- Symptoms: usually contracture of entire side of the face, often with closing of the ipsilateral eye.
- Findings: unilateral, involuntary tonic or clonic contraction of the facial muscles.

Differential Diagnosis

early essential blepharospasm, facial myokymia (see Benign Essential Blepharospasm, Section 13.6.1).

Management

- Workup: MRI of cerebellopontine angle to rule out mass lesion.
- Treatment: carbamazepine or baclofen may be helpful but usually elicit a poor response; botulinum toxin injection, surgical decompression of the facial nerve.

13.7 Myasthenia Gravis

chronic autoimmune disorder associated with reduced number of acetylcholine receptors at neuromuscular junctions resulting in weakness and fatiguability of muscles.

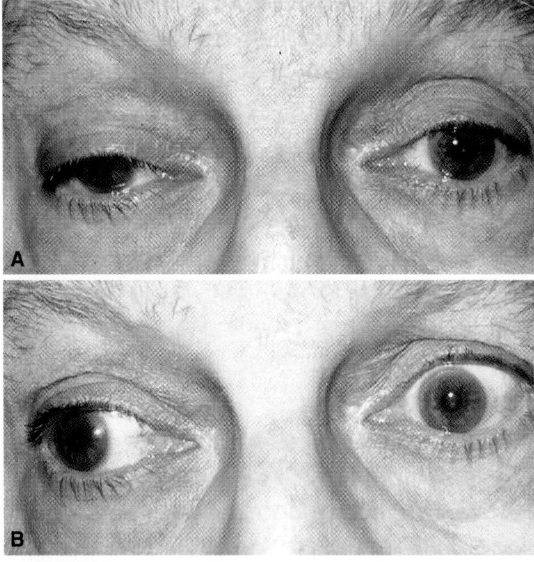

FIGURE 13.7a Myasthenia gravis with ptosis before Tensilon testing.
FIGURE 13.7b Elevation of eyelid after Tensilon testing.

Etiology antibodies to acetylcholine receptors.

Presentation

- Symptoms: droopy eyelids, diplopia worse as day progresses, improved with rest; often with weakness of other facial or ocular muscles, proximal limb muscles, or difficulty breathing and/or swallowing.

- Findings: variable ptosis and weakness of extraocular muscles, sometimes with weakness of other muscles; normal pupils. May imitate other single or combined extraocular muscle palsies or gaze palsies with the following signs: ptosis, extraocular muscle palsies, pseudo-gaze palsies, pseudoconvergence palsies, quiver movements, pseudo–internuclear ophthalmoplegia, lid twitch, orbicularis weakness, nystagmus. Variability and fatiguability are hallmarks of this disease.

Differential Diagnosis

Eaton-Lambert (paraneoplastic) syndrome; medication-induced myasthenia-like syndrome; CPEO; Kearns-Sayre syndrome; third, fourth, or sixth nerve palsy; Horner's syndrome; levator muscle dehiscence or disinsertion; Grave's orbitopathy; myotonic dystrophy.

Management

- Workup: do signs and symptoms fluctuate throughout day or with fatigue? Assess for worsening of symptoms, ptosis on sustained upgaze. Assess orbicularis function, proximal muscle strength, pupillary response, and swallowing.

  Sustained upgaze for 1 minute: Look for increased ptosis or diplopia indicating fatiguability.

  Sleep test: have the patient sleep or rest quietly for 20 minutes and then awake the patient and look for improvement of findings (suggestive of myasthenia).

  Check for serum antibodies for acetylcholine receptor (50% sensitivity). If positive, the tensilon test may be avoided.

  Tensilon test: 0.2 ml IV endrophonium chloride test dose, followed by 0.4 ml IV up to two times if necessary. Have atropine (0.5 mg IV) available for bradycardia or respiratory arrest. The endpoint is resolution of the findings.

Check thyroid function test results (increased association) and consider ANA and RF. Consider chest CT to rule out thymoma.

- Treatment:

  If mild: observe.

  If moderate: consider oral anticholinesterases (e.g., physostigmine, 60 mg PO qid), systemic steroids, immunosuppressives, thymectomy. Treat thyroid disease if present.

  If severe (i.e., compromised swallowing or breathing): hospitalization is warranted and consider plasmapharesis and supportive measures (e.g., respirator).

13.8 Eye Movement Disorders

13.8.1 Acquired Nystagmus—involuntary, rhythmic oscillatory ocular movements.

Etiology

tumor, stroke, trauma, multiple sclerosis, hemorrhage, toxic or metabolic disturbances (such as anticonvulsants, mood stabilizers, sedatives, including alcohol), Wernicke's encephalopathy, thiamine deficiency, acute labrynthitis, benign positional vertigo, peripheral vestibular disorder.

Presentation

- Symptoms: none if congenital or acquired before 8 years of age. Otherwise, environment may appear to move (oscillopsia) corresponding to nystagmus.
- Findings: pendular or jerk oscillatory movements horizontally, vertically, or torsionally.

  Pendular movements have approximately equal speeds with both phases of movement.

  Jerk movements have a slow phase in one direction, followed by a fast corrective movement back to the original position.

  Direction is named for the fast component. Differentiation between peripheral and central causes is important.

Central	Peripheral
May be purely vertical or torsional	Never purely vertical; may be mixed vertical and horizontal
Fixation has no effect	Fixation dampens
Pursuit and saccade abnormalities	Hearing loss or tinnitus common
Direction may change with direction of gaze	Direction does not change
	Amplitude increases on gaze toward fast component

- Specific types may indicate etiology:

  See-saw nystagmus: one eye rises and intorts while the other descends and extorts; usually secondary to chiasmal or third ventricle lesion with accompanying bitemporal hemianopsia. If the torsional component is absent or opposite, may be congenital in origin.

  Convergent–retraction nystagmus: on upgaze, eyes converge and retract into orbit. Seen in Parinaud's syndrome secondary to dorsal midbrain lesion or pineal gland tumor. Accompanied by limitation of upgaze, retraction of eyelids, dilated pupils that constrict to accommodation but not to light, and occasionally by optic nerve swelling.

  Gaze-evoked nystagmus: not present in primary gaze with increased nystagmus with gaze in the direction of the fast phase. Most commonly is physiologic, associated with gaze paresis (e.g., recovering from a third or sixth nerve palsy) or drug induced [(e.g., tranquilizers or anticonvulsants, especially Dilantin (phenytoin)].

  Upbeat nystagmus: fast component upward. If present in the primary position, it is secondary to a brainstem or cerebellar vermis lesion. If present only in upgaze, it is secondary to drug effect. It is nonspecific.

  Downbeat nystagmus: fast component downward. Finding localized to the cervicomedullary junction. Other causes include Arnold-Chiari malformation, alcohol, lithium or Dilantin (phenytoin) toxicity, Wernicke's encephalopathy.

Rebound nystagmus: a horizontal jerk nystagmus after eyes have returned from eccentric to primary gaze, lasting less than 1 minute. Type I is a gaze-evoked nystagmus that slows and reverses to jerk nystagmus toward the primary position with fatigue. Seen in cerebellar hemispheric degeneration secondary to alcohol abuse and other cerebellar disease.

Periodic alternating nystagmus: jerk movements in one direction for 1 to 1 ½ minutes with reversal to the other direction and so forth. Seen in congenital and acquired blindness or cervicomedullary junction lesions.

Vertigo present with nystagmus: etiologies include lesions of membranous labyrinth, eighth nerve, and vestibular nuclear complex, including Wallenberg's lateral medullary syndrome.

Differential Diagnosis

voluntary eye movements, dysmetria, flutter, opsoclonus, myoclonus, spasmus nutans, optic nerve glioma, superior oblique myokymia, myasthenia gravis (quiverlike movements), ocular bobbing.

Management

- Workup: assess whether oscillations were present in the first 3 months of life and whether null point, face turn, compensatory head movements, or oscillopsia are present. Inquire about family history of nystagmus and albinism. Complete an ophthalmic examination including careful examination of optic nerves and a visual field examination, if possible. Consider drug, toxic, or dietary screens and CT or MRI as indicated by the type of nystagmus.
- Treatment: treat the underlying etiology. Baclofen (15 to 80 mg/day in three divided doses) may be helpful.

Consider retrobulbar botulinum toxin in severe, disabling cases.

13.8.2 Congenital Nystagmus—oscillatory eye movements at birth or within the first 3 months of life.

Etiology idiopathic, albinism, aniridia, bilateral cataracts, Leber's congenital amaurosis, any decrease in afferent visual system function.

Presentation congenital nystagmus is associated with age of onset of 2 to 3 months and is associated with afferent visual system dysfunction in most cases. It usually begins with wide-swinging eye movements that decrease to small pendular movements by 4 to 6 months and that then convert to jerk nystagmus with a null point by 6 to 12 months. It is often associated with compensatory head movement (nodding or shaking) or face turn (to bring null point straight ahead). Movement is mostly horizontal, with decreased movement on convergence resulting in better reading than distance vision. Vertical movement is only rarely congenital; torsion may be seen on upgaze.

- *Latent nystagmus* is congenital nystagmus that occurs only when one eye is closed or occluded. It is a jerk nystagmus with slow phase toward the covered eye and is associated with lower visual acuity when each eye is tested individually. It may not present until much later in life.
- *Manifest latent nystagmus* occurs when suppression of one eye (usually due to strabismus) leads to spontaneous nystagmus. The suppression is analogous to covering the eye in latent nystagmus.
- *Monocular nystagmus* is small amplitude and associated with optic atrophy, decreased vision, and an APD. It is usually caused by a chiasmal glioma.
- *Spasmus nutans* is a benign, fine, rapid, bilateral but highly asymmetric nystagmus associated with head bobbing. It resolves by age 5 or 6 years. Since it may be

difficult to distinguish from monocular nystagmus, imaging is indicated.

Management

- Workup: determine the cause and treat appropriately. Any bilateral occlusive disease should be treated as soon as possible.
- Treatment: prism therapy may be used to stimulate convergence. Bilateral recession and resection may be helpful in congenital nystagmus to bring near point to center. Multiple recessions may also be used.

13.8.3 Gaze Palsies/Paresis—weakness or inability of conjugate or vergent movements of both eyes caused by deficits in the supranuclear pathways of the ocular motor system and not defects in individual muscles, nerves, or nuclei.

Etiology

any defect in the supranuclear pathways of the ocular motor system, including developmental anomaly, tumor, hemorrhage, stroke, demyelinating disease, infection, trauma, toxic effect. May be associated with psychosocial stress especially with spasm of near reflex.

Presentation

- Symptoms: inability to gaze in one or more directions. May be asymptomatic, but patients may complain of inappropriate glasses, double vision, blurring or difficulty with vision only with reading or only at distance
- Findings: lack of volitional gaze in one or more directions. Eyes will often move into defective gaze position in response to vestibulo-optic or oculocephalic (doll's eyes) maneuvers. May be a defect in saccadic, pursuit, or vergence movements.

  Horizontal: either PPRF or VI nerve nucleus is affected. If paresis cannot be overcome by doll's head or caloric maneuvers, it is a VI nuclear lesion.

  Vertical: see progressive supranuclear palsy.

Differential Diagnosis

myasthenia gravis, chronic progressive external ophthalmoplegia, optic nerve paresis, infiltrative or restrictive disease of extraocular muscles including thyroid orbitopathy and muscle entrapment, Parkinson's disease.

Management

- Workup: test ductions and versions in response to verbal commands (saccades) and in following a visual stimulus (pursuit). Test convergence. Attempt to move the patient's eyes in the direction of the gaze palsy by using oculocephalic or caloric maneuvers. Forced duction testing is necessary if the preceding do not succeed in moving eyes into the defective gaze position. Evaluate the patient for nystagmus and consider testing with optic kinetic stimulus. Consider MRI to assess the presence of the causative lesion; LP to assess the presence of RBCs, oligoclonal bands, and inflammatory cells; the Tensilon test and tests for neurosyphilis and thiamine deficiency. Assess whether the patient is taking central-acting medications or drugs (consider testing).
- Treatment: as per etiology with neurologic or neurosurgical consultation.

13.8.4 Internuclear Ophthalmoplegia—lag or inability to adduct the eye when attempting conjugate gaze movement in the opposite direction of the affected eye; associated with lesion of the ipsilateral medial longitudinal fasciculus between the VI and III nerve nuclei. If internuclear ophthalmoplegia is present with an ipsilateral VI nucleus or PPRF lesion, it is called a one-and-a-half syndrome (gaze paresis to the ipsilateral side and decreased contralateral gaze of the ipsilateral eye, leaving only abduction of the contralateral eye).

Etiology

multiple sclerosis, brainstem infarction (especially if the patient is older than 50 years).

Presentation

- Symptoms: binocular horizontal double vision or blurred vision that clears with closing one eye.
- Findings: adduction lag on conjugate gaze contralateral to the affected eye (worse with repeated movements into that field of gaze). Abduction nystagmus of the other eye is commonly associated but is not necessary

for the diagnosis. Less commonly, the patient has skew deviation or upbeat nystagmus; usually unilateral but may be bilateral, especially in multiple sclerosis ("wall-eyed").

Differential Diagnosis

myasthenia gravis, infiltrative or inflammatory orbital disease (usually nystagmus is absent).

Management

- Workup: assess the age of the patient and history of presence of other neurologic signs. Carefully examine ocular motility. Consider MRI of brainstem or midbrain and consider the tensilon test.
- Treatment: treat underlying disease (multiple sclerosis, CVA) with neurologic consultation.

13.8.5 Progressive Supranuclear Palsy—a degenerative disease affecting the supranuclear pathways of the optic motor system associated with neck and trunk rigidity, dementia, and dysarthria; also called Steele-Richardson-Olszewski syndrome.

Presentation

- Symptoms: difficulty walking downstairs, reading, eating food from dinner plate, and so on.
- Findings: initial slowing and then cessation of downward saccades (downgaze), followed by defects in upward saccades (upgaze), horizontal saccades, and then pursuit. Oculocephalic reflexes remain intact until late in the disease but may be hard to assess secondary to associated neck and trunk rigidity. Apraxia of lid opening and decreased blinking may be present. Dementia, dystonia, and dysarthria may develop. Age of onset is the 50s and 60s. The disease is unfortunately progressive, with average survival only 8 to 10 years. In middle-aged men, it is associated with Whipple's disease. *Oculogyric crisis* is a tonic deviation of the eyes, usually upward, due to postencephalic Parkinson's disease or phenothiazine toxicity (see also Parinaud's syndrome, Section 13.8.6).

Differential Diagnosis Parkinson's disease, chronic progressive external ophthalmoplegia, myasthenia gravis, brainstem lesions, cavernous sinus syndrome.

Management workup is similar to that for other gaze palsies. In middle-aged men, work up for Whipple's disease (i.e., jejunal biopsy). No effective treatment.

13.8.6 Parinaud's Syndrome

—lesion of the periaqueductal gray matter of the dorsal midbrain with resultant loss or decrease in upward saccades.

Etiology pineal gland tumor or other neoplasm affecting the dorsal midbrain, stroke, hydrocephalus, hemorrhage, infection (including encephalitis, neurosyphilis), multiple sclerosis, trauma, Wernicke's syndrome.

Presentation

- Symptoms: lid retraction, binocular diplopia, headache, transient obscurations of vision.
- Findings: slowed or absent upward saccades, middilated pupil which constricts to accommodation, convergence–retraction nystagmus (see the section on acquired nystagmus), papilledema secondary to obstruction of sylvian aqueduct, Collier's sign (lid retraction in the primary position, which increases with upgaze). Loss of upward pursuit and downward saccades will often follow. Skew deviation and fourth cranial nerve palsy can also be found late.

Differential Diagnosis thyroid orbitopathy, cavernous sinus syndrome, myasthenia gravis.

Management

- Workup: as with other gaze palsies. MRI to assess midbrain structures. LP to assess intracranial pressure.

- Treatment: as per etiology. Neurologic or neurosurgical consult as needed.

13.8.7 Chronic Progressive External Ophthalmoplegia (CPEO)—gradual, progressive EOM weakness and ptosis.

Presentation

- Symptoms: droopy lids, occasional diplopia.
- Findings: partial to complete EOM weakness, ptosis; occasional family history (maternal mitochondrial inheritance); weak orbicularis muscles; no restriction of forced ductions; normal pupil responses. Selected syndromes:

  Kearns-Sayre syndrome: CPEO with retinal pigment epithelial degeneration, onset before age 20, and one or more of the following: cardiac conduction abnormality, increased CSF protein (>100 mg/dl), cerebellar dysfunction. Muscle biopsy shows characteristic "ragged red fibers." Other associations include short stature, hearing loss, mental retardation, vestibular dysfunction, diabetes.

  Abetalipoproteinemia (Bassen-Kornzweig): associated retinitis pigmentosa and lipid abnormalities.

  Presumed mitochondrial: facial, bulbar, and limb myopathy, ataxia, spasticity, maternal inheritance.

  Oculopharyngeal dystrophy: autosomal dominant, dysphagia, onset in 50s or 60s, temporalis wasting, French-Canadian descent.

  Myotonic dystrophy: autosomal dominant, retinal pigment epitheliopathy, abnormal EMG, Christmas tree cataract, frontal balding.

  Refsum's disease: retinitis pigmentosa, polyneuropathy, enlarged corneal nerves.

Differential Diagnosis

multiple cranial neuropathies (e.g., cavernous sinus thrombosis), myasthenia gravis, thyroid orbitopathy.

Management Workup: careful history (family history, age of onset, rate of progression), tensilon test (see myasthenia gravis). Look for retinal pigment epithelial changes.

- For Kearns-Sayre syndromes: EMG, lumbar puncture for CSF protein, EKG.
- For Refsum's disease: serum phytanic acid level.
- For abetalipoproteinemia: lipoprotein electrophoresis and blood smear.

Chapter 14
OPHTHALMIC PHARMACOLOGY

Scott Anagnoste, Michael B. Starr

14.1 ANTIBIOTICS

14.1.1 Bacitracin

Brand Name AK-Tracin.

Solution/ Ointment ointment, 500 U/g.

Mechanism bactericidal against gram-positive organisms by interfering with cell wall synthesis.

Warnings pregnancy category C.

14.1.2 Chloramphenicol

Brand Names AK-Chlor, Chloromycetin, Chloroptic, Ocu-Chlor.

Solution/ Ointment 0.5% solution, 1% ointment.

Mechanism bacteriostatic by inhibition of protein synthesis.

Susceptible Organisms *Staphylococcus aureus*, streptococci, *Escherichia coli*, *Haemophilus influenzae*, *Klebsiella*, *Moraxella*, *Neisseria*.

Indications serious infections in which less potentially dangerous drugs cannot be used.

Warnings aplastic anemia and death have been reported after topical administration.

Preservatives none.

14.1.3 Ciprofloxacin

Brand Name Ciloxan.

Solution/ Ointment 0.3% solution; ointment not yet available but expected.

Mechanism fluoroquinolone—bactericidal by interference with the enzyme DNA gyrase.

Susceptible Organisms broad spectrum; poor coverage of *Pseudomonas cepacia, Pseudomonas maltophilia, Bacteroides, Clostridium,* and most anaerobes and variable activity against streptococcal species.

Warnings pregnancy category C (maternal weight loss and increased incidence of abortion in animal studies). Safety not established in patients less than 1 year old; 17% rate of crystalline precipitate formation on corneal surface.

Preservative benzalkonium chloride.

Dosage

- Corneal ulcer: q15min for 6 hours, q30min for the next 18 hours, q1h for the following 24 hours, and then q4h (depending on severity).
- Bacterial conjunctivitis: q2h while awake for 2 days and then q4h for 5 days.

14.1.4 Erythromycin

Brand Names AK-Mycin, Ilotycin.

Solution/ Ointment 0.5% ointment.

Mechanism inhibits bacterial protein synthesis by binding to the 50S ribosomal subunit.

Susceptible Organisms most gram-positive and some gram-negative bacteria, actinomycetes, mycoplasmas, spirochetes, chlamydiae, rickettsiae.

Warnings pregnancy category B.

14.1.5 Gentamicin

Brand Names Garamycin, Genoptic, Gentacidin, Gentak.

Solution/ Ointment 0.3% solution, 0.3% ointment.

Mechanism aminoglycoside.

Susceptible Organisms *S. aureus, Staphylococcus epidermidis, Enterobacter, E. coli, H. influenzae, Klebsiella, Neisseria gonorrhoeae, Pseudomonas aeruginosa, Serratia marcescens.*

Contraindications not for intraocular use.

Warnings pregnancy category C (harmful effects in study animals; use only if benefits outweigh risks). Ocular surface toxicity with prolonged use.

Preservatives

- Solution: benzalkonium chloride.
- Ointment: methylparaben, propylparaben.

14.1.6 Norfloxacin

Brand Name Chibroxin.

Solution/ Ointment 0.3% solution.

Mechanism fluoroquinolone—bactericidal by inhibiting bacterial DNA gyrase.

Susceptible Organisms *S. aureus, S. epidermidis,* variable activity against streptococcal species, *Acinetobacter calcoaceticus, Aeromonas hydrophila, H. influenzae, Proteus mirabilis, P. aeruginosa, S. marcescens.*

Indications conjunctivitis caused by the above organisms.

Warnings pregnancy category C.

Preservative benzalkonium chloride.

14.1.7 Ofloxacin

Brand Name Ocuflox.

Solution/ Ointment 0.3% solution.

Mechanism fluoroquinolone—bactericidal by inhibition of bacterial DNA gyrase.

Susceptible Organisms *S. aureus, S. epidermidis, S. pneumoniae, Enterobacter cloacae, H. influenzae, P. mirabilis, P. aeruginosa.*

Indications conjunctivitis, corneal ulcer.

Warnings pregnancy category C.

Preservative benzalkonium chloride.

14.1.8 Sulfacetamide

Brand Names AK-Sulf, Bleph-10, Cetamide, Isopto Cetamide, Ophthacet, Sodium Sulamyd, Sulf-10.

Solution/ Ointment 10%, 15%, 30% solution; 10% ointment.

Mechanism bacteriostatic by restriction of synthesis of folic acid.

Susceptible Organisms *E. coli, S. aureus* (many strains resistant), streptococci, *H. influenzae, Klebsiella, Enterobacter.*

Warnings pregnancy category C.

Preservatives
- Solution: benzalkonium chloride.
- Ointment: phenylmercuric acetate.

14.1.9 Sulfisoxazole

Brand Name Gantrisin.

Solution/ Ointment 4% solution, 4% ointment.

Mechanism bacteriostatic by restriction of synthesis of folic acid.

Susceptible Organisms *E. coli, S. aureus* (many strains resistant), streptococci, *H. influenzae, Klebsiella, Enterobacter.*

Warnings pregnancy category C.

Preservatives
- Solution: benzalkonium chloride.
- Ointment: phenylmercuric acetate.

14.1.10 Tobramycin

Brand Names Defy, Tobrex, AKTOB.

Solution/ Ointment 0.3% solution, 0.3% ointment.

Mechanism aminoglycoside.

Susceptible Organisms staphylococci, variable activity against streptococci, *P. aeruginosa, Enterobacter, E. coli, Klebsiella, Morganella, H. influenzae, Haemophilus aegyptus, Moraxella,* some *Neisseria.*

Contraindications hypersensitivity.

Warnings pregnancy category B (no evidence of harm to fetus in animals but no human studies).

Preservatives
- Solution: benzalkonium chloride.
- Ointment: chlorobutanol.

14.1.11 Polymyxin B–Bacitracin

Brand Name AK-Poly-Bac.

Solution/ Ointment 10,000 U of polymyxin B and 500 U of bacitracin per gram.

14.1.12 Polymyxin B–Neomycin–Bacitracin

Brand Names AK-Spore, Neosporin.

Solution/ Ointment 10,000 U of polymyxin B, 3.5 mg of neomycin, and 400 U of bacitracin per gram.

Mechanism
- Polymyxin B: bactericidal by interference with cell wall synthesis.
- Neomycin: interferes with bacterial protein synthesis.

Susceptible Organisms *Proteus, Klebsiella, S. aureus, E. coli, H. influenzae, P. aeruginosa, diphtheria bacilli.*

Contraindications hypersensitivity.

Warnings neomycin can cause cutaneous sensitization.

Preservatives none.

Size Available 3.5 g.

14.1.13 Polymyxin B–Neomycin–Gramicidin

Brand Names AK-Spore, Neosporin.

Solution/ Ointment 10,000 U of polymyxin B, 1.75 mg of neomycin, and 0.025 mg of gramicidin per milliliter.

Mechanism bactericidal by interference with cell wall synthesis.

Susceptible Organisms *Proteus, Klebsiella, S. aureus, E. coli, H. influenzae, P. aeruginosa, diphtheria bacilli.*

Contraindications hypersensitivity.

Warnings neomycin can cause cutaneous sensitization.

Preservatives alcohol, thimerosal.

Sizes Available 2 ml, 10 ml.

14.1.14 Polymyxin B–Oxytetracycline

Brand Names Terramycin, Terak.

Solution/ Ointment 10,000 U of polymyxin B and 5 mg of oxytetracycline per gram.

Susceptible Organisms gram-positive and gram-negative bacteria, rickettsiae, spirochetes. Particularly effective against *P. aeruginosa* and Koch-Weeks bacillus.

Contraindications hypersensitivity.

Size Available 3.5 g.

Dosage Frequency bid to qid.

14.1.15 Polymyxin B–Trimethoprim

Brand Name Polytrim.

Solution/ Ointment 10,000 U of polymyxin B and 1 mg of trimethoprim per milliliter.

Mechanism

- Trimethoprim: inhibits dihydrofolate reductase, preventing synthesis of tetrahydrofolic acid from dihydrofolic acid.

- Polymyxin B: increases cell membrane permeability by interacting with the phospholipid component.

Susceptible Organisms *S. aureus, S. pneumoniae, Streptococcus viridans, H. influenzae,* and possibly *P. aeruginosa.*

Warnings pregnancy category C.

Preservative benzalkonium chloride.

Size Available 10 ml.

14.2 Fortified Antibiotics

14.2.1 Cefazolin

Brand Names Ancef, Kefzol.

Solution 50 mg/ml; add 10 ml of artificial tears to 500-mg sterile vial (refrigerate).

Mechanism first-generation cephalosporin—bactericidal due to damage to cell wall.

Susceptible Organisms gram-positive cocci and bacilli.

Indications susceptible corneal ulcers and infectious scleritis.

Warnings epithelial toxicity with prolonged use.

Dosage Frequency see Section 5.1.4, Bacterial Corneal Ulcer.

14.2.2 Tobramycin

Brand Name Nebcin.

Solution 14 mg/ml; use standard ophthalmic preparation 5-ml bottle (0.3%) and sterilely add 2 ml of parenteral solution, 40 mg/ml (refrigerate).

Mechanism aminoglycoside.

Susceptible Organisms gram-negative bacilli, including *P. aeruginosa*.

Indications susceptible corneal ulcers and infectious scleritis.

Warnings epithelial toxicity.

Dosage Frequency see Section 5.1.4, Bacterial Corneal Ulcer.

14.2.3 Vancomycin

Brand Name Vancocin.

Solution 25 to 50 mg/ml; add 10 to 20 ml of artificial tears to 500-mg sterile vial.

Mechanism bactericidal due to damage to cell wall.

Susceptible Organisms gram-positive cocci and bacilli.

Indications susceptible corneal ulcers and infectious scleritis.

Warnings epithelial toxicity with prolonged use.

Dosage Frequency see Section 5.1.4, Bacterial Corneal Ulcer.

14.3 Intravitreal Antibiotics and Endophthalmitis

see Chapter 10, Endophthalmitis.

14.4 Antivirals

14.4.1 Idoxuridine

Brand Name Herplex.

Solution/ Ointment 0.1% solution.

Mechanism thymidine analogue, inhibitor of thymidine kinase.

Susceptible Organisms Herpes simplex virus.

Indications Herpes simplex keratitis.

Warnings pregnancy category C. Should not be used concomitantly with boric acid.

Preservative benzalkonium chloride.

Size Available 15 ml.

Dosage Frequency either (1) qh while awake and q2h at night or (2) one drop every minute for 5 minutes, repeated q4h.

14.4.2 Vidarabine

Brand Name Vira-A.

Solution/ Ointment 3.0% ointment.

Mechanism purine nucleoside believed to interfere in an early step in viral DNA synthesis.

Susceptible Organisms herpes simplex virus 1 and 2, herpes zoster virus.

Indications keratoconjunctivitis and keratitis due to herpes simplex virus.

Warnings pregnancy category C.

Size Available 3.5 g.

Dosage Frequency 5 times a day at 3-hour intervals.

14.4.3 Trifluridine

Brand Name Viroptic.

Solution/ Ointment 1.0% solution.

Mechanism fluorinated pyrimidine, inhibitor of thymidine kinase.

Susceptible Organisms herpes simplex virus 1 and 2, vaccinia virus.

Indications keratoconjunctivitis and keratitis due to herpes simplex virus.

Warnings pregnancy category C.

Preservative thimerosal.

Size Available 7.5 ml.

Dosage Frequency 9 times a day.

14.4.4 Acyclovir

Brand Name Zovirax.

Solution/ Ointment 5% ointment, 200-mg capsules.

Mechanism fluorinated pyrimidine, inhibitor of viral DNA synthesis.

Susceptible Organisms herpesviruses.

Indications herpes simplex and herpes zoster (treatment and prophylaxis).

Dosage

- Mucocutaneous lesions: ointment tid.
- Herpes zoster: 800 mg 5 times a day.
- Herpes simplex prophylaxis: 400 mg bid.

14.4.5 Ganciclovir

Brand Name Cytovene.

Solution/ Ointment 500-mg vials, intravitreal implant, tablets.

Mechanism nucleoside analogue, inhibitor of viral DNA synthesis.

Susceptible Organisms herpesviruses (especially cytomegalovirus).

Indications cytomegalovirus retinitis.

Warnings granulocytopenia, thrombocytopenia, pregnancy category C, caution in decreased renal function.

Dosage 5 to 10 mg/kg/day, 2 doses per day for 14 to 21 days; then 5 mg/kg daily for maintenance.

14.4.6 Foscarnet

Brand Name Foscavir.

Solution/ Ointment solution, 24 mg/ml.

Mechanism inhibits viral DNA polymerases and reverse transcriptases.

Susceptible Organisms herpesviruses (especially cytomegalovirus).

Indications cytomegalovirus retinitis.

Warnings renal toxicity in most patients, altered electrolytes and seizures, anemia, pregnancy category C.

Dosage 60 mg/kg q8h for 14 to 21 days; then 90 to 120 mg/kg daily for maintenance. Adjust for renal function.

14.5 Antifungals

14.5.1 Natamycin

Brand Name Natacyn.

Solution/ Ointment 5% solution.

Mechanism polyene that binds to sterol of the fungal cell membrane, increasing permeability.

Susceptible Organisms *Candida, Aspergillus, Cephalosporium, Fusarium, Penicillium.*

Warnings pregnancy category C.

Preservative benzalkonium chloride.

Size Available 15 ml.

Dosage Frequency initially q 1 to 2h; gradual reduction in frequency every 4 to 7 days for the next 14 to 21 days.

14.5.2 Amphotericin B

Brand Name Fungizone.

Solution/ Ointment 50-mg vials; topically prepare 2 mg/ml in distilled water, or 0.15%.

Mechanism polyene that binds to sterol of the fungal cell membrane, increasing permeability.

Susceptible Organisms *Candida, Aspergillus, Cephalosporium, Fusarium, Penicillium.*

Warnings pregnancy category C, very toxic subconjunctivally, epithelial toxicity.

Dosage Frequency see Section 5.1.6, Fungal Keratitis.

14.5.3 Flucytosine

Brand Name Ancobon.

Solution/ Ointment 250 to 500-mg capsules; 250 mg in 25 ml of distilled water makes 1% solution.

Mechanism pyrimidine—blocks thymidine synthesis.

Susceptible Organisms *Candida,* few strains of *Aspergillus, Penicillium.*

Warnings renal toxicity, marrow suppression, epithelial toxicity topically.

Dosage Frequency

- Oral: 150 mg/kg/day.
- Topically up to q1h. See Section 5.1.6, Fungal Keratitis.

14.5.4 Miconazole

Brand Name Monistat IV.

Solution/ Ointment vials 10 mg/ml (1%); topical concentration also.

Mechanism imidazole—blocks fungal lipid synthesis.

Susceptible Organisms *Candida, Aspergillus, Cephalosporium, Fusarium, Penicillium.*

Warnings Stevens-Johnson syndrome, epithelial toxicity topically.

Dosage Frequency topical. See Section 5.1.6, Fungal Keratitis.

14.5.5 Fluconazole

Brand Name Diflucan.

Solution/ Ointment tablets, 50, 100, and 200 mg; vials (IV), 2 mg/ml (2%); topical concentration also.

Mechanism imidazole—blocks fungal lipid synthesis.

Susceptible Organisms *Candida, Aspergillus, Cephalosporium, Fusarium, Penicillium.*

Warnings

- Oral: hepatic toxicity, rash, seizures, leukopenia, hypokalemia, GI upset, Stevens-Johnson syndrome.
- Topical: epithelial toxicity.

Dosage Frequency topical. See Section 5.1.6, Fungal Keratitis.

14.6 Antiparasitics

see Section 5.1.5, *Acanthamoeba*.

14.7 Steroids

14.7.1 Dexamethasone

Brand Name Decadron Phosphate 0.1%.

Contraindications acute herpetic keratitis, fungal infection, vaccinia, varicella and most other viral keratoconjunctivitis, ocular manifestations of tuberculosis.

Warnings can cause increased intraocular pressure. Can worsen thinning disorders of the sclera or cornea. Pregnancy category C (teratogenic in mice).

Preservatives benzalkonium chloride, phenylethanol, sodium bisulfite.

Size Available 5 ml.

14.7.2 Medrysone

Brand Name HMS.

Solution/ Ointment 1% solution.

Mechanism synthetic corticosteroid.

Indications allergic conjunctivitis, vernal conjunctivitis, episcleritis, epinephrine sensitivity.

Contraindications herpes simplex, ocular tuberculosis, ocular fungal disease.

Warnings pregnancy category C.

Preservative benzalkonium chloride.

Sizes Available 5 ml, 10 ml.

Dosage Frequency up to every 4 hours.

14.7.3 Prednisolone Acetate

Brand Names Econopred 0.125%, Econopred Plus 1% Suspension, Pred Forte 1%.

Indications inflammation, surface or intraocular.

Contraindications acute herpetic keratitis, fungal infection, vaccinia, varicella and most other viral keratoconjunctivitis, ocular manifestations of tuberculosis.

Warnings can cause increased intraocular pressure. Can worsen thinning disorders of the sclera or cornea. Pregnancy category C (teratogenic in mice).

Sizes Available 5 ml, 10 ml.

Preservative benzalkonium chloride.

14.7.4 Prednisolone Sodium Phosphate

Brand Name AK-Pred. Inflammase Forte.

Solution/ Ointment 0.125%, 1%.

Indications inflammation, surface or intraocular.

Contraindications acute herpetic keratitis, fungal infection, vaccinia, varicella and most other viral keratoconjunctivitis, ocular manifestations of tuberculosis.

Warnings can cause increased intraocular pressure. Can worsen thinning disorders of the sclera or cornea. Pregnancy category C (teratogenic in mice).

Preservative benzalkonium chloride.

Sizes Available 5 ml, 10 ml.

Dosage Frequency qid.

14.7.5 Fluorometholone

Brand Names Flarex, FML.

Solution/ Ointment
- Solution: Flarex 0.1%, FML 0.1%, FML Forte 0.25%.
- Ointment: FML 0.1%.

Indications inflammation.

Contraindications acute herpetic keratitis, fungal infection, vaccinia, varicella and most other viral keratoconjunctivitis, ocular manifestations of tuberculosis.

Warnings can cause increased intraocular pressure. Can worsen thinning disorders of the sclera or cornea. Pregnancy category C (teratogenic in mice).

Preservative benzalkonium chloride.

Sizes Available 2.5 ml, 5 ml, 10 ml.

Dosage Frequency qid.

14.7.6 Rimexolone

Brand Name Vexol 1%.

Indications equivalent anti-inflammatory action to 1% prednisolone with intraocular pressure rise similar to fluorometholone.

Contraindications acute herpetic keratitis, fungal infection, vaccinia, varicella and most other viral keratoconjunctivitis, ocular manifestations of tuberculosis.

Warnings can cause increased intraocular pressure. Can worsen thinning disorders of the sclera or cornea. Pregnancy category C (teratogenic in rabbits).

Preservative benzalkonium chloride.

Sizes Available 2.5 ml, 5 ml, 10 ml.

Dosage Frequency qh to qid.

14.8 Antibiotic–Steroid Combinations

14.8.1 Tobramycin–Dexamethasone

Brand Name Tobradex.

Solution/ Ointment suspension and ointment: 0.3% tobramycin, 0.1% dexamethasone.

Mechanism aminoglycoside and steroid.

Susceptible Organisms see Tobramycin, Section 14.1.10.

Contraindications acute herpetic keratitis, fungal infection, vaccinia, varicella and most other viral keratoconjunctivitis, ocular manifestations of tuberculosis.

Warnings can cause increased intraocular pressure. Can worsen thinning disorders of the sclera or cornea. Pregnancy category C (teratogenic in mice).

Preservatives
- Suspension: benzalkonium chloride.
- Ointment: chlorobutanol.

Sizes Available
- Suspension: 2.5 ml, 5 ml.
- Ointment: 3.5 g.

Dosage Frequency usually q 4 to 6h.

14.8.2 Neomycin–Polymyxin B–Dexamethasone

Brand Name Maxitrol.

Solution/ Ointment suspension and ointment: 3.5 mg of neomycin, 10,000 U of polymyxin B, and 0.1% dexamethasone.

Susceptible Organisms see Neomycin–Polymyxin B.

Contraindications acute herpetic keratitis, fungal infection, vaccinia, varicella and most other viral keratoconjunctivitis, ocular manifestations of tuberculosis.

Warnings can cause increased intraocular pressure. Can worsen thinning disorders of the sclera or cornea. Not studied in pregnancy.

Preservatives
- Suspension: benzalkonium chloride.
- Ointment: methylparaben, propylparaben.

Sizes Available
- Suspension: 5 ml.
- Ointment: 3.5 g.

Dosage Frequency usually q 4 to 6h.

14.8.3 Neomycin–Polymyxin B–Prednisolone Acetate

Brand Name Polypred.

Solution/ Ointment prednisolone acetate 0.5%, neomycin 0.35%, and 10,000 U of polymyxin B per milliliter.

Contraindications acute herpetic keratitis, fungal infection, vaccinia, varicella and most other viral keratoconjunctivitis, ocular manifestations of tuberculosis.

Warnings can cause increased intraocular pressure. Can worsen thinning disorders of the sclera or cornea. Not studied in pregnancy.

Preservative thimerosal.

Sizes Available 5 ml, 10 ml.

Dosage Frequency usually q 3 to 4h.

14.8.4 Sulfacetamide–Prednisolone Acetate

Brand Names Blephamide,Vasocidin.

Solution/ Ointment prednisolone acetate, 0.2%, sulfacetamide 10%.

Contraindications acute herpetic keratitis, fungal infection, vaccinia, varicella and most other viral keratoconjunctivitis, ocular manifestations of tuberculosis.

Warnings can cause increased intraocular pressure. Can worsen thinning disorders of the sclera or cornea. Pregnancy category C.

Preservatives

- Solution: benzalkonium chloride.
- Ointment: phenylmercuric acetate.

Sizes Available

- Solution: 2.5 ml, 5 ml, 10 ml.
- Ointment: 3.5 g.

Dosage Frequency usually qid.

14.8.5 Sulfacetamide–Prednisolone

Brand Name AK-Cide.

Solution/ Ointment 5 mg of prednisolone acetate and 100 mg of sulfacetamide per gram of ointment or milliliter of solution.

Susceptible Organisms *S. aureus, S. pneumoniae, S. viridans, Pseudomonas, H. influenzae, Klebsiella, E. coli, Enterobacter.*

Indications inflammatory conditions with risk of infection.

Contraindications hypersensitivity.

Warnings Stevens-Johnson syndrome reported.

Preservatives
- Solution: phenylethyl alcohol, benzalkonium chloride.
- Ointment: methylparaben, propylparaben.

Sizes Available
- Ointment: 3.5 g.
- Solution: 5 ml.

Dosage Frequency tid to qid.

14.8.6 Neomycin–Polymyxin B–Dexamethasone

Brand Name AK-Trol.

Solution/ Ointment 3.5 mg of neomycin, 10,000 U of polymyxin B, and 0.1% dexamethasone per gram of ointment or milliliter of solution.

Susceptible Organisms *S. aureus, Neisseria, Pseudomonas, H. influenzae, Klebsiella, E. coli, Enterobacter.*

Indications inflammatory conditions with risk of infection.

Contraindications as with all steroids, hypersensitivity.

Warnings can raise intraocular pressure.

Preservatives
- Solution: benzalkonium chloride.
- Ointment: methylparaben, propylparaben.

Sizes Available
- Ointment: 3.5 g.
- Solution: 5 ml.

Dosage Frequency q1h to qid.

14.9 Decongestants

14.9.1 Naphazoline

Brand Names AK-Con, Albalon, Clear Eyes, Degest 2, Naphcon, Opcon, Vasoclear, Vasocon.

Solution/ Ointment up to 0.1% solution.

Mechanism vasoconstrictor—imidazoline sympathomimetic.

Indications temporary relief of ocular irritation.

Warnings pregnancy category C, rebound hyperemia.

Preservative benzalkonium chloride.

Dosage Frequency up to q4h.

14.9.2 Phenylephrine

Brand Names AK-Nefrin, Efricel, Eye Cool, Isopto Efrin, Prefrin Liquifilm, Relief, Tear-Efrin, Velva-Kleen.

Solution/ Ointment 0.12% solution.

Mechanism vasoconstrictor.

Indications temporary relief of ocular irritation.

14.9.3 Tetrahydrozoline

Brand Names Collyrium, Murine Plus, Soothe, Tetracon, Visine.

Preservative benzalkonium chloride.

14.10 Antiallergics

14.10.1 Lodoxamide

Brand Name Alomide.

Solution/ Ointment 0.1% solution.

Mechanism mast cell stabilizer.

Indications vernal conjunctivitis, keratoconjunctivitis, keratitis.

Warnings pregnancy category B (no evidence of fetal harm in animals but no human studies).

Preservative benzalkonium chloride.

Size Available 10 ml.

Dosage Frequency qid for up to 3 months.

14.10.2 Cromolyn Sodium

Brand Name Crolom.

Solution/ Ointment 4% solution.

Mechanism mast cell stabilizer.

Indications vernal conjunctivitis, keratoconjunctivitis, keratitis.

Warnings pregnancy category B (no evidence of fetal harm in animals but no human studies).

Preservative benzalkonium chloride.

Sizes Available 2.5 ml, 10 ml.

Dosage Frequency 4 to 6 times a day.

14.11 Nonsteroidals

14.11.1 Diclofenac

Brand Name Voltaren.

Solution/ Ointment 0.1% solution.

Mechanism cyclooxygenase inhibition.

Indications postoperative inflammation.

Contraindications concomitant soft contact lens wear.

Warnings pregnancy category B.

Preservatives boric acid, edetate disodium.

Sizes Available 2.5 ml, 5 ml.

Dosage Frequency qid.

14.11.2 Ketorolac

Brand Name Acular.

Solution/ Ointment 0.5% solution.

Mechanism inhibition of prostaglandin synthesis.

Indications seasonal allergic conjunctivitis.

Contraindications concomitant soft contact lens wear.

Warnings pregnancy category C. Use with caution in patients with bleeding disorders.

Preservative benzalkonium chloride.

Size Available 5 ml.

Dosage Frequency qid.

14.11.3 Suprofen

Brand Name Profenal.

Solution/ Ointment 1% solution.

Mechanism cyclooxygenase inhibition.

Indications inhibition of intraoperative miosis.

Contraindications herpes simplex keratitis.

Warnings pregnancy category C.

Preservative thimerosal.

Size Available 2.5 ml.

Dosage Frequency either hourly for 3 hours prior to surgery or q4h on the day before surgery.

14.11.4 Flurbiprofen

Brand Name Ocufen.

Solution/ Ointment 0.03% solution.

Mechanism cyclooxygenase inhibition.

Indications inhibition of intraoperative miosis.

Warnings pregnancy category C. Use with caution in patients with bleeding tendencies. May cause delayed wound healing.

Preservative thimerosal.

Size Available 2.5 ml.

Dosage Frequency every half-hour for 2 hours prior to surgery.

14.12 Mydriatics–Cycloplegics

14.12.1 Tropicamide

Brand Names Mydriacyl, Tropicacyl, 0.5%, 1.0%.

Mechanism parasympatholytic.

Indications short-acting mydriasis.

Onset of Action 20 to 40 minutes.

Duration of Action 4 to 6 hours.

Warnings use with caution in patients with narrow angles.

Preservative 0.01% benzalkonium chloride.

Sizes Available 3 ml, 15 ml.

14.12.2 Phenylephrine

Brand Names 2.5% and 10% solution: AK-Dilate, Efricel, Mydfrin, Neo-Synephrine HCl, Phenoptic.

Onset of Action 30 to 60 minutes.

Duration of Action 3 to 5 hours.

Indications short-acting mydriasis.

Contraindications low birth weight infants; elderly patients with arteriosclerotic disease or cerebrovascular disease.

Warnings not for intraocular use. Use with caution in patients on MAO inhibitors. May cause tachycardia when used with atropine, especially in infants. Contains sulfites.

Preservative 0.01% benzalkonium chloride.

Sizes Available 3 ml, 5 ml.

14.12.3 Cyclopentolate

Brand Names AK-Pentolate, Cyclogyl, 0.5%, 1%, 2%.

Onset of Action 30 to 60 minutes.

Duration of Action 1 day.

Indications short-acting mydriasis and cycloplegia.

14.12.4 Atropine

Brand Names Atropisol, Atropine-Care, Isopto Atropine, 0.5%, 1%, 2%, 3%; 0.5% and 1% ointment.

Onset of Action 45 to 120 minutes.

Duration of Action 7 to 14 days.

Indications mydriasis and cycloplegia.

Contraindications narrow-angle glaucoma.

Warnings pregnancy category C. Use with extreme caution in children and patients with spastic paralysis, brain damage, or Down syndrome.

Preservative chlorobutanol.

Size Available 15 ml.

Dosage Frequency up to tid.

14.12.5 Scopolamine

Brand Name Isopto Hyoscine 0.25%.

Onset of Action 30 to 60 minutes.

Duration of Action 4 to 7 days.

Indications mydriasis and cycloplegia.

Contraindications narrow-angle glaucoma.

Warnings use with extreme caution in children and patients with spastic paralysis, brain damage, or Down syndrome.

14.12.6 Homatropine

Brand Name Isopto Homatropine 2%, 5%.

Onset of Action 30 to 60 minutes.

Duration of Action 3 days.

Indications mydriasis and cycloplegia.

Contraindications narrow-angle glaucoma.

Warnings pregnancy category C. Use with extreme caution in children and patients with spastic paralysis, brain damage, or Down syndrome.

14.13 Anesthetics

14.13.1 Proparacaine

Brand Names Ak-Taine, Alcaine, Ophthaine, Ophthetic, Ocu-Caine.

Onset of Action 12.9 seconds.

Duration of Action 20 minutes.

Indications topical anesthesia.

Warnings prolonged use is not recommended.

Preservative 0.01% benzalkonium chloride.

Sizes Available 2 ml, 15 ml.

14.13.2 Tetracaine

Brand Name Pontocaine.

Onset of Action 30 seconds.

Duration of Action 20 minutes.

Indications topical anesthesia.

Warnings prolonged use is not recommended.

Sizes Available 1 ml, 15 ml.

14.13.3 Lidocaine

Brand Name Xylocaine 1%, 2%, 4%.

Onset of Action 4 to 6 minutes (applied topically).

Duration of Action 40 to 60 minutes.

Indications topical or infiltrative anesthesia.

Warnings no more than 0.5 g should be used during one procedure.

14.13.4 Cocaine

Onset of Action 30 seconds.

Duration of Action 8 minutes.

Indications topical anesthesia and vasoconstriction, especially in nasal surgery, evaluation of Horner's syndrome (use 4 to 10%).

Contraindications use in patients taking MAO inhibitors, reserpine, guanethidine, or methyldopa.

Warnings severe reactions have occurred at doses of 20 mg; 1 g is lethal.

14.13.5 Bupivacaine

Brand Name Marcaine 1%, 2%.

Onset of Action 5 to 10 minutes.

Duration of Action 8 to 12 hours.

Indications infiltrative anesthesia.

14.14 Glaucoma Medications

14.14.1 Osmotic Agents

14.14.1.1 Glycerin

Brand Name Osmoglyn (50% glycerin).

Indications short-term reduction of intraocular pressure.

Duration of Action maximum effect 1 to 1 ½ hours; effective for 5 to 6 hours.

Contraindications anuria, dehydration, pulmonary edema, cardiac decompensation.

Warnings *use with caution in diabetics.* Pregnancy category C. Frequent nausea as a side effect.

Preservative potassium sorbate.

Dosage 2 to 3 ml/kg; serve over ice.

14.14.1.2 Isosorbide

Brand Name Ismotic 45%.

Indications short-term reduction of intraocular pressure.

Duration of Action maximum effect 1 to 1 ½ hours; effective for 5 to 6 hours.

Contraindications anuria, dehydration, pulmonary edema, cardiac decompensation.

Warnings pregnancy category B. Frequent nausea as a side effect.

Dosage 1.5 g/kg (equivalent to 1.5 ml/lb); serve over ice.

14.14.1.3 Mannitol

Brand Name Osmitrol.

How Supplied 5%, 10%, 15%, 20%, 25% solution.

Indications short-term reduction of intraocular pressure.

Duration of Action maximum effect 1 to 1 ½ hours; effective for 5 to 6 hours.

Contraindications anuria, dehydration, pulmonary edema, cardiac decompensation.

Warnings pregnancy category B. Headaches, confusion, hypotension.

Dosage 1.5 to 2.0 mg/kg IV.

14.14.2 Oral Carbonic Anhydrase Inhibitors

14.14.2.1 Acetazolamide

Brand Name Diamox.

How Supplied 125-mg tablets, 250-mg tablets, 500-mg sustained-release capsules.

Mechanism carbonic anhydrase inhibitor.

Indications glaucoma.

Contraindications kidney or liver disease, adrenal dysfunction, sensitivity to sulfonamides.

Warnings Stevens-Johnson syndrome and hematologic disorders reported. Baseline CBC and platelet count recommended. Pregnancy category C. Use with caution in patients receiving high-dose aspirin.

Side Effects GI distress, renal stones, fatigue, acidosis, hypokalemia, paresthesias of extremities.

Dosage Frequency 250 to 1000 mg/day in divided doses.

14.14.2.2 Methazolamide

Brand Names MZM, Neptazane, Glaucatabs.

How Supplied 25-mg and 50-mg tablets.

Mechanism carbonic anhydrase inhibitor.

Half-Life 14 hours.

Indications glaucoma.

Contraindications kidney or liver disease, adrenal dysfunction, sensitivity to sulfonamides.

Warnings Stevens-Johnson syndrome and hematologic disorders reported. Baseline CBC and platelet count recommended. Pregnancy category C (teratogenic in animal studies—skeletal anomalies).

Side Effects GI distress, fatigue, acidosis, hypokalemia, paresthesias of extremities.

Dosage Frequency 50 to 100 mg bid to tid.

14.14.2.3 Dichlorphenamide

Brand Name Daranide.

How Supplied 50-mg tablets.

Mechanism carbonic anhydrase inhibitor.

Indications glaucoma.

Contraindications kidney or liver disease, adrenal dysfunction, sensitivity to sulfonamides.

Warnings pregnancy category C (teratogenic in animal studies—skeletal anomalies).

Dosage Frequency 25 to 50 mg qd to tid.

14.14.3 Topical Carbonic Anhydrase Inhibitors

14.14.3.1 Dorzolamide

Brand Name Trusopt 2%.

Mechanism carbonic anhydrase inhibitor.

Contraindications sulfonamide sensitivity.

Warnings pregnancy category C. Has not been studied in patients with renal or hepatic failure.

Side Effects metallic taste.

Preservative benzalkonium chloride.

Sizes Available 5 ml, 10 ml.

Dosage Frequency tid.

14.14.4 Topical α-Agonist

14.14.4.1 Apraclonidine

Brand Name Iopidine 0.5% and 1% solution.

Indications

- 1%: postsurgical intraocular pressure control.
- 0.5%: short-term adjunctive therapy for glaucoma.

Contraindications concomitant MAO inhibitor use.

Warnings pregnancy category C (embryocidal in rabbits)).

Side Effects mydriasis, eyelid retraction, vasovagal attack.

Preservative benzalkonium chloride.

Sizes Available

- 1%: 0.1 ml.
- 0.5%: 5 ml.

Dosage Frequency tid.

14.14.4.2 Brimonidine

Brand Name Alphagan 0.2%

Indications intraocular pressure control.

Contraindications concomitant MAO inhibitor use.

Side Effects reduced heart rate, reduced blood pressure, irritation.

Sizes Available
- 1%: 0.1 ml.
- 0.5%: 5 ml.

Dosage Frequency bid.

14.14.5 Topical Sympathomimetics

14.14.5.1 Dipivefrin

Brand Name Propine 0.1%.

Mechanism pro-drug of epinephrine, sympathomimetic—decreases aqueous production and increases outflow.

Warnings pregnancy category B.

Side Effects irritation, rebound hyperemia, up to 30% rate of macular edema in aphakic patients on epinephrine. Use with caution in patients with narrow angles, adenochrome deposits. or hypertension.

Preservative benzalkonium chloride.

Sizes Available 5 ml, 10 ml, 15 ml.

Dosage Frequency bid.

14.14.5.2 Epinephrine

Brand Name Epifrin 0.5%, 1%, 2%.

Mechanism sympathomimetic—decreases aqueous production and increases outflow.

Warnings pregnancy category C. Use with caution in patients with narrow angles, hypertension, cardiovascular disease, or coronary artery disease. Contains sodium metabisulfite, which may cause reaction in patients with sulfite sensitivities.

Side Effects irritation, rebound hyperemia, macular edema in aphakic patients, adenochrome deposits, hypertension.

Preservative benzalkonium chloride.

Size Available 15 ml.

Dosage Frequency qd to bid.

14.14.6 Topical β-Blockers

14.14.6.1 Betaxolol

Brand Names Betoptic 0.5% solution, Betoptic S 0.25% suspension.

Mechanism β_1-adrenergic blocker.

Contraindications sinus bradycardia, greater than first-degree AV block, cardiac failure. Use with caution in asthmatics.

Warnings pregnancy category C (evidence of postimplantation loss in animals, not found to be teratogenic in animals).

Side Effects irritation, blurring, bradycardia, heart block, bronchospasm, depression, impotence, dry eye.

Preservative benzalkonium chloride.

Sizes Available 2.5 ml, 5 ml, 10 ml, 15 ml.

Dosage Frequency bid.

14.14.6.2 Carteolol

Brand Name Ocupress 1%.

Mechanism nonselective β-adrenergic blocker with intrinsic sympathomimetic activity.

Contraindications sinus bradycardia, greater than first-degree AV block, cardiac failure. Use with caution in asthmatics.

Warnings pregnancy category C.

Side Effects irritation, blurring, bradycardia, heart block, bronchospasm, depression, impotence, dry eye.

Preservative benzalkonium chloride.

Size Available 5 ml.

Dosage Frequency bid.

14.14.6.3 *Levobunolol*

Brand Names Betagan, AK-Beta 0.25%, 0.5%.

Mechanism nonselective β-adrenergic blocker equally potent at β_1- and β_2-adrenergic receptors.

Contraindications sinus bradycardia, greater than first-degree AV block, cardiac failure. Use with caution in asthmatics.

Warnings pregnancy category C.

Side Effects irritation, blurring, bradycardia, heart block, bronchospasm, depression, impotence, dry eye.

Preservative benzalkonium chloride.

Sizes Available 2 ml, 5 ml, 10 ml, 15 ml.

Dosage Frequency qd to bid.

14.14.6.4 *Metipranolol*

Brand Name Optipranolol 0.3%.

Mechanism nonselective β-adrenergic blocker.

Contraindications sinus bradycardia, greater than first-degree AV block, cardiac failure. Use with caution in asthmatics.

Warnings pregnancy category C.

Side Effects irritation, blurring, bradycardia, heart block, bronchospasm, depression, impotence, dry eye.

Preservative benzalkonium chloride.

Sizes Available 2 ml, 5 ml, 10 ml.

Dosage Frequency bid.

14.14.6.5 Timolol

Brand Names Timoptic 0.25%, 0.5%; Timoptic XE 0.25% 0.5%.

Mechanism nonselective β-adrenergic blocker.

Contraindications sinus bradycardia, greater than first-degree AV block, cardiac failure, use with caution in asthmatics.

Warnings pregnancy category C.

Side Effects irritation, blurring, bradycardia, heart block, bronchospasm, depression, impotence, dry eye.

Preservative benzalkonium chloride.

Sizes Available 2.5 ml, 5 ml, 10 ml, 15 ml.

Dosage Frequency

- Timoptic: bid.
- Timoptic XE: qd.

14.14.7 Topical Direct Cholinergic Agents

14.14.7.1 Carbachol

Brand Name Isopto Carbachol 0.75% 1.5%, 2.25%, 3%.

Mechanism cholinergic agent—stimulates motor end plate of muscle cells and partially inhibits cholinesterase.

Contraindications iritis.

Warnings pregnancy category C. Associated with retinal detachment in susceptible individuals.

Side Effects miosis, nyctalopia, myopia, brow ache, decreased vision due to cataract, retinal tear.

Preservative benzalkonium chloride.

Sizes Available 15 ml, 30 ml.

Dosage Frequency tid.

14.14.7.2 Pilocarpine

Brand Names Isopto Carpine 0.25%, 0.5%, 1%, 2%, 3%, 4%, 5%, 6%, 8%, 10%; Ocusert.

Mechanism direct stimulation of muscarinic receptors producing miosis and reducing outflow resistance.

Contraindications iritis, pupillary block.

Warnings pregnancy category C. Associated with retinal detachment in susceptible individuals.

Side Effects miosis, nyctalopia, variable myopia, brow ache, decreased vision, retinal tear.

Preservative benzalkonium chloride.

Sizes Available 15 ml, 30 ml.

Dosage Frequency tid to qid.

14.14.8 Topical Cholinesterase Inhibitors

14.14.8.1 Demecarium

Brand Name Humorsol 0.125%, 0.25%.

Mechanism cholinesterase inhibitor.

Contraindications iritis.

Warnings use with caution in patients with myasthenia gravis.

Preservative benzalkonium chloride.

Size Available 5 ml.

Dosage Frequency 1 to 2 drops twice per week to twice per day.

14.14.8.2 Echothiophate Iodide

Brand Name Phospholine Iodide 0.03%, 0.06%, 0.125%, 0.25%.

Mechanism long-acting cholinesterase inhibitor.

Contraindications iritis. Discontinue prior to general anesthesia.

Warnings use with caution in patients with myasthenia gravis, history of retinal detachment, exposure to insecticides, and other conditions sensitive to vagotonic medications.

Side Effects miosis, nyctalopia, myopia, brow ache, decreased vision due to cataract, retinal tear, iris cysts, cataract, punctal stenosis, abdominal cramps.

Preservative chlorobutanol.

Size Available 5 ml.

Dosage Frequency bid.

14.14.8.3 Isoflurophate

Brand Name Floropryl 0.025% ointment.

Mechanism cholinesterase inhibitor.

Contraindications iritis. Discontinue prior to general anesthesia.

Warnings use with caution in patients with myasthenia gravis, history of retinal detachment, exposure to insecticides, and other conditions sensitive to vagotonic medications.

Side Effects miosis, nyctalopia, myopia, brow ache, decreased vision due to cataract, retinal tear.

Size Available 3.5 g.

Dosage Frequency ¼ inch every 8 to 72 hours.

14.14.8.4 Physostigmine

Brand Name Eserine 0.25% ointment.

Mechanism cholinesterase inhibitor.

Contraindications iritis. Discontinue prior to general anesthesia.

Warnings use with caution in patients with myasthenia gravis, history of retinal detachment, exposure to insecticides, and other conditions sensitive to vagotonic medications.

Side Effects miosis, nyctalopia, myopia, brow ache, decreased vision due to cataract, retinal tear.

Size Available 3.5 g.

14.14.9 Prostaglandin Analogue

14.14.9.1 Latanaprost

Brand Name Xalatan 0.005% solution.

Mechanism prostaglandin analogue—increases uveoscleral outflow.

Warnings pregnancy category C (embryocidal in rabbits). Gradually causes increased pigmentation of the iris by increasing the number of melanosomes within melanocytes; this is more noticeable in persons with light irides.

Side Effects hyperemia, darkening of iris.

Preservative benzalkonium chloride.

Size Available 2.5 ml.

Dosage Frequency qhs.

14.14.10 Antimetabolite

14.14.10.1 5-Fluorouracil

Mechanism inhibits fibroblastic proliferation.

Warnings pregnancy category C (embryocidal in rabbits). Gradually causes increased pigmentation of the iris by increasing the number of melanosomes within melanocytes; this is more noticeable in persons with light irides.

Side Effects keratitis, wound leaks.

Size Available 500 mg/10 ml. Use 5-mg (0.1 ml) injections subconjunctivally.

Dosage Frequency up to qd as tolerated, as needed up to 2 weeks.

14.15 Diagnostic Medications

14.15.1 Glycerol

Brand Name Ophthalagan.

Mechanism osmotically dehydrates the cornea, reducing corneal haze due to edema.

Indications ophthalmoscopic and gonioscopic examination of patients with corneal edema.

Contraindications hypersensitivity.

Warnings pregnancy category C (no animal or human studies—use only if clearly needed).

Preservative chlorobutanol 0.55%.

Size Available 7.5 ml.

14.15.2 Fluorescein

14.15.2.1 Topical

Brand Names Fluor-I-Strip, many others.

Solution/Ointment 9-mg strips.

Indications delineating corneal injuries, fitting contact lenses, Seidel's testing, lacrimal drainage testing.

Contraindications hypersensitivity.

Warnings do not use with soft contact lenses, because they will stain.

Preservative chlorobutanol.

14.15.2.2 Intravenous

Brand Names AK-Fluor, many others.

Solution/Ointment 10% and 20% solution.

Indications angiography.

Contraindications hypersensitivity.

Warnings avoid use in pregnancy, although **no** reports of fetal abnormality.

Preservatives none.

Sizes Available 2 ml 250 mg/ml; 5 ml 100 mg/ml.

14.15.3 Hydroxyamphetamine

Brand Name Paremyd 1% (with Tropicamide).

Onset of Action 15 to 60 minutes.

Duration of Action 3 to 4 hours.

Indications mydriasis.

Contraindications has rarely caused CNS disturbances in the elderly, infants, and children.

Warnings use with caution in patients with narrow angles. Pregnancy category C.

Preservative benzalkonium chloride.

Size Available 15 ml.

14.15.4 Dapiprazole

Brand Name Rev-Eyes.

Solution/ Ointment 0.5% solution.

Indications reversal of diagnostic mydriasis caused by phenylephrine or tropicamide.

Contraindications hypersensitivity.

Warnings 80% of patients have conjunctival injection lasting for 20 minutes. Pregnancy category B.

Preservative benzalkonium chloride.

Size Available 5 ml.

14.16 Botulinum Toxin

Brand Name Botox.

Solution/ Ointment 100-U vials.

Mechanism sterilized botulinum toxin A—blocks neuromuscular receptors.

Indications blepharospasm, facial spasms, strabismus management.

Contraindications hypersensitivity.

Side Effects ptosis, diplopia.

Dose blepharospasm—1.25 to 2.5 U after proper dilution (see package insert for dilution instructions).

Chapter 15

OCULAR MANIFESTATIONS OF SYSTEMIC DISEASE

David Leventer, Mary Gilbert Lawrence

15.1 Diabetes Mellitus

a multisystem disorder of insulin production or action. Type I insulin-dependent diabetes mellitus (juvenile onset) occurs as a result of loss of insulin producing β cells. Type II non-insulin-dependent diabetes mellitus (adult onset) is characterized by insufficient insulin secretion and abnormal peripheral tissue action.

Presentation systemic complaints include polydipsia, polyuria, weight loss, and fatigue; chronic complications such as nephropathy, peripheral neuropathy, cardiac and cerebrovascular disease, and recurrent infections may result.

Ocular complaints include decreased vision, transient visual obscurations, and diplopia (refer to Section 9.2 for Diabetic Retinopathy). Cataracts, especially posterior subcapsular, are more common and occur earlier in diabetics. Transient visual changes occur with hyperopic and myopic shifts due to lens swelling secondary to an osmotic gradient created by the accumulation of sorbitol during acute, hyperglycemic episodes. There is an increased risk of primary open-angle glaucoma. Secondary glaucoma resulting from iris neovascularization due to PDR may lead to blindness in diabetics. Corneal neurotrophic changes and epitheliopathy may occur. Isolated, pupil-sparing CN III, IV, or VI palsies (Section 13.1) resulting from microvascular disease may occur. Disc edema is usually benign and resolves spontaneously. Mucormycosis, a potentially life-threatening, ocular emergency, presents as orbital cellulitis (Section 3.2.1); necrosis of the nasal mucosa and skin may rapidly occur.

Management laboratory testing includes fasting plasma glucose, oral glusose tolerance test, and urine dipstick for glucose and ketones. Encourage tight blood sugar control in all patients; the Diabetes Control and Complications Trial recommends tight control for type I diabetes mellitus to decrease new retinopathy or progression of existing disease. Do not prescribe new glasses during periods of poor blood sugar control. Avoid β-blockers for glaucoma treatment, because they may mask hypoglycemic warning symptoms.

15.2 Acquired Immune Deficiency Syndrome (AIDS)

HIV is the retrovirus responsible for AIDS. Worldwide, unprotected heterosexual intercourse is the main risk factor; in the United States, however, anal intercourse and IV drug abuse are the most frequent modes of transmission.

Presentation viremia followed by a period of latency of 5 to 10 years. Viral replication continues until CD4 helper cells are depleted. External diseases include dry eye syndrome, microsporidiosis (persistent epithelial infection), corneal ulcers, HSV and HZV, molluscum contagiosum (see Chapters 2 and 4) and Kaposi's sarcoma. The retina is the most common site of ocular HIV infection. HIV retinopathy is a microvasculopathy that consists of cotton-wool spots, intraretinal heme, microaneurysms and telangiectasias, and areas of capillary nonperfusion on FA (refer to Chapter 6 for CMV Retinitis). Toxoplasmosis, candida retinitis, herpetic retinitis, and progressive outer retinal necrosis, PCP choroidopathy, TB and atypical mycobacterial infection, and *Histoplasma capsulatum* may all occur. In addition, cryptococcal infection may cause papilledema. Other neuro-ophthalmic manifestations include cranial nerve palsies, pupillary abnormalities, optic neuritis, or visual field defects. Non-Hodgkin's lymphoma is more common in HIV and may be found in the orbit.

Management diagnose disease with ELISA and Western blot test. Monitor CBC, CD4 count, and screen for syphilis, toxoplasmosis, and TB. Coordinate treatment with the appropriate infectious disease specialist.

15.3 Varicella (VZV) and Herpes Zoster (HZV)

a highly contagious DNA virus spread by airborne droplets as well as infected secretions. Dormant virus resides in the neuronal ganglia and may become activated, causing classic, dermatomal involvement.

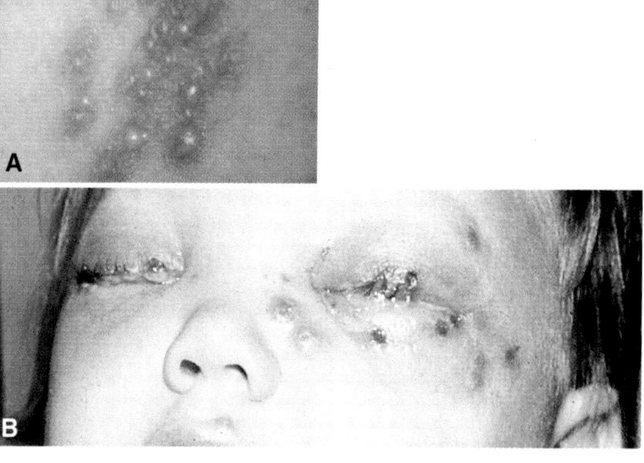

FIGURE 15.3a Early vesicles on an erythematous base ("dew drops on a rose petal") in Varicella

FIGURE 15.3b Blepharoconjunctivitis after autoinnoculation in a case of varicella

Presentation

- VZV: chickenpox occurs most commonly at age 1 to 14 years. A flulike prodrome occurs 24 to 48 hours prior to the eruption of erythematous, maculopapular vesicles (at different stages), which break and crust. Healing occurs after 10 to 14 days. Ocular involvement may include an acute conjunctivitis, secondary bacterial infection, pseudodendritic corneal epithelial defects, stromal keratitis, anterior uveitis, optic neuritis, retinitis, and ophthalmoplegia. Potential systemic complications include pneumonia, cerebellar ataxia, and encephalitis. A live attenuated vaccine is available.

- HZV: this commonly occurs in immunocompromised or aged patients. A flulike prodrome progresses to burning, itching, or tingling, eventually erupting into an acute vesicular rash in the affected dermatomal distribution, which obeys the midline. Thoracic dermatomes are most commonly affected while cranial, cervical, lumbar, and sacral zones follow in that order. Ocular involvement is as noted with VZV. In HZV ophthalmicus, the upper eyelid is commonly involved (CN V_1) but the lower lid (CN V_2) and the jaw (CN V_3) may become involved (Section 5.1.2). Late manifestations include scarring and postherpetic neuralgia.

Management in patients less than 40 years of age, perform a general systemic workup for an immunocompromised state, including HIV, TB, and diabetes testing. Treat systemically with acyclovir or related compounds (IV in immunocompromised states). Prednisone, cimetidine, and antidepressants may be used to minimize postherpetic neuralgia.

15.4 Rheumatoid Arthritis (RA)

a chronic multisystem disease of unknown etiology; the most common rheumatologic disorder, affecting 1% of adults. Association with HLA-DW4/DR4 occurs in Caucasians.

Presentation a 3 : 1 female–male predominance; insidious disease with onset in the third to fourth decades. Fever, malaise, and weight loss may progress to morning stiffness, joint pain and inflammation, and limitation of movement. Ulnar deviation and swan-neck deformities are classic; bursal effusion, Baker's cysts, and hallux valgus may also result. Extra-articular manifestations are more common with severe joint disease and RF-positive disease; superficial rheumatoid nodules may occur on the extensor surfaces of the forearms, olecranon, and the Achilles' tendon; pericarditis and pleural effusions, Caplan's syndrome (RA, intrapulmonary nodules, and pneumoconiosis), and Felty's syndrome (RA, anemia, splenomegaly, and leukopenia) may occur.

Ocular findings include keratoconjunctivitis sicca (25 to 40% of RA patients also have Sjögren's Syndrome), episcleritis, scleritis (including scleromalacia perforans), and peripheral ulcerative keratitis.

Management laboratory testing of RF (positive in 80%), ANA, and CBC with differential; rheumatologic consultation. Oral NSAIDs may be used. Hydroxychloroquine use requires monitoring for retinal toxicity (Section 9.18.3), and chronic prednisone use requires IOP checks and cataract screening.

15.5 Systemic Lupus Erythematosis

a multisystem disease of unknown etiology, characterized by B-cell hyperreactivity and hypergammaglobulinemia.

Presentation a 9 : 1 female–male ratio, generally in the third to fourth decades of life. Common presenting symptoms include fever, fatigue, and weight loss. Musculoskeletal, cutaneous (classic butterfly malar rash, alopecia, and photosensitivity), renal, neurologic, pulmonary and cardiac, and hematologic manifestations may occur. Raynaud's phenomenon occurs in 20% of these patients.

Ocular findings include keratoconjunctivitis sicca; episcleritis and scleritis; retinal sequelae such as cotton-wool spots, hemorrhages, Roth's spots, hyperviscosity

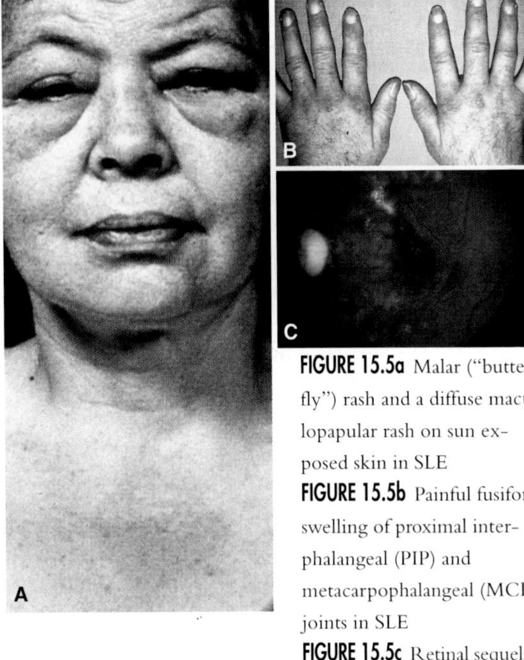

FIGURE 15.5a Malar ("butterfly") rash and a diffuse maculopapular rash on sun exposed skin in SLE
FIGURE 15.5b Painful fusiform swelling of proximal interphalangeal (PIP) and metacarpophalangeal (MCP) joints in SLE
FIGURE 15.5c Retinal sequelae.

syndrome, and vascular occlusions; and neuro-ophthalmic manifestations such as ischemic optic neuropathy, internuclear ophthalmoplegia, and cranial nerve palsies.

Management diagnosis is based on four or more of the American Rheumatologic Association criteria. Skin or renal biopsy may also aid in the diagnosis. Laboratory tests include CBC with differential, ANA, double-stranded and single-stranded DNA, SSA/SSB (Sjögren's), ESR, antiphospholipid antibody, and lupus anticoagulant.
Therapy is directed at specific manifestations. Manage with medicine and/or rheumatology.

15.6 Sjögren's Syndrome (SS)

a multisystem disorder of autoimmune etiology commonly affecting the lacrimal and salivary glands.

Presentation a 9 : 1 predilection for women and most common in the fourth to fifth decades. Systemically, primary SS includes xerostomia and xerophthalmia; SS is termed secondary if associated with a connective tissue disorder such as RA or SLE. Immune-complex deposition may lead to thyroid, GI, renal, and pulmonary complications. Hypergammaglobulinemia occurs in 50% and anemia in 33% of patients, and there is an increased risk of malignancy, especially lymphoma.

Ocular findings include keratoconjunctivitis sicca (90%), filamentary keratitis, staphylococcal blepharoconjunctivitis, pannus formation with symblepharon, peripheral ulcerative keratitis, and corneal perforation.

Management laboratory tests include CBC with differential, RF (positive in 90%), ANA (positive in 70%), autoantibodies to Ro (SSA) and La (SSB), cryoglobulins (Raynaud's disease), circulating immune complexes, gammaglobulins, and antithyroglobulin antibody (positive in 35%). Diagnosis can often be made with a minor salivary gland biopsy. Therapy is directed at specific manifestations. Dry eye symptoms may require aggressive lubrication and punctal plugs. Comanage with medicine and/or rheumatology.

15.7 Lyme Disease

the most common vectorborne infection in the United States; the spirochete *Borrelia Burgdorferi* is usually transmitted by the *Ixodides dammini* tick. Most commonly reported in the northeast.

Presentation viral prodrome, photophobia, skin rash, decreased vision, double vision, arthralgia and myalgia, stiff neck, and palpitations:

- Stage 1: erythema chronica migrans (pathognomonic), fever, lymphadenopathy.

- Stage 2: cardiac arrhythmia, myocarditis, arthralgias, meningitis, cranial nerve palsies (especially CN VII), encephalitis.
- Stage 3: acrodermatitis chronica atrophicans, arthritis, demyelinatiing encephalomyelitis, dementia.

Ocular findings are rare, even in endemic areas:

- Stage 1 (local): conjunctivitis.
- Stage 2 (disseminated): iridocyclitis, pars planitis, vitritis, choroiditis, panophthalmitis, macular edema, exudative retinal detachment, optic disc edema, AION, optic neuritis, neuroretinitis, blepharospasm, cranial nerve palsies, Horner's syndrome, Argyll Robertson pupil.
- Stage 3 (persistant): IK, episcleritis, orbital myositis.

Management history of tick bite, exposure, or characteristic rash, and perform a thorough dermatologic, neurologic, and ocular examination. Immunofluorescence and ELISA for antibodies are notoriously unreliable, with both false-negative and false-positive results. There is cross-reactivity with syphilis. Use Western blot for confirmation. Lumbar puncture may be necessary. Consider medical consultation. Treat specific ocular findings. Treat systemically with tetracycline, doxycycline, amoxicillin, ceftriaxone, or penicillin G.

15.8 Leprosy and Hansen's Disease

Mycobacterium leprae causes two types of disease: tuberculoid with granulomas and lepromatous with suppressed immunity and bacteremia.

Presentation tuberculoid disease presents with well-demarcated, paresthetic, hypopigmented plaques on the skin, peripheral nerve involvement with paresthesias, and muscular atrophy and contracture. Lepromatous disease presents with poorly demarcated plaques, erythema nodosa, and bacteremia.

Ocular findings include anterior uveitis, iris atrophy and granulomas, episcleritis and scleritis, IK, prominent corneal nerves, corneal anesthesia, vasculitis, optic nerve atrophy, lid granulomas, madarosis, and lagophthalmos.

Management treat specific ocular findings. Systemic treatment is dapsone for several years.

15.9 Leukemia

a WBC proliferative disorder, characterized as acute or chronic and labeled according to cell type (B cell, T cell, or myeloid).

Presentation acute leukemias present with constitutional symptoms (fever), lymphadenopathy, hepatosplenomegaly, epistaxis, or easy bruisability. CNS involvement occurs in 70% of cases, and secondary infection, often with atypical organisms, is common.

Patients present with blurred vision, pain and infection. Although thickening of the choroid is the most common ocular finding, marginal ulcers and peripheral corneal infiltrates may be the presenting signs in acute or chronic myeloid leukemia. In addition, bilateral subconjunctival hemorrhages may be a presenting sign with profound thromboctyopenia. A granulocytic sarcoma (a chloroma) may involve the orbit in acute myeloid leukemia (see Section 11.1.7). Retinal changes include vascular sheathing and tortousity, nerve fiber layer hemorrhages, cotton-wool spots and exudates, and neovascularization. Secondary infection of the retina and vitreous may masquerade as posterior vitritis. Papillitis and papilledema may also occur.

Management definitive diagnosis is made by bone marrow aspiration and biopsy with immunocytologic markers. CT scan and lumbar puncture are sometimes warranted for CNS involvement. Supportive therapy including antimicrobial precautions, antibiotics, transfusions, and radiotherapy, along with chemotherapeutic agents must be coordinated by a hematology/oncology specialist. Emergent irridation can sometimes save vision when retrolaminar invasion occurs.

15.10 Lymphoma

a malignant neoplasm caused by a proliferation of monoclonal lymphoid tissue.

Presentation elderly adults may present with weakness, headache, disorientation in cases of CNS lymphoma. Visceral lymphoma usually presents with systemic symptoms before ocular involvement; in contrast, CNS lymphoma (typically reticulum cell sarcoma, a B-cell lymphoma) commonly presents with ocular complaints of painless decrease in visual acuity with floaters. Unilateral disease often becomes bilateral in months to years. Anterior granulomatous or nongranulomatous inflammation with or without hypopyon; large vitreal cells in sheets, veils and clumps; white or gray fluffy retinal infiltrates, often perivascular and with hemorrhages; choroidal infiltrates; cystoid macular edema; and optic nerve head infiltration may be found.

Management diagnosis should be considered in all cases of vitritis in older individuals, especially if refractory to treatment. In addition, there may be an initial response to steroids. Consider vitreous biopsy with a 20-gauge needle or diagnostic vitrectomy with high-quality cytologic preparations. Granulomatous inflammation is often found on initial biopsy, and repeat biopsies may be required. Further workup includes CT scan or MRI of the brain and lumbar puncture. Treatment should be coordinated by an oncologist and includes radiation therapy, chemotherapy, and corticosteroids; the prognosis is variable but poor.

15.11 Pregnancy

includes various physiologic and hormonal and vascular changes, many of which can manifest as ocular symptoms and pathology.

Presentation blurred vision secondary to refractive shifts, difficulty reading, headache, visual field complaints, and contact lens discomfort are common complaints. Retinal changes include hypertensive retinopathy with preeclampsia or eclampsia after 20 weeks' gestation, CSC, and exudative retinal detachments. Preexisting diabetic retinopathy may progress during pregnancy, but gestational diabetes is not a risk factor. Migraine headaches may worsen during and immediately following pregnancy. Choroidal, retinal, and orbital hemangiomas, meningiomas, uveal melanomas, and cortical blindness can occur in association with pregnancy. Pituitary tumors may present or enlarge, causing headache and bitemporal hemianopia or other visual field defects. Blepharoptosis and eyelid hypopigmentation have been reported.

Management treatment is directed at specific pathologic state and must be coordinated with the patient's obstetrician. In cases of refractive shift, do not prescribe new glasses until 6 weeks postpartum, when vision typically normalizes. In terms of hypertensive and diabetic retinopathy, a delay of FA and laser photocoagulation may be warranted, as spontaneous regression may occur. On the other hand, PDR may require treatment, and C-section is often recommended to avoid VH during labor and delivery.

15.12 Down's Syndrome

Trisomy 21 is the most common cause of congenital mental retardation, occurring in 1 per 600 births.

Presentation diagnosis is usually made at birth with recognition of typical physical findings: prominent epicanthal folds and abnormal palpebral fissures with upward temporal slant, single palmar crease, and hypotonia. Later findings include various degrees of mental retardation, short stature, adrenal and pituitary abnormalities, hypothyroidism, endocardial cushion defects, duodenal atresia, and abnormal development of genitalia and reproductive organs.

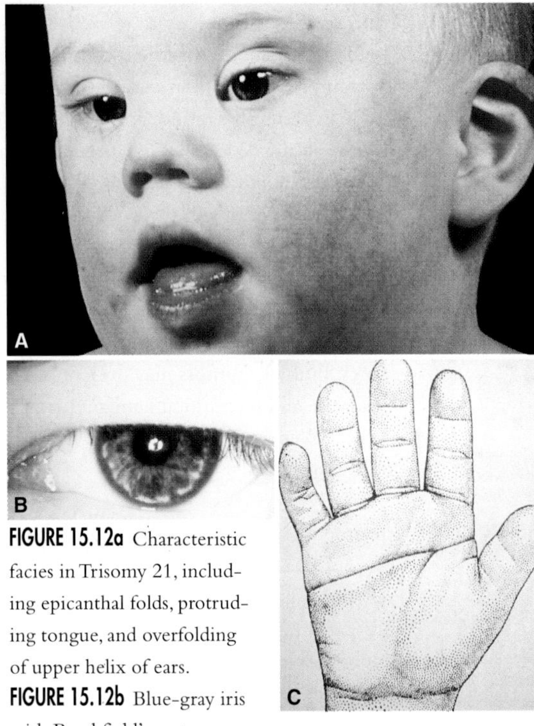

FIGURE 15.12a Characteristic facies in Trisomy 21, including epicanthal folds, protruding tongue, and overfolding of upper helix of ears.
FIGURE 15.12b Blue-gray iris with Brushfield's spots.
FIGURE 15.12c Diagram of short metacarpals and phalanges and single palmar crease (Simean crease).

Several ocular findings may be present: blepharitis, strabismus (most commonly esodeviations) and nystagmus (most commonly horizontal), astigmatism and KC (up to 15% of patients), a typical blue-gray color to the irides with Brushfield's spots (found in 20% of normals and up to 90% of patients with Down's; see Chapter 11, cataracts, and myopia.

Management appropriate chromosomal studies must be obtained, along with a complete systemic evaluation including cardiac, endocrine, and hematologic workup. Intelligence testing may be performed later. Strabismus and resultant amblyopia and myopia must be appropriately treated; cycloplegic refraction is usually necessary. In cases of KC, PK may be entertained at an earlier stage because these patients are generally not candidates for contact lens wear.

15.13 Albinism

a group of heritable disorders characterized by defective biosynthesis and distribution of melanin. There are three major forms described.

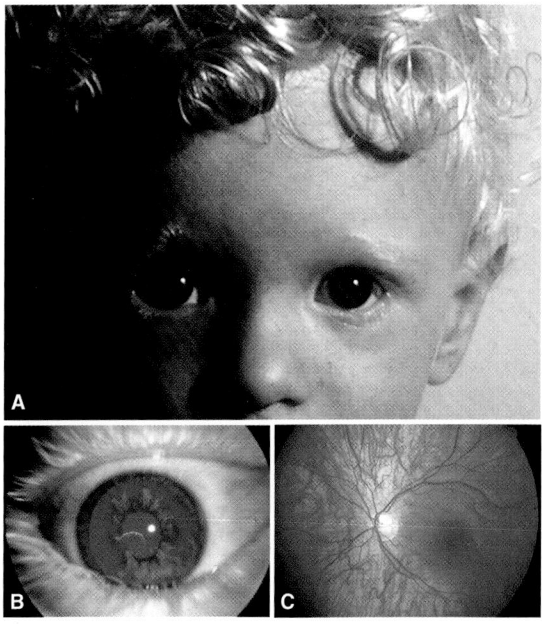

FIGURE 15.13a Partial albinism in a child.
FIGURE 15.13b Iris transillumination in albinism.
FIGURE 15.13c Fundus in albinism.

Presentation

- Oculacutaneous albinism (OCA): usually autosomal recessive. Tyrosinase-negative patients have pink skin, white hair, skin photosensitivity, and severe photophobia. Visual acuity is 20/80 or worse due to foveal hypoplasia. Blue-gray irides that transilluminate, lack of fundus pigmentation or foveal light reflex, pendular nystagmus, and lack of binocularity due to abnormal visual pathways may be found. Tyrosinase-positive patients generally have milder symptoms than the tyrosinase-negative group; vision may improve with age as patients acquire more pigment. This type of albinism is associated with two autosomal recessive disorders: Hermansky-Pudlak syndrome is a bleeding diathesis due to platelet defects most commonly in patients of Puerto Rican descent, and Chediak-Higashi syndrome is a disorder of impaired WBC function leading to infection, lymphadenopathy, and death.
- Ocular albinism (OA): albinism is limited to the eyes. Patients have normal skin pigmentation, light hair color, and ocular signs including nystagmus, iris transillumination, absent foveal reflex and macular pigmentation, and hypopigmented fundus. Female carriers may be detected by translucent irides and a mosaic pigmentation pattern of the fundi. Several forms have been described, including x-linked nettleship falls variant. Autosomal recessive variant is similar, but females are affected.
- Partial albinism (also pie baldism or albinoidism) denotes autosomal dominant, cutaneous disease without photophobia, nystagmus, or foveal hypoplasia. Hair and skin are devoid of pigment in localized areas.

Management

the tyrosinase test may be performed to differentiate types; hematology consultation should be obtained if either Hermansky-Pudlak syndrome or Chediak-Hiashi syndrome is suspected. ERG may aid in diagnosis but is rarely necessary.

No treatment is currently available; dark glasses, low-vision aides, and genetic counseling may be helpful. As abnormal neuronal connections exist, binocular vision is rarely achieved after strabismus surgery. Retinal detachment surgery usually fails because of inadequate RPE to retinal adhesions.

15.14 Marfan Syndrome

an autosomal dominant, connective tissue disease with skeletal, cardiac, and ocular manifestations; 15% of cases are sporadic.

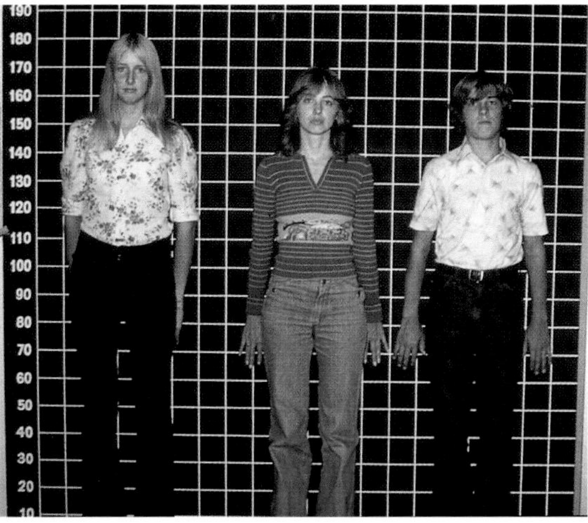

FIGURE 15.14 Three children, ages 14, 12, and 10 years, with Marfan's syndrome.

Presentation systemic findings include joint deformities, lengthening of extremities with arm span exceeding height, marfanoid habitus with kyphoscoliosis and pectus carinatum (funnel chest) or pectus excavatum (pigeon chest), high-arched palate, and cardiac abnormalities such as mitral valve prolapse, aortic arch dissection, cardiomyopathy, and bacterial endocarditis.

Ocular complaints include decreased visual acuity and monocular diplopia. Lens subluxation occurs in 50 to 80% of patients; it is typically bilateral, superotemporal in orientation, with an associated iridodonesis. Lens opacification with corneal touch and endothelial decompensation may occur. In addition, severe myopia due to an increased axial length, retinal detachment, megalocornea, and poor dilation may occur. Glaucoma is infrequent unless related to lens subluxation.

Management obtain a family history and rule out other causes of lens subluxation. Treat subluxation if the patient is symptomatic (see Chapters 1 and 7). Consider cardiology consultation and echocardiogram.

15.15 Homocystinuria

an autosomal recessive inborn error of methionine metabolism; there is a deficiency of cystathionine B synthase (which catalyzes the conversion of homocystine to cystathionine) leading to an increase in plasma homocystine levels.

Presentation clinical manifestations are heterogeneous with variation in severity and age of onset. A slowly progressive mental retardation is common, although 50% of patients retain average intelligence. Patients are often tall with light-colored hair, have skeletal abnormalities with lengthening of long bones, and can suffer from seizures. Thrombosis and thromboembolism are the most common causes of death, with a 50% mortality before 20 years of age and 75% by age 30; general anesthesia, surgery, and angiography pose a significant risk.

Decreased vision and monocular diplopia are common ocular complaints. Bilateral, symmetric lens subluxation, in an inferonasal orientation, is typical; 30% of patients develop subluxation at infancy, whereas 80% manifest it by age 15. Complete dislocation of the lens into the anterior chamber with resultant acute glaucoma is found more commonly than in Marfan syndrome. Spontaneous retinal detachments and BRAOs and CRAOs have been reported.

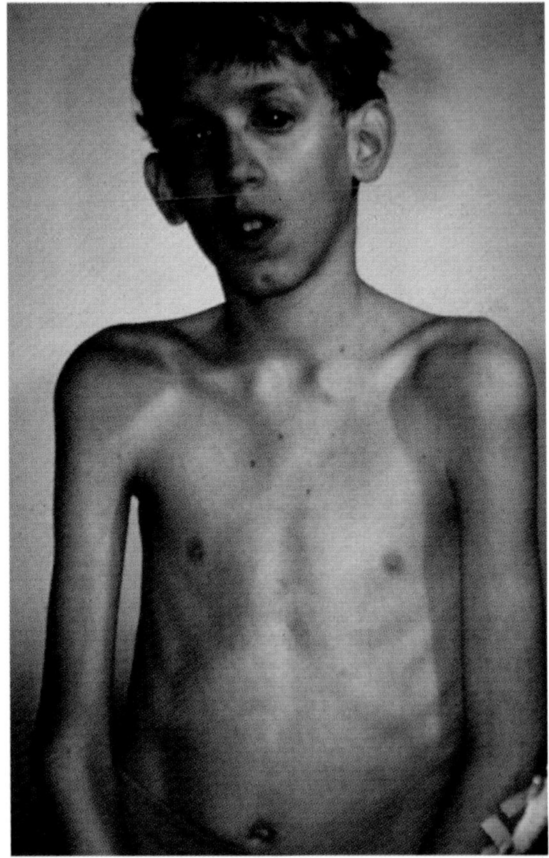

FIGURE 15.15 Thin skeletal build and pectus excavatum in homocystinuria.

Management

the sodium nitroprusside test or urine chromatography can confirm the diagnosis. Consider intelligence testing and imaging of the vertebrae. Limit dietary methionine and increase cysteine intake. Consider aspirin and vitamin-B_6 (cofactor of cystathione synthase) to reduce the incidence of thromboembolism. Rule out other causes of lens subluxation. Treat subluxation if the patient is symptomatic (see Chapters 1 and 7).

15.16 Weill-Marchesani Syndrome

an autosomal recessive connective tissue disorder due to an unknown metabolic defect. Penetrance is variable and consanguinity is often present.

Presentation pyknic physique with brachycephaly, brachydactyly, short stature, limitation of joint mobility (hand, wrist), and seizures are common; affected individuals are of normal intelligence.

Patients complain of decreased vision, monocular diplopia, and difficulty reading. Lenticular myopia occurs commonly in the first decade with a −3.00 to −20.00 refractive error. Microspherophakia (increased anteroposterior lens diameter, decreased equatorial diameter, and elongated, irregular zonules) may cause refractive error or lead to lens subluxation. Glaucoma is common and may be secondary to pupillary block with or without lens dislocation.

Management radiography of the metacarpals is essential. Treat angle-closure glaucoma with cycloplegics and laser iridotomy (see Chapter 8). Rule out other causes of lens subluxation. Treat subluxation if the patient is symptomatic (see Chapters 1 and 7).

15.17 Paget's Disease

Osteitis deformans is a chronic, progressive bone disorder characterized by abnormal osteoclastic activity with anomalous bone resorption, production, and deposition.

Presentation patients may complain of bone pain, change in hat size, headache, or hearing difficulty. Bone fractures are common, and compressive skull abnormalities may cause trigeminal neuralgia, hemifacial spasm, brainstem and cerebellar dysfunction, and spinal cord compression. Renal and cardiac symptoms may also occur.

Orbital and periorbital bony destruction may cause exophthalmos, superior orbital fissure compression with

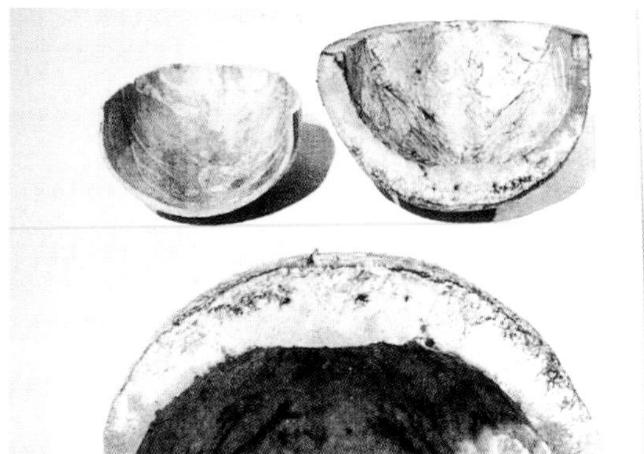

FIGURE 15.17 Normal skull and two others demonstrating abnormal thickening in Paget's disease

extraocular muscle palsies, or lacrimal duct obstruction with epiphora. Angioid streaks occur in 8 to 15% of cases and may lead to subretinal neovascularization. Optic neuropathy has also been reported.

Management laboratory testing for serum calcium, alkaline phosphatase, and urine calcium is recommended. Radiologic studies, especially skull films, may be performed. If symptomatic, patients may be treated with calcitonin as well as osteoclast inhibitors (etidronate and pamidronate). Surgical debulking procedures may be required if compressive skull abnormalities occur. Rule out other causes of angioid streaks (see Section 9.10).

15.18 Pseudoxanthoma Elasticum

a rare connective tissue disorder of elastic fiber production and calcification with cutaneous, cardiovascular, and/or ocular manifestations; inherited in an autosomal dominant or recessive pattern, depending on disease type.

Presentation cutaneous findings include yellow, xanthomatous lesions occurring in the intertriginal areas with *peau d'orange* and

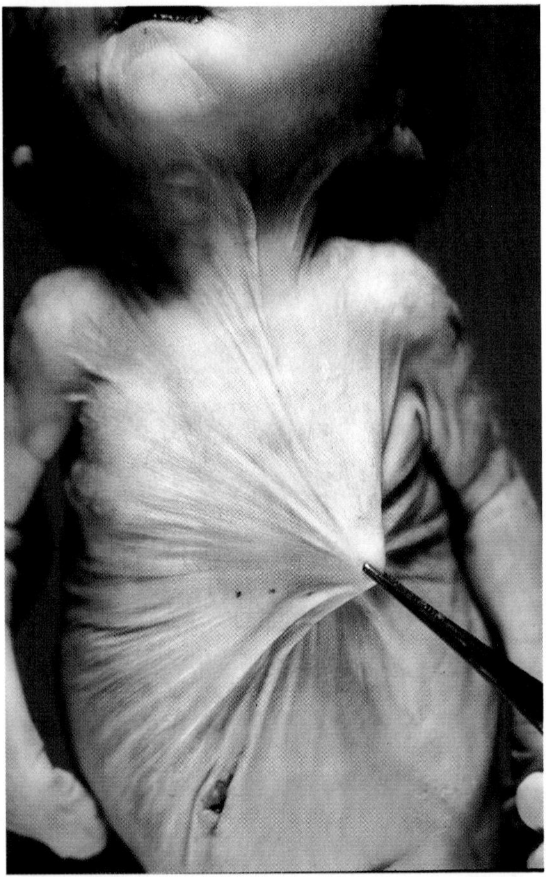

FIGURE 15.18 Lax, inelastic folds of skin in pseudoxanthoma elasticum

scattered yellow papules. Hypertension, mitral valve prolapse, myocardial infarction, peripheral vascular disease, and GI bleeding may occur.

Patients may complain of decreased vision and metamorphopsia. Angioid streaks are the most common ocular finding, occurring in 85% of patients (see Section 9.10). Secondary complications such as macular hemorrhage and scarring and choroidal or RPE atrophy may occur.

The macula has a *peau d'orange* appearance. White, crystalline deposits may occur in the retina and the corneal stroma. Myopia and a blue discoloration of the sclera have also been described.

Management skin biopsy may be diagnostic. If metamorphopsia is present, FA may help to detect angioid streaks and a possible choroidal neovascular membrane. Sickle cell preparation and hemoglobin electrophoresis are recommended to rule out other causes of angioid streaks. Patients are instructed to use an Amsler's grid daily to detect macular involvement.

15.19 Phakomatoses

a group of disorders known as neurocutaneous syndromes.

15.19.1 Neurofibromatosis (von Recklinghausen's Disease)

—an autosomal dominant disorder with high penetrance of neurofibromatous, cutaneous and ocular lesions composed of neural crest mesenchyme. Two heritable forms are now recognized: neurofibromatosis type I (NF1), carried on chromosome 17, and neurofibromatosis type II (NF2), carried on chromosome 22.

Presentation

- NF1: Cutaneous involvement includes café au lait spots and nodular neurofibromas (sometimes plexiform). Seizures and mental retardation may occur, and there is an increased risk of malignancy and pheochromocytoma. Visual acuity is generally unaffected. Lisch iris nodules are pathgnomonic (see Section 11.1.10). Optic nerve gliomas occur in 25% of patients (see Section 13.5.1). Retinal hamartomas may also occur, and patients are predisposed to uveal melanoma. Glaucoma may also occur.
- NF2: There is a decreased incidence of cutaneous neurofibromas. Bilateral acoustic neuromas are the hallmarks. Other CNS tumors may occur. Visual acuity is often compromised early in life (age 10 to 20 years) due to posterior subcapsular cataract. No mental retardation is seen.

Management CT scan of brain and yearly blood pressure checks.

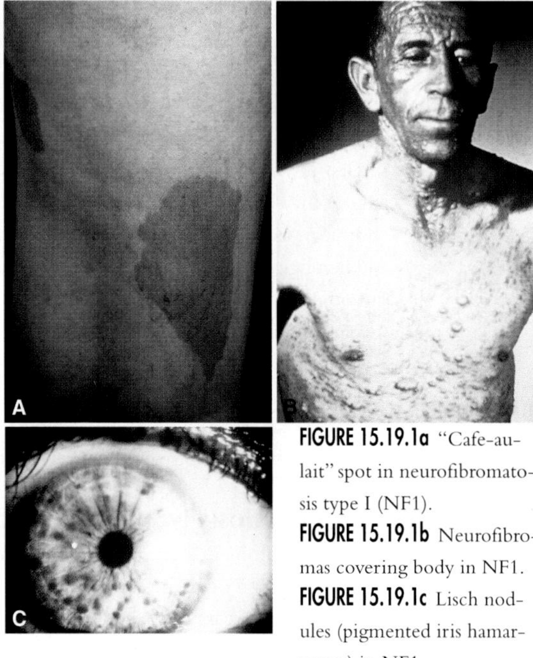

FIGURE 15.19.1a "Cafe-au-lait" spot in neurofibromatosis type I (NF1).
FIGURE 15.19.1b Neurofibromas covering body in NF1.
FIGURE 15.19.1c Lisch nodules (pigmented iris hamartomas) in NF1.

15.19.2 Tuberous Sclerosis (Bourneville's Disease)—an autosomal dominant disease with incomplete penetrance with cutaneous, CNS, and ocular manifestations.

Presentation *Adenoma sebaceum* is the most common cutaneous lesion, found in 70% of patients over the age of 4 years; it is an angiofibroma distributed in a butterfly pattern over the cheeks, chin, and forehead. Other findings include "white revi" over trunk and limbs, seen best with a wood's lamp, lumbosacral "shagreen pattern" and, less commonly, café au lait spot. CNS findings include infantile spasm or seizures (in 80 to 90% of patients, it may be a presenting sign), subependymal hamartomas, and cortical tubers (found on CT scan or at autopsy). Severe mental retardation is present in 50% of cases. Renal angiomyolipomata, cardiac rhabdomyoma, and pulmonary fibrosis may also occur.

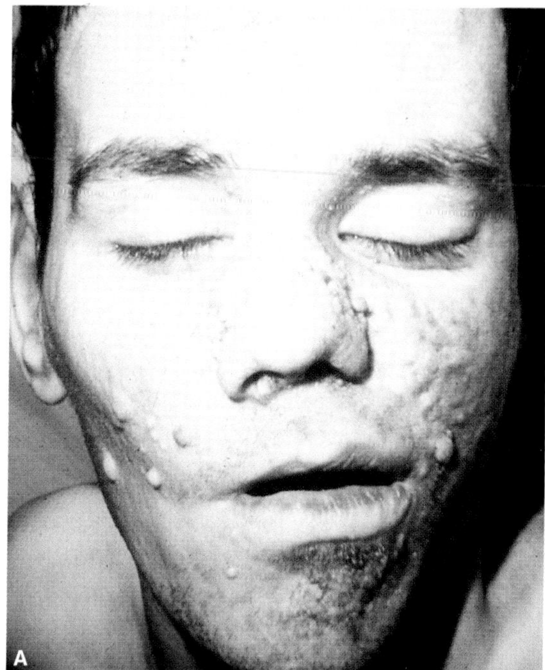

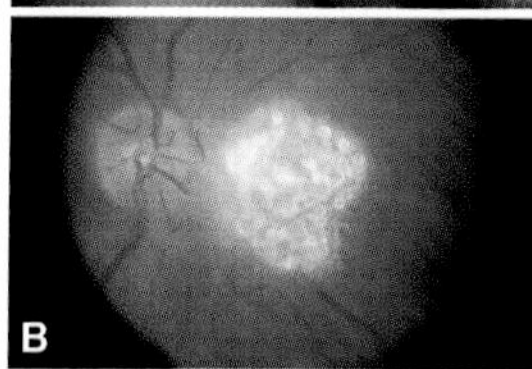

FIGURE 15.19.2a Adenoma sebaceum (facial angiofibromas) in tuberous sclerosis **FIGURE 15.19.2b** Optic disc astrocytoma.

Visual acuity is rarely affected by the astrocytic retinal or optic disc hamartoma (see Chapter 11), the most common ocular finding, present in over 50% of patients. These lesions are usually 1 to 2 disc diameters and are bilateral in one-third to one-half of cases. The term *giant drusen* represents optic nerve head involvement. Peripheral punched-out areas of retinal depigmentation, iris hypopigmentation, and angiofibromata of the eyelids and conjunctiva may occur.

Management

prognosis is poor, with death by the second or third decade. Retinal astrocytomas require no intervention. CT scan of the brain and orbits is recommended, along with cardiac and GI evaluation. Genetic counseling is important.

15.19.3 Sturge-Weber Syndrome (Encephalofacial Cavernous Hemangiomatosis)

15.19.3 Sturge-Weber Syndrome (Encephalofacial Cavernous Hemangiomatosis)—a congenital disorder with no definite inheritance pattern and presumed to be caused by an anomaly of the primordial vasculature during early development.

Presentation facial hemangioma (*nevus flammeus* or port-wine stain) is commonly found at birth in the distribution of the second division of the trigeminal nerve (unilaterally). Cranial hemangiomas, cerebral calcification, mental retardation (intelligence may be normal), and jacksonian seizures may also occur.

Visual symptoms may be absent until adulthood, when progressive hyperopia, RPE degeneration with visual field defects, and serous retinal detachments may occur. Diffuse choroidal hemangiomas ("tomato-catsup" fundus) occur in 40 to 50% of cases. These are slow-growing, yellow-orange, elevated lesions with greatest height at the macula. In addition, unilateral glaucoma occurs in 30% of patients; iris heterochromia, megalocornea, and episcleral telangiectasias may occur.

Management facial angiomas may be masked with makeup or treated with laser surgery. Choroidal lesions are treated only when visual acuity worsens due to tumor growth; photocoagulation, diathermy, cryotherapy, and local irradiation may be necessary. Glaucoma often requires surgical intervention. CT scan and electroencephalography should also be performed.

15.19.4 Von Hippel-Lindau Syndrome (Retinocerebellar Capillary Hemangiomatosis)—a rare, heterogeneous autosomal dominant disorder of the vasculature of the retina and the CNS with incomplete penetrance.

Presentation cerebellar hemangioblastoma (Lindau's tumor) is the most common cause of death, with symptoms beginning in the mid-30s with headache, vertigo, gait disturbance, slurred speech, and nystagmus. Renal cell carcinoma (25% of cases) and pheochromoctyoma (10% of cases) may also occur. Intelligence is normal.

Retinal capillary hemangiomas (a focal collection of capillaries that enlarges to form a red tumor 1 to 3 disc diameters in size, supplied by a feeder artery) may be present at birth but evade detection until the second or third decade. Most commonly found in the inferotemporal, midperiphery, these tumors are bilateral in 50% of cases. Lipid exudation and hemorrhage may progress to retinal detachment, neovascularization, rubeosis iridis, glaucoma, and blindness.

Management systemic complications require head CT scan testing, annual abdominal ultrasound, and urine catecholamine testing (see Retinal Capillary Hemangioma, Section 11.5.2).

15.19.5 Wyburn-Mason Syndrome (Racemose Hemangiomatosis)

—a sporadic disease characterized by one or more anomalous AV anastomoses between the retina and the brain (usually the midbrain).

Presentation a unilateral, intracerebral vascular malformation may present in the second to third decades with headache, nausea, vomiting, nuchal rigidity, and loss of consciousness, secondary to cerebral or subarachnoid hemorrhage. Ipsilat-

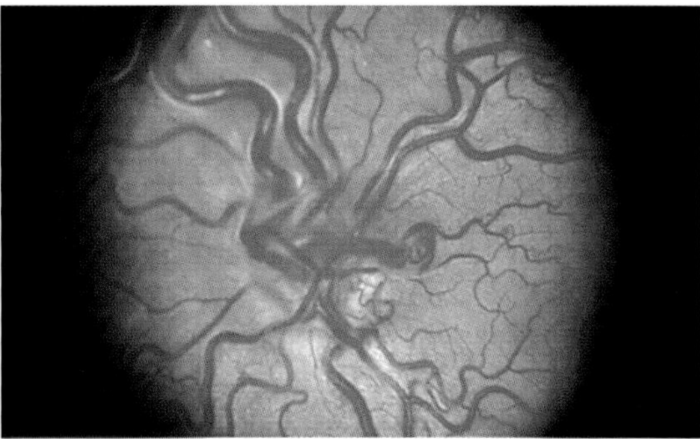

FIGURE 15.19.5 Racemose hemangioma of retina.

eral vascular nevi and facial angiomata may mimic Sturge-Weber syndrome. Congenital defects of bone, muscle, and GI tract have also been reported.

Visual acuity may range from 20/20 to NLP secondary to complications of the direct communication between the engorged, nonpulsating artery and vein (most commonly in the temporal retina) (see Section 11.5.4, AV Malformation). Vitreoretinal hemorrhage or spontaneous thrombosis, papilledema or optic atrophy, and rubeosis iridis with neovascular glaucoma may occur. Proptosis, orbital bruits, and ophthalmoplegia may be found.

Management obtain a CT scan of the brain and orbits with neurosurgical consultation. Laser photocoagulation of symptomatic lesions may be risky. CNS lesions may benefit from embolization or radiotherapy. The prognosis is generally poor, with early mortality.

15.19.6 Ataxia–Telangiectasia (Louis-Bar Syndrome)—a rare, autosomal recessive disorder characterized by neurologic, ocular, and immune system abnormalities.

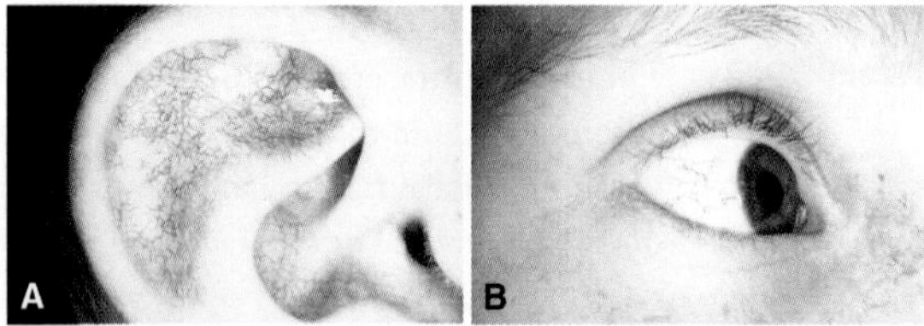

FIGURE 15.19.6a Telangiectasias in ear in Ataxia-telangiectasia.
FIGURE 15.19.6b Telangiectasias in bulbar conjunctiva.

Presentation progressive cerebellar ataxia is the first presenting sign, manifesting as the child begins to walk, and progressing to choreoathetosis, dysarthria, and mental retardation (in adolescence). There is an increased incidence of endocrine disorders and sinopulmonary and otic infections. Telangiectasias of the malar area, ears, and palate, and antecubital and popliteal fossae appear during childhood.

Other abnormalities including premature graying of hair, vitiligo, seborrheic and atopic dermatitis, and testicular and ovarian atrophy may occur.

Bulbar conjunctival telangiectasias usually present in childhood and eventually develop in all patients; strabismus, oculomotor apraxia, nystagmus, and abnormal saccadic function may later become evident.

Management

CT scan or brain MRI shows cerebellar cortical atrophy with diffuse fibrillary gliosis. Treat infection aggressively because more than one-half of patients die of recurrent pulmonary infection. Others die of malignancy, including leukemia and lymphoma. Genetic counseling should be offered to the family.

Chapter 16
CONTACT LENSES

Paul E. Beade, David H. Haight

16.1 FITTING

16.1.1 Soft Hydrogel Contact Lenses—flexible, water and oxygen permeable lenses.

Advantages increased comfort, ease of fitting, little spectacle blur, and ease of adaptation. Extended-wear lenses provide convenience but with an increased risk of corneal ulcers and allergic reactions. Disposable lenses decrease problems of cleaning and deposits.

Drawbacks fragility, tendency to develop deposits, increased susceptibility to infection, limitations to the degree of astigmatic correction achievable (rarely more than 1.00 D), meticulous care and replacement schedule, intolerance for patients with dry eyes or allergies.

16.1.1.1 Selecting Lens Parameters

Diameter a medium diameter can be selected as a first trial, or a lens 0.5 to 1.0 mm larger than the horizontal corneal measurement. Available diameters include small (12.0 to 13.5 mm), average (13.8 to 14.5 mm), and large (14.8 to 15.0 mm).

Base Curve keratometry readings should be obtained. A relatively straightforward method is to take the corneal curvature measurements in diopters, average them, and then convert this average K to radius of curvature using Table 16.1. Choose about 1 mm flatter than this K.

TABLE 16.1. Diopter to radius of curvature conversion

Diopters (D)	Radius (mm)	Diopters (D)	Radius (mm)	Diopters (D)	Radius (mm)	Diopters (D)	Radius (mm)
36.00	9.37	40.37	8.36	44.75	7.54	49.12	6.87
36.12	9.34	40.50	8.33	44.87	7.52	49.25	6.85
36.25	9.31	40.62	8.30	45.00	7.50	49.37	6.84
36.37	9.27	40.75	8.28	45.12	7.48	49.50	6.82
36.50	9.24	40.87	8.25	45.25	7.46	49.62	6.80
36.62	9.21	41.00	8.23	45.37	7.44	49.75	6.78
36.75	9.18	41.12	8.20	45.50	7.42	49.87	6.77
36.87	9.15	41.25	8.18	45.62	7.40	50.00	6.75
37.00	9.12	41.37	8.16	45.75	7.38	50.12	6.73
37.12	9.09	41.50	8.13	45.87	7.36	50.25	6.72
37.25	9.06	41.62	8.10	46.00	7.34	50.37	6.70
37.37	9.03	41.75	8.08	46.12	7.32	50.50	6.68
37.50	9.00	41.87	8.06	46.25	7.30	50.62	6.67
37.62	8.97	42.00	8.03	46.37	7.28	50.75	6.65
37.75	8.94	42.12	8.01	46.50	7.26	50.87	6.63
37.87	8.91	42.25	7.99	46.62	7.24	51.00	6.62
38.00	8.88	42.37	7.96	46.75	7.22	51.12	6.60
38.12	8.85	42.50	7.94	46.87	7.20	51.25	6.58
38.25	8.82	42.62	7.92	47.00	7.18	51.37	6.57
38.37	8.79	42.75	7.89	47.12	7.16	51.50	6.55
38.50	8.76	42.87	7.87	47.25	7.14	51.62	6.54
38.62	8.73	43.00	7.85	47.37	7.12	51.75	6.52
38.75	8.70	43.12	7.82	47.50	7.10	51.87	6.50
38.87	8.68	43.25	7.80	47.62	7.08	52.00	6.49
39.00	8.65	43.37	7.78	47.75	7.06	52.12	6.47
39.12	8.62	43.50	7.76	47.87	7.05	52.25	6.46
39.25	8.59	43.62	7.74	48.00	7.03	52.37	6.44
39.37	8.57	43.75	7.71	48.12	7.01	52.50	6.43
39.50	8.54	43.87	7.69	48.25	6.99	52.62	6.41
39.62	8.51	44.00	7.67	48.37	6.98	52.75	6.40
39.75	8.49	44.12	7.65	48.50	6.96	52.87	6.38
39.87	8.46	44.25	7.63	48.62	6.94	53.00	6.36
40.00	8.43	44.37	7.61	48.75	6.92		
40.12	8.41	44.50	7.58	48.87	6.91		
40.25	8.38	44.62	7.56	49.00	6.89		

Example: K = 44.00/45.00 @180°
choose K = (44.00 + 45.00)/2 = 44.50
base curve (radius of curvature from table) = 7.58
7.58 + 1.00 = 8.58 mm (choose lens closest to this base curve).

Power obtain a manifest refraction in minus-cylinder form. The cylinder (1.00 diopter or less) is omitted from the refraction. If the remaining spherical magnitude is greater than 4.00 D, a vertex distance conversion must be performed (see Table 16.1.1.1).

16.1.1.2 Trial Lens—selected based on the three lens parameters (diameter, base curve, and power). Some latitude is permissible in both the diameter and base curve parameters, as different brands vary in fit.

16.1.1.3 Evaluating Fit—done at the slit lamp with white light illumination. The contact lens should exhibit good centration relative to the limbus and should recenter after every blink. In general, the lens should follow the eye on upward or lateral gaze, usually lagging behind the eye by up to 1 mm. The lens should move upward with gentle pressure on the lower lid.

Tight Fit poor movement on blinking and with upward or lateral gaze. The patient may report that the vision clears briefly with blinking or that the lens becomes progressively less comfortable during wear. Complaints of a burning sensation followed by redness (especially circumcorneal) are seen.

Loose Fit excessive movement in all fields of gaze and with blinking, and poor centration. The patient will report lens awareness, variable vision, or the lens that frequently slides out of place.

16.1.1.4 Overrefraction—fine-tune refraction after fit is acceptable.

16.1.2 Rigid Gas Permeable Contact Lenses—a nonporous, semirigid lens.

TABLE 16.1.1.1 Vertex distance conversion

Spectacle lens power (D)	10	11	12	13	10	11	12	13
	Plus lenses				Minus lenses			
4.00	4.12	4.12	4.25	4.25	3.87	3.87	3.87	3.75
4.50	4.75	4.75	4.75	4.75	4.25	4.25	4.25	4.25
5.00	5.25	5.25	5.25	5.37	4.75	4.75	4.75	4.75
5.50	5.75	5.87	5.87	5.87	5.25	5.12	5.12	5.12
6.00	6.37	6.37	6.50	6.50	5.62	5.62	5.62	5.50
6.50	7.00	7.00	7.00	7.12	6.12	6.00	6.00	6.00
7.00	7.50	7.62	7.62	7.75	6.50	6.50	6.50	6.37
7.50	8.12	8.12	8.25	8.25	7.00	6.87	6.87	6.87
8.00	8.75	8.75	8.87	8.87	7.37	7.37	7.25	7.25
8.50	9.25	9.37	9.50	9.50	7.87	7.75	7.75	7.62
9.00	9.87	10.00	10.12	10.25	8.25	8.25	8.12	8.00
9.50	10.50	10.62	10.75	10.87	8.62	8.62	8.50	8.50
10.00	11.12	11.25	11.37	11.50	9.12	9.00	8.87	8.87
10.50	11.75	11.87	12.00	12.12	9.50	9.37	9.37	9.25
11.00	12.37	12.50	12.75	12.87	9.87	9.75	9.75	9.62
11.50	13.00	13.12	13.37	13.50	10.37	10.25	10.12	10.00
12.00	13.62	13.87	14.00	14.25	10.75	10.62	10.50	10.37
12.50	14.25	14.50	14.75	15.00	11.12	11.00	10.87	10.75
13.00	15.00	15.25	15.50	15.62	11.50	11.37	11.25	11.12
13.50	15.62	15.87	16.12	16.37	11.87	11.75	11.62	11.50
14.00	16.25	16.50	16.75	17.12	12.25	12.12	12.00	11.87
14.50	17.00	17.25	17.50	17.87	12.62	12.50	12.37	12.25
15.00	17.75	18.00	18.25	18.62	13.00	12.87	12.75	12.50
15.50	18.25	18.75	19.00	19.37	13.50	13.25	13.00	12.87
16.00	19.00	19.37	19.75	20.25	13.75	13.62	13.50	13.25
16.50	19.75	20.25	20.50	21.00	14.12	14.00	13.75	13.62
17.00	20.50	21.00	21.50	22.00	14.50	14.25	14.12	14.00
17.50	21.25	21.75	22.25	22.75	14.87	14.75	14.50	14.25
18.00	22.00	22.50	23.00	23.50	15.25	15.00	14.75	14.62
18.50	22.75	23.25	23.75	24.50	15.62	15.37	15.12	14.87
19.00	23.50	24.00	24.75	25.25	16.00	15.75	15.50	15.25

Vertex distance in millimeters (columns 10–13).

Advantages

RGP contact lenses are the choice for patients with moderate amounts of astigmatism (up to 3.00 D), keratoconus, dry eye syndrome, and other external disease

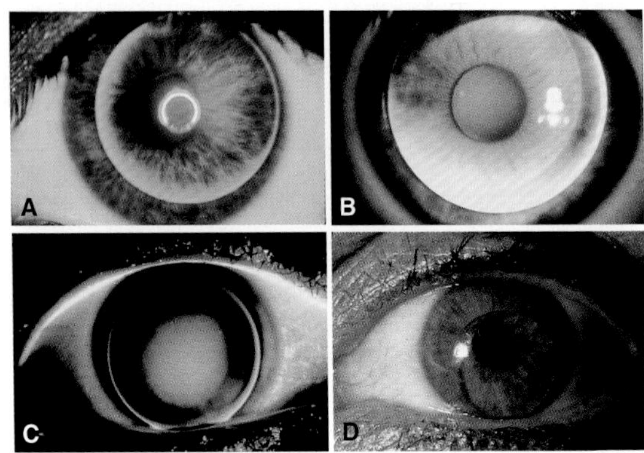

FIGURE 16.1.2a Good fit by fluorescein for RGP lens.
FIGURE 16.1.2b Good fit for RGP lens for with-the-rule astigmatism.
FIGURE 16.1.2c Tight fit for RGP lens.
FIGURE 16.1.2d Loose fit with excessive RGP lens motion.

problems. They also tend to last longer and require less daily care.

Drawbacks less comfort, difficulties adjusting to image movement on blink, more difficulty achieving a good fit, and spectacle blur due to temporary corneal warpage.

16.1.2.1. Selecting Lens Parameters

Diameter lens diameter is selected by taking the iris diameter and subtracting 2.3 mm or selecting a medium-range diameter for the given lens brand.

Base Curve if the difference in curvature between the two Ks is greater than 1.50 D, the base curve can be selected by taking the difference between the two Ks and adding one-quarter of their difference to the flatter K (the "mean of the means" technique).

Example: K = 43.50/45.50 @90°
45.50 − 43.50 = 2.00
2.00/4 = 0.50
Thus select base curve = 43.50 + 0.50 =
44.00 = K_{eff}.

This effective K value (K_{eff}) is then converted to radius of curvature using Table 16.1. In low astigmatics (difference between Ks ≤ 1.50 D) fit for a base curve of 0.50 D flatter than the flattest K reading.

Power refraction is noted in minus-cylinder form, and then cylindrical power is ignored. Again, vertex distance must be corrected for all refractive errors greater than 4.00 D.

16.1.2.2 Evaluating Fit

16.1.2.2 Evaluating Fit—assessed at the slit lamp with fluorescein staining and the cobalt-blue lighting source. Topical anesthetic may be required. Fluorescein will pool in areas of greater lens–cornea clearance and appear highly fluorescent. In areas of less clearance, there will be less fluorescence, and in cases where there is lens–corneal touch, the area will appear dark (no fluorescence).

Alignment Fitting the lens should position slightly high on the cornea with its superior aspect tucked just underneath the upper lid. Alignment fitting works best for with-the-rule astigmatics. The properly fitting RGP lens should move as one with the upper lid and on blink should move smoothly downward and tuck underneath the lower lid. With fluorescein staining in primary position of gaze, there should be clearance demonstrated in the optical zone that stains lightly, no staining in the midperiphery, and a band of staining around the lens periphery to indicate edge lift.

Interpalpebral Fit works best for patients whose upper lids are at or above the superior limbus, precluding an alignment fit, and in against-the-rule and oblique astigmatics. Smaller-diameter, steeper apical clearance lenses are selected to keep the lens well centered and away from contact with the lids.

Tight Fit lens will move poorly in all directions of gaze and may slide out of place. Symptoms of lens awareness, variable vision, redness, and pain may occur. Staining shows a large degree of apical clearance with central pooling extending into the midperiphery, with no staining in the periphery due to tight lens–cornea contact. To correct the fit, flatten the base curve, decrease the lens diameter, or decrease the posterior optical zone.

Loose Fit excessive lens movement. The patient will have lens awareness, unstable vision, and the lens may not stay in the eye. Staining will demonstrate poor apical clearance with absence of fluorescein centrally (no staining) and pooling of fluorescein under the edges of the lens. To correct a loose fit, steepen the lens diameter, or increase the posterior optical zone.

16.1.2.3 *Final Refraction*—if it becomes necessary to alter lens base curve for fit, one must either overrefract the trial lens or alter the refraction according to the "steeper-add-minus, flatter-add-plus rule" (SAM FAP). This involves changing the refraction by 0.25 D for every 0.05-mm change in base curve.

Example: Refraction is − 3.00 − 1.50 × 180
A trial lens with parameters of K = 44.50 (base curve = 7.58), power = −3.00, and diameter = 9.5 mm is fitted.
If the lens fits too tightly and you wish to increase the radius of curvature to 7.63 mm (flatten by 0.05 mm), change the spectacle refraction to −2.75 D ("flatter add plus" of 0.25 D).

16.1.3 Soft Toric Contact Lens Fitting—soft lenses with the astigmatic correction built-in and that require one of various means to keep the axes properly aligned on the cornea. Most toric lenses have a prism at the 6-o'clock periphery that works with gravity to ballast the lens

and maintain proper orientation. In patients with more than 3.00 D of astigmatism, lenticular astigmatism, or moderate astigmatism who cannot tolerate RGP lenses, toric lenses should be considered.

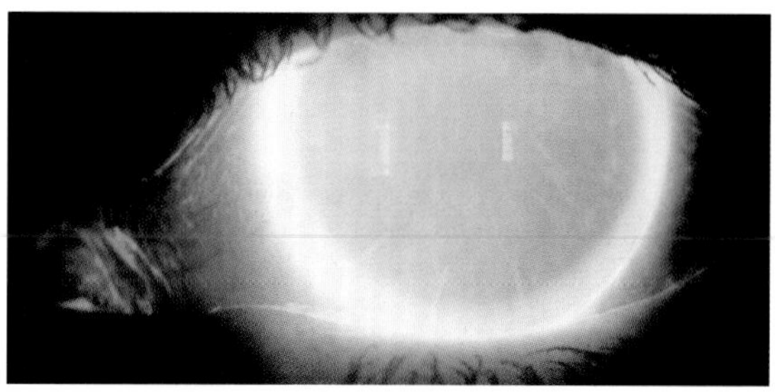

FIGURE 16.1.3 Toric lens with clockwise rotation.

16.1.3.1 Selecting Lens Parameters

Base Curve select a medium base curve to start.

Power with refraction written in minus-cylinder form, choose the spherical component (with appropriate vertex conversion). Cylindrical power should be equal to or up to 0.75 D less than the cylindrical refraction. Axis should be as close to the patient's as possible.

16.1.3.2 Evaluating Fit—trial lens should be in place for at least 10 minutes before checking the fit. At the slit lamp, fit as for a soft hydrogel lens (see Soft Hydrogel Contact Lenses). The rotation (axis) of the lens is evaluated during the blink cycle by monitoring the movement of lens markings, the middle of which ideally rests at the 6-o'clock position. Any rotation from this position is corrected with the mnemonic LARS (left add, right subtract) as follows:

Example: For a refraction of +2.00 −2.50 × 090
Lens rotating 15° to the **R**ight (counterclockwise).
LA**RS**—Subtract 15° from the axis
Choose + 2.00 −2.50 × 075° (or try less cylinder, such as −2.00).

16.1.3.3 Overrefract—with sphere as with soft lenses.

16.1.4 Presbyopic Lens Designs—specialty lenses recommended only for highly motivated patients who are willing to give up some visual acuity for the convenience of simultaneous presbyopic correction.

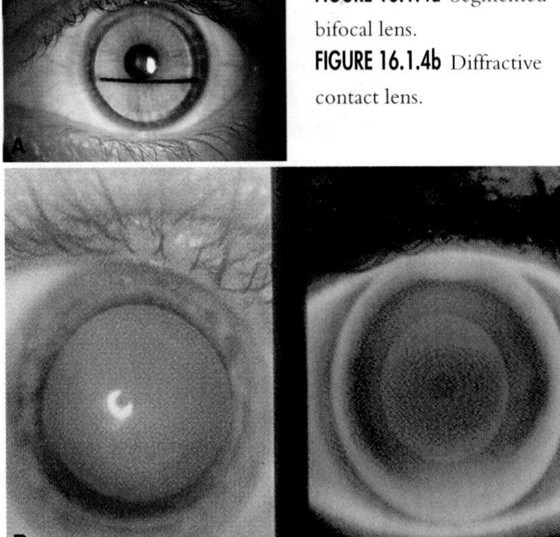

FIGURE 16.1.4a Segmented bifocal lens.
FIGURE 16.1.4b Diffractive contact lens.

- *Alternating vision* (segmented or concentric) design involves lens movement in the upward direction with downward gaze so that the optical axis and the presbyopic add coincide.
- *Simultaneous vision* (concentric, aspheric, and diffractive) design allows vision of near and far objects coincidentally, with the patient choosing which image to consider
- *Monovision* presbyopic correction is a method of fitting the dominant eye for full distance correction and the nondominant eye for near. The advantages of this method are cost and ease of fitting, whereas disadvantages include difficulty in adapting to this method, loss

of stereopsis at distance, and glare with night vision. The modified monovision technique involves using a single vision lens for the dominant eye and a bifocal lens for the nondominant eye for increased stereopsis in distance vision.

Fitting

to fit bifocal contact lenses, one first needs to determine the distance refraction and necessary near add. If the astigmatism is more than 1.00 to 1.25 D, the patient will likely require a RGP lens; otherwise a soft lens is usually preferred. Fit lenses as for soft or hard lenses (see Soft Hydrogel Contact Lenses and Rigid Gas Permeable Contact Lenses) with the following considerations applied to each lens type. Overrefract using handheld trial lenses as opposed to a phoropter to achieve optimum results.

- Segmented bifocal lenses: patients should have pupillary size of greater than 3 mm in normal light illumination. The base curve for your trial lens should be fit 0.50 to 1.00 D flatter than K. The lens should move well as previously outlined and must move upward on downward gaze to allow presbyopic alignment in the reading position. The lens may rotate no more than 1 clock hour in either direction during the blink cycle to allow for stable vision. If the patient has difficulty with near vision, consider increasing the reading segment height, trying a flatter base curve, decreasing the prism, overrefracting, or increasing the add in small increments. If poor distance vision is the problem, try decreasing reading segment height, steepening the base curve, or overrefracting.
- Concentric (multifocal) and aspheric lenses have similar fitting guidelines. Patients with narrow interpalpebral fissure width tend to do well with aspheric and concentric (simultaneous) lenses, whereas patients with large fissure width (>8.5 mm) tend to prefer concentric (alternating) designs. Fit for a base curve 0.50 to 1.00 D flatter than K. For aspheric lenses, select lens diameter with respect to pupil size, with less eccentricity of fit allowed for large pupils and vice versa. If the patient complaints of poor

near vision, flatten the base curve, and recheck the over-refraction. If distance vision is the problem, steepen the base curve, and check the overrefraction.

16.1.5 Keratoconus Considerations—keratoconus (see Section 5.9.1) introduces some special fitting considerations. The corneal apex is usually displaced downward and somewhat temporally, and there is a high degree of irregular corneal astigmatism.

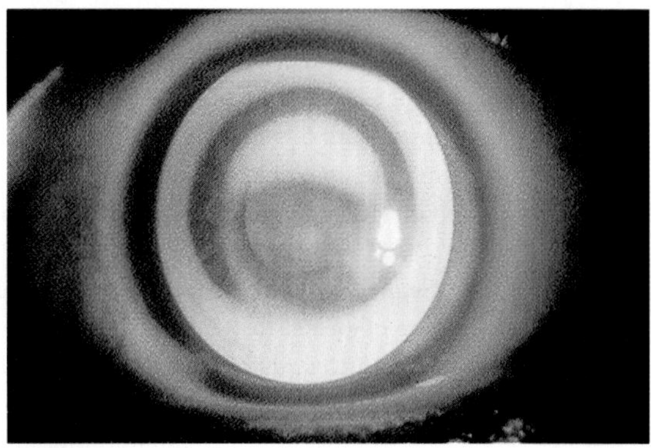

FIGURE 16.1.5 Good RGP keratoconic fit with apical touch and edge lift.

Keratometric classification is as follows: mild (K <45.00 D), moderate (K between 45.00 and 52.00 D in both meridians), advanced (between 52.00 and 60.00 D), and severe (>60.00 D).

- Mild KC: may tolerate spectacle correction or special soft or rigid lenses. Fitting of rigid lenses should allow minimal apical touch, with the remaining lens demonstrating peripheral touch. Apical touch can lead to recurrent corneal abrasions and scarring. If a proper apical fit cannot be achieved, another method of fitting should be tried.
- Moderate KC: should be fit with aspheric RGP lenses with a flatter superior alignment fit. Superior alignment utilizes the more normal superior cornea (above the

cone). The superior aspect of the lens is tucked underneath the upper lid. The inferior lens edge exhibits slight edge lift, which enhances tear circulation and allows for better oxygenation. On slit-lamp fluorescein evaluation, there should be vaulting over the cone and good tear exchange underneath the cone. Once the lens has stabilized, an overrefraction should be performed. Frequent follow-up is necessary.

- Advanced KC: may require specialty contact lenses such as a multicurve lens or a piggyback-type lens. The multicurve lenses are of numerous types, including the Soper, Menicon, McGuire, and NiCone types. The piggyback method makes use of both soft and RGP lenses, with the soft lens placed posteriorly to stabilize the lens system and an RGP lens placed anteriorly. The thin soft lens should sit and move as previously described (see Soft Hydrogel Contact Lenses). Usually a slightly myopic −1.00 to −2.00 soft lens is placed. The RGP lens should be fit flatter than K over the soft lens, and they should move independently during the blink cycle.
- Severe KC (or those who no longer tolerate contact lenses): usually require keratoplasty.

16.2 Complications of Contact Lens Wear

16.2.1 Damaged Contact Lens—lenses of all types are susceptible to damage and can lead to a painful red eye.

Presentation pain; red eye; tearing on lens insertion, usually with immediate relief of symptoms on lens removal; corneal abrasion; SPK; conjunctival injection; RGP lenses with cracks or chipping; soft lenses with fissurelike defects, rips, or missing pieces.

Differential Diagnosis poorly finished lens surface, dry eye syndrome, blepharitis, corneal abrasion, keratoconjunctivitis, chemical injury,

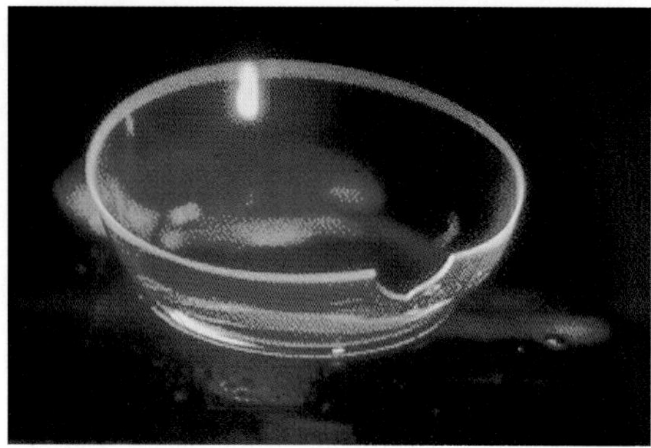

FIGURE 16.2.1 Torn soft contact lens.

hypersensitivity/toxic reactions, other forms of infectious keratitis, lens deposits.

Management

- Slit-lamp examination of anterior segment with and without fluorescein. Examine lens (no fluorescein with soft lenses).
- Discontinue lens wear until cornea is healed completely. Fluoroquinolone (Ciloxan, Ocuflox) 4 to 6 times a day until any abrasion is healed. Soft lenses are discarded, and the patient is refit. Hard lenses with poor finish may be polished in some circumstances.

16.2.2 Lens Deposits

16.2.2 Lens Deposits—protein deposits found on contact lenses that consist of either round elevated bumps or a thin film on the lens surface.

Presentation symptoms range from asymptomatic to redness, irritation, foreign-body sensation, tearing, blurry vision, and lid swelling: SPK, GPC (see Section 16.2.3), lid edema, corneal abrasion or erosion, excess lens movement, deposits as seen on examining the lens.

Differential Diagnosis infectious keratitis (bumplike deposits on lens must be differentiated from fungal infection), dry eye syndrome,

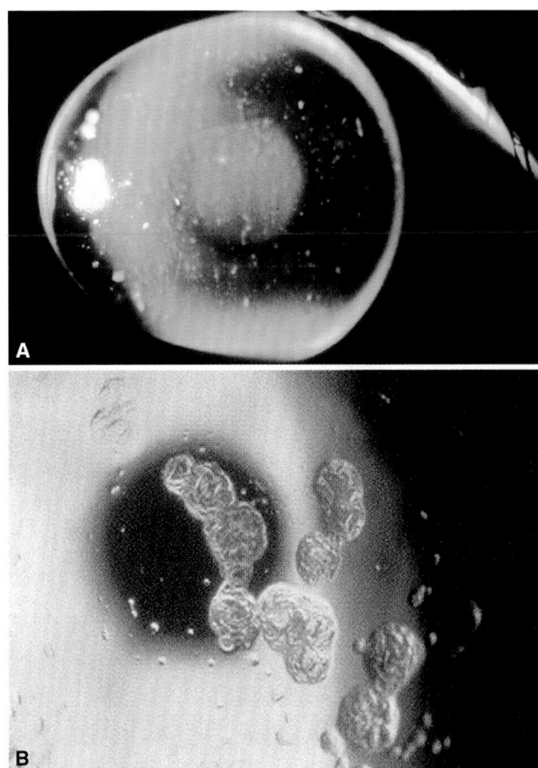

FIGURE 16.2.2a RGP lens deposits.
FIGURE 16.2.2b Soft contact lens with elevated deposits.

blepharitis, GPC, hypersensitivity/toxic keratoconjunctivitis, lens damage, corneal abrasion/erosion.

Management

- History and slit-lamp examination. Examine lenses for deposits.
- Replace the soft lens for significant deposits, and consider switching to disposable lenses. Increase frequency of enzyme cleaning. RGP lenses may sometimes be cleaned with polishing compound. Reinforce importance of daily cleaning regimen. If problem persists,

may need to switch from current soft lens to low water content soft or RGP lens.

16.2.3 Giant Papillary Conjunctivitis—the most common soft contact lens–associated complication, which is believed to be an inflammatory reaction to protein deposits on the lens or secondary to mechanical aspects of lens design. Seen more often in extended-wear than in daily-wear lenses. GPC is also seen with rigid contact lens wear or related to ocular foreign body such as a suture (usually nylon) or ocular prosthesis.

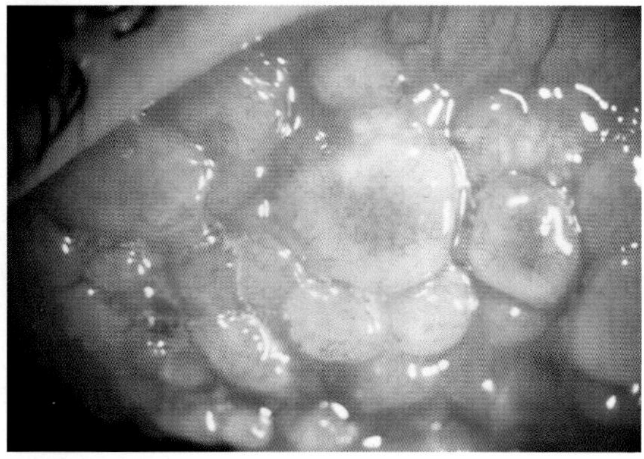

FIGURE 16.2.3 GPC.

Presentation symptoms range from asymptomatic to itching, upper eyelid edema, red eye, mucoid discharge, decreased acuity (usually from coating of lens with mucus), and progressive contact lens intolerance. Eversion of upper eyelid reveals large papillae (>0.3 mm) identical to those found in vernal conjunctivitis, conjunctival and corneal inflammation is usually minimal, contact lens almost always found to have deposits, high-riding lens, upper eyelid edema/ptosis.

Differential Diagnosis vernal conjunctivitis.

Management

- History must include details of contact lens wear, such as age of current lenses and cleaning and enzyme regimen. Slit-lamp examination of anterior segment with special attention to examination of everted upper lids and contact lens.

- Decrease lens wearing time; temporarily discontinue lens wear in severe cases. Lodoxamide, one drop 4 times a day. Follow-up in 2 to 4 weeks, tapering lodoxamide as signs and symptoms improve. Patient is instructed to clean lenses more thoroughly with preservative-free solutions and to increase enzyme use. In some cases, it may be necessary to switch to higher water content, thinner, smaller-diameter lenses, and occasionally a change to RGP lenses is warranted. Extended-wear lens wearers should be advised to switch to daily wearing practices. In cases in which discontinuation of lens wear is deemed necessary, restart lens wear when condition resolves (usually 1 month or more).
- Exposed suture: removal is indicated with proper technique and antibiotic coverage.
- Prosthesis-related GPC: prosthesis should be carefully cleaned and polished. Special coatings are also available for prostheses to minimize GPC. Lodoxamide may also be helpful.
- Severe GPC: a short course of topical steroids may be indicated.

16.2.4 Overwear/Hypoxia—corneal decompensation due to hypoxia has become less common with the advent of RGP and soft lenses mostly supplanting the use of PMMA lenses.

Presentation

- Acute hypoxia: the patient typically complains of redness, tearing, mild blurriness, and irritation. Conjunctival injection and a corneal erosion may be noted on slit-lamp examination.
- Chronic hypoxia: may be asymptomatic or may involve increasing redness and progressive discomfort with time of lens wear, as well as tearing and varying degrees of blurriness. Findings include SPK, epithelial microcysts, stromal edema, corneal neovascularization, and conjunctival injection.

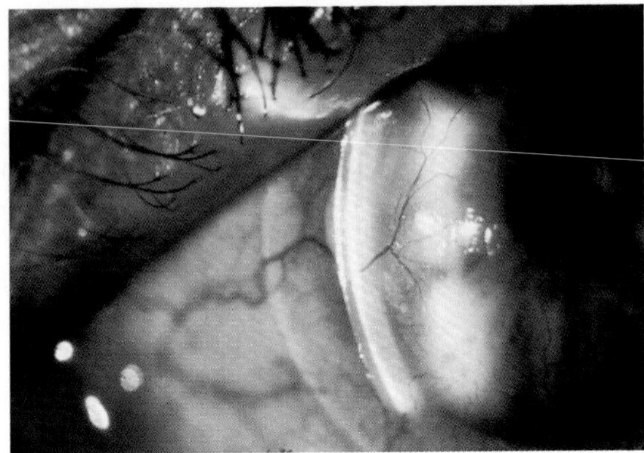

FIGURE 16.2.4 Contact lens overwear with marked neovascularization/pannus.

Differential Diagnosis

tight contact lens fit, dry eye syndrome, blepharitis, infectious keratitis, hypersensitivity/toxic reaction, corneal abrasion/erosion.

Management

- Slit-lamp examination and typical history in contact lens wearer, especially in PMMA or other low oxygen transmitting lens wearers.
- Acute hypoxia is treated by immediately discontinuing lens wear and use of prophylactic antibiotic drops with good *Pseudomonas* coverage (fluoroquinolone [Ocuflox, Ciloxan]qid). On resolution of signs and symptoms, the patient may be refit with higher oxygen transmitting lenses.
- Chronic hypoxia with or without neovascularization (see Section 16.2.5) should be treated by discontinuing lens wear until discomfort and corneal edema resolve. The patient may be refit with higher oxygen transmitting contact lenses with reduced daily wearing time. If the patient does not improve with this method of treatment, contact lenses may be discontinued indefinitely to protect the corneal integrity.

16.2.5 Contact Lens–Induced Corneal Neovascularization/Pannus Formation

16.2.5 Contact Lens–Induced Corneal Neovascularization/Pannus Formation—new vessels occurring superficially along the limbus or invading the corneal stroma in more severe cases. Seen more often with extended wear and less often with RGP lenses.

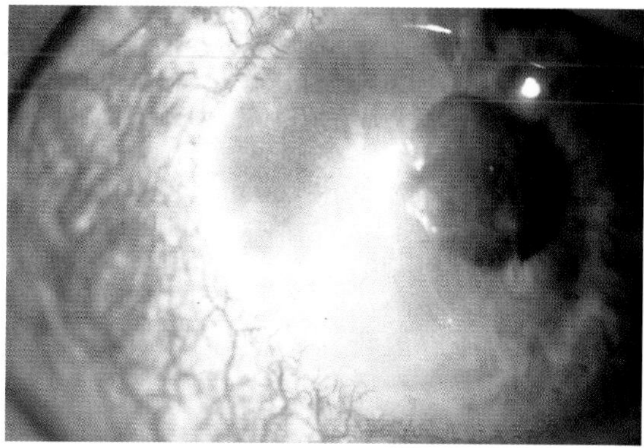

FIGURE 16.2.5 Intracorneal hemorrhage due to neovascularization.

Presentation usually asymptomatic. Less than 2 mm of corneal neovascularization is often seen in soft contact lens wear (micropannus); however, if vessels extend more than 2 mm, serious consequences such as lipid keratopathy, corneal scarring and opacification, and even intracorneal hemorrhage may result. Stromal ghost vessels, perivascular fibrotic vascular sheathing, and corneal edema may be present.

Differential Diagnosis neovascularization secondary to trauma from damaged contact lens, hypersensitivity/toxic reactions, chemical injury, tight lens.

Management

- Slit-lamp examination, especially using retroillumination in patient with history of chronic lens overwear.
- Contact lens wear should be discontinued until the vessels are less than 2 mm in size. Weak topical steroids

(e.g., Pred Mild, FML) may be used. When patient meets above criteria, new lenses with higher oxygen transmission (flatter, thinner, or higher water content soft or RGP). Extended-wear lenses should be changed to daily wear, and further restrictions to lens wear may ultimately be necessary. Particular care should be taken in refitting new lenses, being careful that they exhibit good movement. Preservative-free contact lens solutions are recommended.

16.2.6 Tight Lens Syndrome

16.2.6 Tight Lens Syndrome—a complication of extended-wear contact lens use in which a well-fitted lens suddenly exhibits lack of movement on the cornea, impinging on the limbal blood vessels and trapping debris and mucus beneath the lens. The etiology is uncertain; theories include lens dehydration and changes in tear pH, which result in corneal hypoxia.

Presentation red eye, especially on wakening in myopes and aphakes; irritation; mild blurriness; conjunctival hyperemia; usually mild anterior chamber reaction (in severe cases may develop sterile hypopyon after days of symptoms); superficial punctate staining; corneal epithelial edema; tight-fitting lens.

Differential Diagnosis tight lens fit, contact lens overwear.

Management

- History and physical examination.
- Contact lens wear should be discontinued immediately for at least 1 week. Once the epithelium has healed and any anterior chamber reaction has resolved, contact lens wear may be resumed. Contact lenses greater than 6 months old should be replaced. Use of antibiotics or topical steroids is controversial.

16.2.7 Corneal Warpage Syndrome—induced warpage of the cornea from long-term PMMA lenses, which account for less than 1% of all types of contact lenses. It is believed to result from long-term hypoxia combined with the mechanical stress of the rigid PMMA lens. This effect is usually temporary, depending on duration of lens wear and severity of corneal distortion.

Presentation usually asymptomatic except for blurriness of vision with contact lenses or spectacle correction, distorted mires on keratometry with or without irregular astigmatism, corneal edema, decreased vision on post–contact lens wear refraction, lens decentration, decreased corneal sensitivity.

Differential Diagnosis KC or other ectatic corneal dystrophy.

Management

- Slit-lamp examination, keratometry, post–contact lens wear refraction in long-term PMMA contact lens wearer.
- Studies have shown that those who are immediately refit with RGP lenses based on keratometry readings taken approximately 15 minutes after PMMA lens removal do well. If the mires are too distorted at this time, then a period of PMMA deadaptation is recommended with gradual decreased wearing time by 1 to 2 hours per day, with 1 week of follow-up for refit with RGP lenses. Immediate discontinuation of lens wear should be discouraged because it has been related to severe changes in corneal curvature and these patients often exhibit poor vision with spectacle correction.
- Some recommend refitting with low oxygen transmission RGP lenses at first with gradual increase in D_k with subsequent lenses. Follow-up should be frequent, and the patient should ultimately have a full anterior segment evaluation at least every 6 months once symptoms have resolved. New spectacle refraction can usually safely be given 3 weeks after stability of vision with RGP lenses.

16.2.8 Corneal Staining Patterns

16.2.8.1 Epithelial Microcysts—formation of corneal intraepithelial cysts seen in association with long-term contact lens wear. They are thought to result from effects of trauma or hypoxia, leading to an abnormality in cellular development.

Presentation usually asymptomatic. Slit-lamp examination demonstrates tiny translucent dots of varying optical densities involving the central and midperipheral corneal epithelium.

Differential Diagnosis epithelial vacuoles, epithelial bullae, preservative toxicity.

Management

- Slit-lamp examination in long-term contact lens wearer; the lenses are typically soft or extended-wear type but may be RGP.
- Refit patient with contact lens of higher oxygen transmissibility. Recommend that the patient use preservative-free contact lens solutions.

16.2.8.2 Corneal Abrasions—see Section 1.1.5, Corneal Abrasions.

Note: Corneal abrasions in contact lens wearers should never be patched, and the patient should be empirically covered with topical antibiotics with good *Pseudomonas* coverage (e.g., fluoroquinolone). Be sure to examine lens for damage or embedded foreign body.

16.2.8.3 Contact Lens–Related Superficial Punctate Keratitis—a common staining pattern seen with contact lens wear, especially related to dehydration in patients wearing thin, high water content hydrogel lenses. Arid environments and poor blinking exacerbate this phenomenon.

Presentation symptoms range from asymptomatic to irritation, tearing, blurry vision, and redness. Slit-lamp examination reveals tiny grayish-white epithelial erosions, especially involving the central cornea, and staining with fluorescein.

Differential Diagnosis dry eye, blepharitis, toxic reactions. Other contact lens–related causes of SPK include 3- and 9-o'clock staining, hypersensitivity/toxic reactions to solutions, lens-related hypoxia, tight fit.

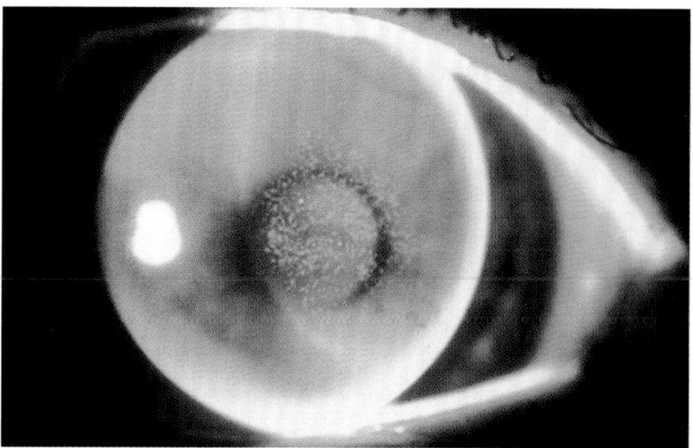

FIGURE 16.2.8.3 Contact lens–related SPK.

Management

- Slit-lamp examination, especially in patient wearing thin, high water content hydrogel lenses.
- Corneal findings may disappear within hours of discontinuing lens wear. Preservative-free tears every 1 to 2 hours. Refitting with thicker, lower water content lenses often eliminates the problem. If there is any question of infection, close follow-up with appropriate antibiotics must be considered.

16.2.8.4 Contact Lens–Related Superior Limbic Keratoconjunctivitis (or Contact Lens Keratoconjunctivitis)—a usually bilateral syndrome of contact lens intolerance occurring more commonly with soft lenses. Believed to result from the absorption of materials such as thimerosal or hypoxia, physical irritation, allergy, or a toxic reaction.

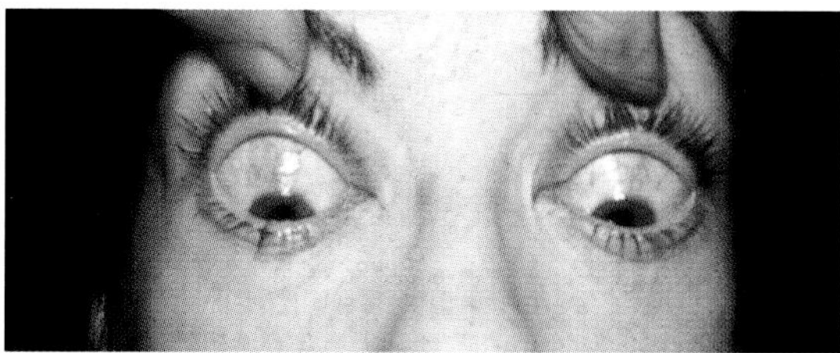

FIGURE 16.2.8.4 Contact lens–related SLK with rose bengal.

Presentation

symptoms range from burning and irritation after progressively shorter periods of comfortable lens wear to more severe complaints of redness, photophobia, and usually mild visual loss (rarely can be 20/200 or less). Crescent- or wedge-shaped area of hazy epithelium separated from superior limbus by small clear zone with the apex of the wedge directed toward the pupil. Usually only upper one-third of cornea involved but occasionally can involve visual axis. Often gray punctate opacities at level of Bowman's layer. Mild hyperemia and thickening of bulbar conjunctiva immediately superior to limbus. Occasional micropannus. Usually fine papillae of upper lid on eversion. On fluorescein or rose bengal staining, SPK is seen superiorly with staining over the involved area of conjunctiva. Corneal filaments may be seen.

Differential Diagnosis

poorly fitting soft contact lens, viral keratitis, GPC, SLK not related to contact lens wear (e.g., thyroid disease).

Management

- Question history of previous episodes. Slit-lamp examination with and without fluorescein or rose bengal staining of cornea, conjunctiva, and superior eyelid with eversion. Gross examination without the slit lamp often aids in diagnosis.
- Discontinue contact lens wear.
- Mild cases: preservative-free artificial tear drops may be used 4 to 6 times a day, with a tear ointment at bedtime.
- More severe cases: chemical cauterization with silver nitrate solution 0.5 to 1.0% in wax ampules (**not** cautery sticks!) may be applied with cotton swab for approximately 15 seconds to the involved areas of bulbar and tarsal conjunctiva after appropriate topical anesthesia. This treatment may be reapplied at weekly follow-up visits.
- Patients should be made aware that lenses should be discontinued at the first symptoms or signs suggestive of previous episode, with immediate follow-up.

16.2.8.5 3- and 9-O'Clock Staining—chronic inflammation and characteristic epithelial staining in a hard contact lens wearer with dry eyes, inadequate or incomplete blinking due to hypoxia.

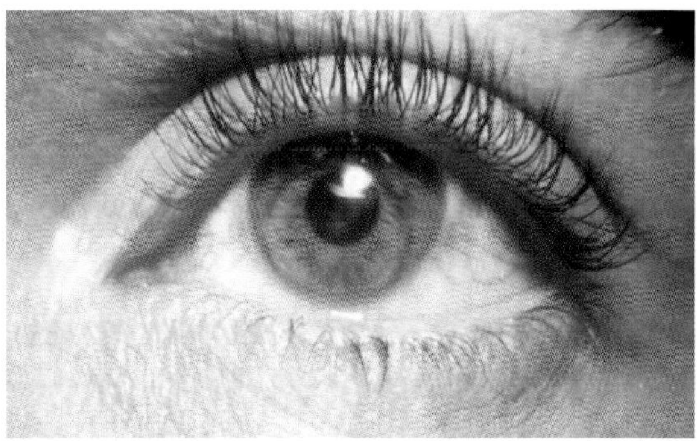

FIGURE 16.2.8.5 Conjunctival injection in 3- and 9-o'clock disease.

Presentation pain, photophobia, red eye, itching, foreign-body sensation, blurry vision, contact lens intolerance. Fluorescein staining of the cornea, especially in the nasal and temporal paralimbal regions. In extreme cases with chronic involvement, a vascular limbal keratitis can result, which presents with a pterygium-like vascularization of the cornea, corneal scarring, epithelial hyperplasia, and dellen formation.

Differential Diagnosis viral keratitis, tight lens syndrome, toxic keratopathy, corneal abrasion, poor lens fit.

Management

- Note degree and type of symptoms, type and age of contact lens, and lens-wearing and hygiene habits. Investigate for signs and symptoms of dry eye or predisposing conditions (see Section 4.4).
- Discontinue contact lens wear. Treat any underlying condition or dry eye with preservative-free artificial tears at least 4 times a day. Depending on severity, follow up in 1 to 4 weeks until resolved. Refitting with a

larger-diameter or higher D_k lens may be helpful, and switching from RGP to soft lenses may alleviate this process in appropriate patients. Use preservative-free contact lens solutions. Inform the patient to discontinue lens wear and seek immediate attention at the first sign of recurrence.

16.2.8.6 Bubble Staining or Dimple Veiling—staining pattern seen more frequently in RGP lenses believed to result from a poor fitting relationship. Bubbles of carbon dioxide trapped under the lens indent the epithelium, leaving tiny depressions.

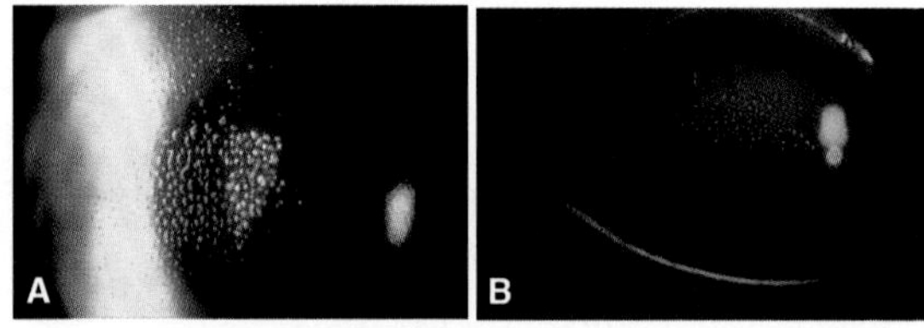

FIGURE 16.2.8.6a Dimple veiling.
FIGURE 16.2.8.6b Dimple staining.

Presentation often asymptomatic, but may be associated with irritation, tearing, and blurry vision (especially with apical involvement). Dimples are seen on the corneal surface, giving it a "golf ball" appearance. The corneal depressions do not stain but are clearly outlined by fluorescein. The lens often displays a poor fit.

Differential Diagnosis corneal microcysts.

Management

- Slit-lamp examination, usually in a patient with history of RGP more often than soft contact lens wear.
- This represents a poor lens–cornea relationship, and thus refitting is the mainstay of treatment. Often resolves with flatter or smaller-diameter lens. May require change from hard to soft lenses if possible. Patients must be checked frequently until signs resolve.

16.3 Contact Lens Infiltrates

16.3.1 Corneal Ulcers—see Section 5.1.4, Bacterial Corneal Ulcer and Fungal Keratitis for a complete discussion.

Note: Contact lens wear is strictly prohibited until complete recovery has occurred (weeks to months) as evidenced by lack of progression or symptoms after antibiotics are discontinued and after examination by a qualified practitioner. The current pair should be cultured in addition to corneal scrapings. Lenses should be discarded and refitted if necessary. Wearing schedules in extended wearers should at least be shortened and more appropriately should restrict routine overnight wear. Oral pain medications such as acetaminophen, aspirin, and NSAIDs may be necessary. Patching is contraindicated in all patients with corneal ulcer; however, when severe thinning occurs, a shield should be worn around the clock.

16.3.2 Contact Lens Sterile Corneal Infiltrates—multiple sterile corneal infiltrates with or without ulceration may be seen in association with hard or soft lens wear (see Chapter 5, Sterile Infiltrates).

Presentation symptoms range from asymptomatic to mild irritation, redness, and tearing, to severe discomfort and loss of vision. Persistent corneal epithelial defect that stains with fluorescein, leading to infiltrate and progressive stromal thinning on slit-lamp examination. Anterior chamber inflammation varies from absent to severe. In severe cases, keratinization of the cornea has been described.

Differential Diagnosis infectious corneal infiltrate or ulcer, neurotrophic ulcer (see Chapter 5, Neurotrophic Ulcer).

Management

- Consider scraping for culture and Gram's stain for significant lesions (>1 mm or central).

- Many contact lens–related corneal ulcers are sterile, but they should be treated empirically for an infectious cause (fluoroquinolone qid in most cases is adequate). Discontinue lens wear until infiltrates completely resolve. Use lubrication, especially in dry eye–related disorders, as needed. Judicious use of steroids after infection is ruled out may hasten recovery.

16.4 Reactions to Preservatives in Solutions

16.4.1 Hypersensitivity Reactions

16.4.1 Hypersensitivity Reactions—allergic inflammatory reactions that occur after reexposure to a substance. One example is thimerosal, a bacteriostatic mercurial preservative still found in some contact lens solutions, which is absorbed by hydrogel lenses and slowly released.

Presentation diffuse redness, lid edema, itching, burning, tearing, photophobia, conjunctival injection, chemosis, eyelid edema, follicles, less commonly SPK, anterior stromal infiltrates, corneal neovascularization, dendritiform lesions.

Differential Diagnosis allergic conjunctivitis, viral conjunctivitis, toxic keratoconjunctivitis.

Management

- Investigate history of using thimerosal-containing contact lens solutions. Typically they have used these lenses at least 3 months prior to presentation.
- Discontinue contact lens wear. Avoid thimerosal and other mercurials in the future. Corticosteroid drops may be used only if infectious etiology can be reasonably excluded (especially bacterial, herpetic, or chlamydial disease). When symptoms resolve completely, may restart with a new pair of contact lenses.

16.4.2 Toxic Reactions—inflammatory reactions to substances without prior exposure to the immune system, leading to rapid tissue in-

needle inferiorly and laterally into the subconjunctival or sub-Tenon's area as shown. Avoid conjunctival blood vessels and make sure that the needle moves freely prior to injection. Pull back on the syringe, to check for heme, prior to injection. Avoid scleral perforation.

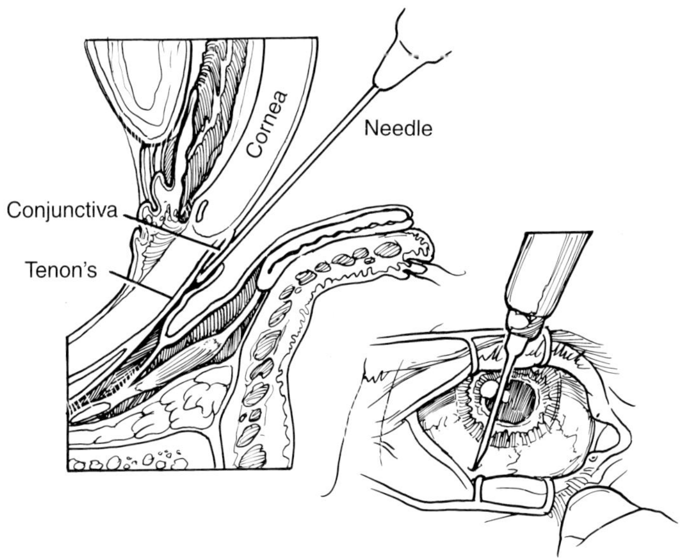

FIGURE 18.5 Subconjunctival injection.

18.6 Retrobulbar Injection

instruct the patient to look straight ahead. Place your finger on the inferior orbital rim midway between the lateral and inferior rectus muscles. Use a blunt-tip, retrobulbar needle with the bevel facing up; follow the path of your finger and insert the needle through the orbital septum to the equatorial region of the globe. Then, as you advance, redirect the needle up toward the apex of the globe. Once the needle is resting in the muscle cone, gently move it from side to side to make sure you have not penetrated the globe, and gently pull back on the syringe, looking for heme. Inject anesthetic, remove the needle, and apply firm

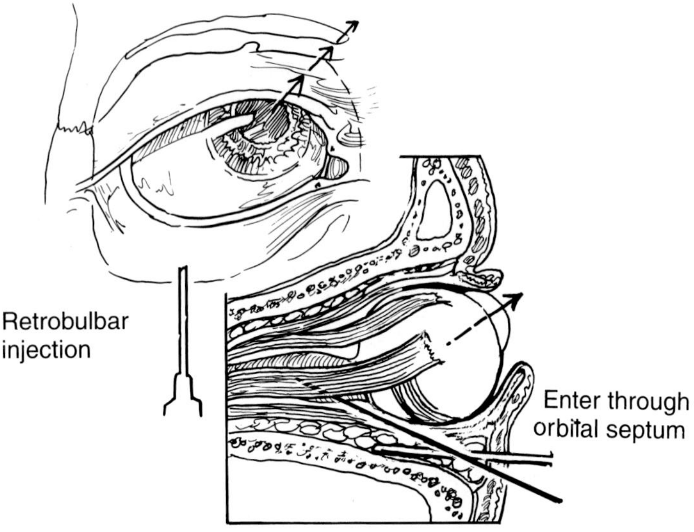

FIGURE 18.6 Retrobulbar injection.

pressure. After 5 to 10 minutes, the eye should be soft and immobile, except for the movement of the superior oblique muscle. A typical solution is a 50 : 50 mixture of 4% lidocaine and .75% bupivicaine, with wydase.

18.7 Anterior Stromal Puncture

instill tetracaine and antibiotics in the eye prior to the procedure. Instill fluorescein to help to visualize the puncture marks. Place a disposable stromal puncture needle or a bent 27-gauge needle on a tuberculin syringe and make sure that the patient is comfortable at the slit lamp. Place the tip of the needle perpendicular to the surface of the cornea and gently penetrate the cornea to the level of the anterior stroma. Cover the entire erosive area with nonconfluent punctures and continue to create a 2-mm margin of punctures into the normal cornea. Try to avoid treatment of the visual axis. Postoperatively, use cycloplegics, topical antibiotics, and nonsteroidals. Consider a pressure patch or a bandage contact lens.

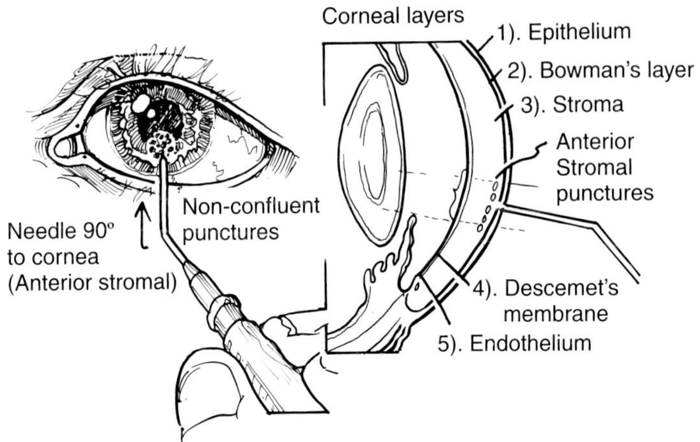

FIGURE 18.7 Anterior stromal puncture.

18.8 Placement of Punctal Plugs

instill tetracaine and place a tetracaine-soaked pledget onto the punctum. Load the punctal plug into the inserter and place the punctal dilator into the punctum. Remove the dilator and promptly insert the plug. The dome of the plug should be visible in the punctum. Hold the dome with a forceps while you remove the inserter.

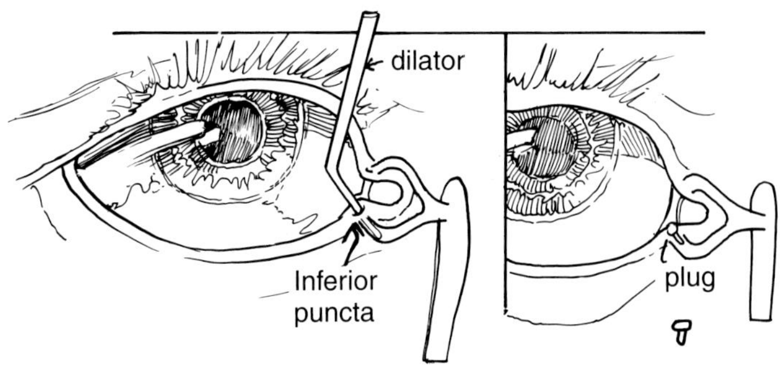

FIGURE 18.8 Punctal plugs.

18.9 Punctal Ectropion Repair

inject 1 to 2% Xylocaine (lidocaine) with epinephrine subconjunctivally below the area of the affected canaliculus. Prepare and drape the patient in the usual sterile fashion. Apply tetracaine and place a scleral shield in the eye. Insert a lacrimal probe into the inferior canaliculus. Excise a 5-mm-long by 3-mm-wide elliptical portion of conjunctiva and tarsus-lid retractor complex from an area 2 mm below the punctum. Remove the lacrimal probe, and close the incision with 7–0 Vicryl (polyglactin 910). Place the interrupted sutures deep enough to bring the edges of the tarsus and lower lid retractors together. Remove the scleral shell and place antibiotic ointment in the eye.

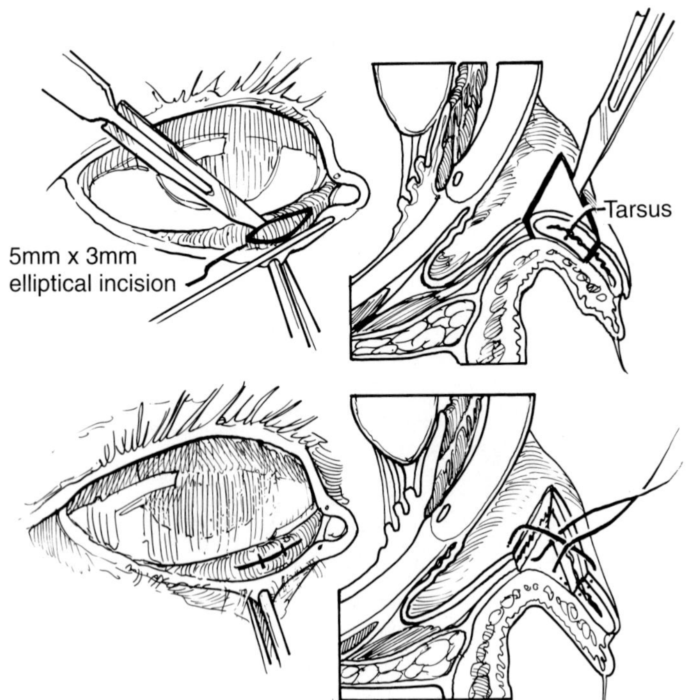

FIGURE 18.9 Punctal ectropion repair.

18.10 Nasolacrimal Duct Irrigation

instill tetracaine drops and place a tetracaine pledget on the punctal area. After inserting the punctal dilator, insert the irrigation probe inferiorly for 2 mm and then rotate it horizontally as you insert it toward the nose. At this point, it helps to stretch the eyelid laterally. Then, inject the irrigating solution. If there is no resistance, ask patients if they can taste the solution. If they say yes, there is no occlusion. If there is resistance, apply gentle pressure. If there is still resistance, the patient has a blockage and you must now determine the level of the blockage. Remember to irrigate both the lower and upper systems.

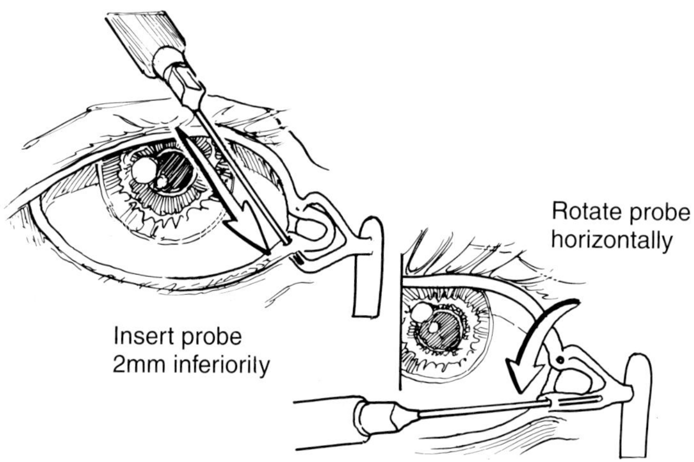

FIGURE 18.10 Nasolacrimal duct irrigation.

18.11 Corneal and Conjunctival Cultures and Scrapings

for conjunctival cultures, try to use a sterile swab in the inferior fornix prior to instilling topical anesthetic. For corneal cultures, instill sterile tetracaine and place the patient at the slit lamp. Use the Kimura spatula to scrape the base of the ulcer so that a portion of the infiltrate is on

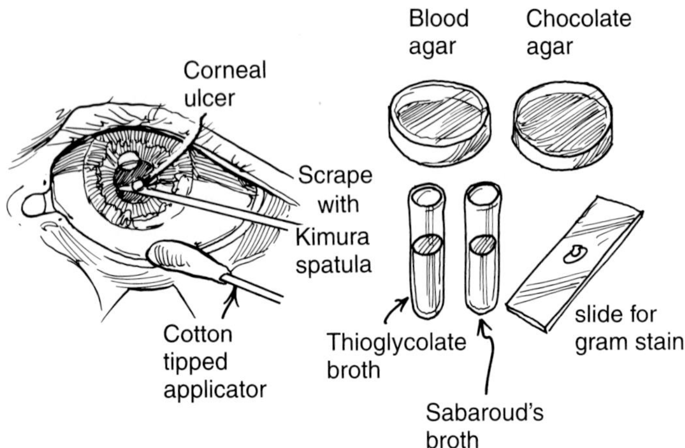

FIGURE 18.11 Cornea and conjunctival cultures.

the instrument. Place the specimen on a slide for Gram's stain or on selected media, such as blood and chocolate agar, Sabouraud's dextrose agar or thioglycolate broth. For each separate specimen, resterilize the spatula over the flame of an alcohol burner. Allow the spatula time to cool prior to touching the conjunctiva or cornea. Alternatively, use sterile gauge needles to scrapte ulcer.

18.12 Eyelid Margin Laceration Repair

place tetracaine and a scleral shell in the eye. Irrigate the eyelid wound and attempt to remove all foreign debris. Anesthetize the eyelid with 1 to 2% Xylocaine (lidocaine) with epinephrine. Debride the frankly necrotic tissue and trim the eyelid margin so that the wound edges are sharp. Initially close the tarsus with interrupted 6–0 Vicryl (polyglactin 910) sutures. Then, reapproximate the margin with three 6–0 silk sutures: place vertical suture through the gray line (Riolan's muscle), a second suture through the lash line, and a third just posterior to the meibomian glands. Each of these three sutures should be 1 to 2 mm deep and 1 to 2 mm lateral to the wound edges. Keep the suture ends long so that they may be secured under the skin sutures. Close the skin with interrupted 6–0 silk or Vicryl sutures.

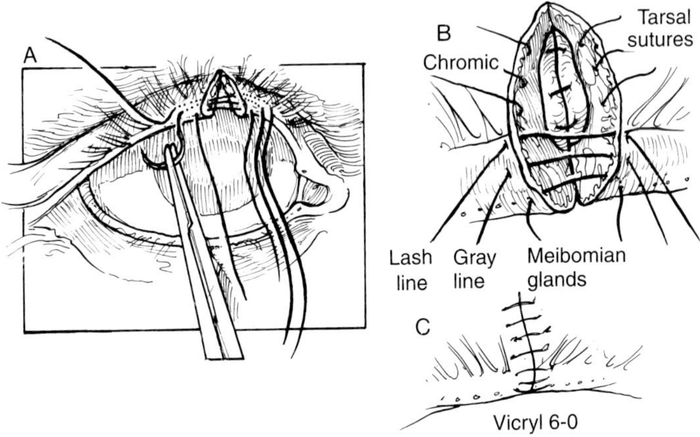

FIGURE 18.12 Eyelid margin repair.

18.13 Pterygium Excision with Conjunctival Graft

the patient should receive a retrobulbar or peribulbar block, and the eye should be prepared and draped in the usual sterile fashion. Place a lid speculum in the eye and inject the pterygium with 3 ml of 1 to 2% Xylocaine (lidocaine) with epinephrine. This helps to determine the extent of the pterygium and to determine your dissection plane. Use the forceps to pull the pterygium gently off the corneal surface as you establish a dissection plane with a 57-Beaver blade. Then use a Westcott scissors to free the scleral portion of the pterygium, leaving bare sclera behind. Hemostasis is then achieved with either electrocautery or wet-field cautery. The 57-Beaver blade may then be used to smooth the corneal surface.

Use calipers to measure the bare scleral area. The donor graft is usually taken from the superior bulbar conjunctiva. Use the cautery to mark the dimensions of the conjunctival graft (usually no larger than 5 to 6 mm in

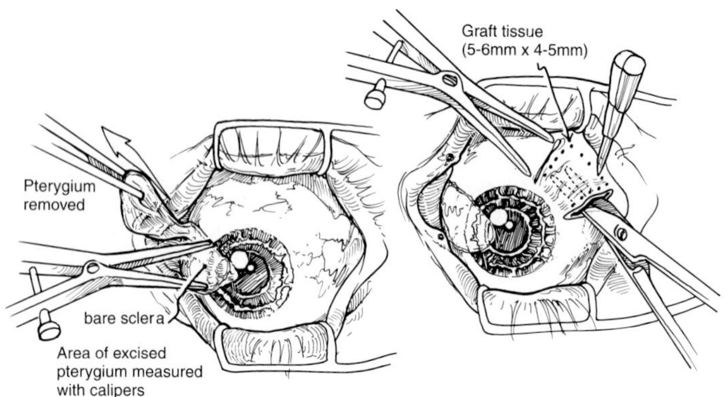

FIGURE 18.13 Pterygium excision with conjunctival graft.

length by 4 to 5 mm in width). Use a Westcott scissors and smooth forceps to dissect the thin conjunctival flap. Be sure to avoid Tenon's capsule and the episclera. Free the limbal edge of the graft and move the superior limbal portion of the graft to the limbal portion of the bare sclera. Leave a 1- to 2-mm clear zone between the limbus and the graft. Anchor the four edges of the graft with either 8–0 Vicryl (polyglactin 910) or 10–0 nylon suture. Apply a topical antibiotic or steroid drop and patch the eye.

Chapter 19
REFRACTIVE SURGERY

Suresh Mandava, Vadim Filatov, John Talamo

19.1 Radial Keratotomy

an incisional keratorefractive procedure involving multiple linear, radial incisions in the paracentral and peripheral cornea to treat myopia or, with the addition of astigmatic keratotomy, myopic astigmatism. "Mini-RK" is a variation with shorter incisions and a larger optical zone (7 or 8 mm). Astigmatic keratotomy involves horizontal or arcuate cuts to relax steepening in the same meridian.

Technique RK has evolved toward the use of a combined (bidirectional) incisional approach with a guarded diamond blade that has only a partial front-cutting surface. This technique combines the safety of an "American style" (centrifugal) incision and a second "Russian style" (centripetal) incision. Nomograms for determining surgical parameters depend on age and desired degree of correction. Parameters include the number of incisions (now typically 4, 6, or 8) and diameter of the central clear zone (usually 3.0 to 5.0 mm). Peripherally, incisions end 1 mm or more from the limbus. The desired depth of incisions is 90 to 95% of the stromal thickness, as determined with intraoperative pachymetry before setting the diamond blade. Postoperative regimen includes topical antibiotics, corticosteroids, and NSAIDs.

19.2 Complications of Radial Keratotomy

19.2.1 Perforation—intraoperative entry into the anterior chamber with the diamond blade.

Presentation microperforations cause a small leak of aqueous, which spontaneously seal; macroperforations cause constant efflux of aqueous and shallowing of the anterior chamber. Rarely, damage to the iris or anterior lens capsule may be seen. Most perforations occur in the inferior and temporal quadrants, where the cornea is thinnest. Sequelae include an increased risk of infection, iridocorneal adhesion, and epithelial downgrowth.

Management

- Microperforation: if the wound is sealed after challenge, the procedure is continued. Pachymetry and diamond blade settings should be rechecked.
- Macroperforation: the wound is sutured and the procedure is aborted until perforation is healed. Perform careful follow-up to rule out infection.

19.2.2 Central Clear Zone Incision—one or more incisions infringe on the intended central clear zone; now rare with bidirectional diamond blade techniques.

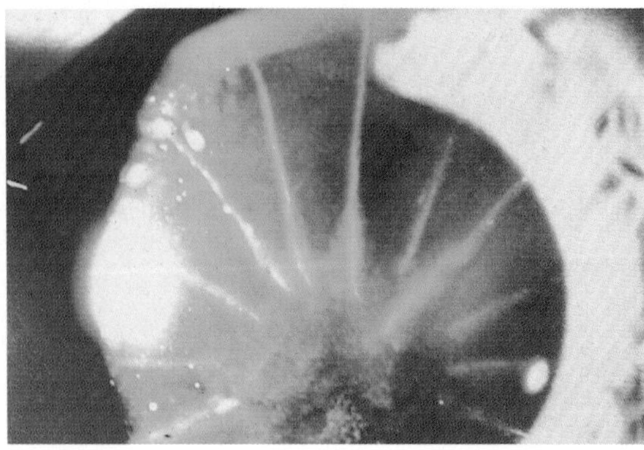

FIGURE 19.2.2 Central clear zone incision after 16-incision RK.

Presentation

- Symptoms: decreased BCVA, increase in glare and haloes.
- Findings: incision may enter the clear zone and cross the visual axis; irregular astigmatism.

Management lamellar keratoplasty or PK for severe visual loss.

19.2.3 Intersecting Incisions—incisions are inadvertently joined or crossed; more common when transverse incisions for astigmatism are combined with radial incisions.

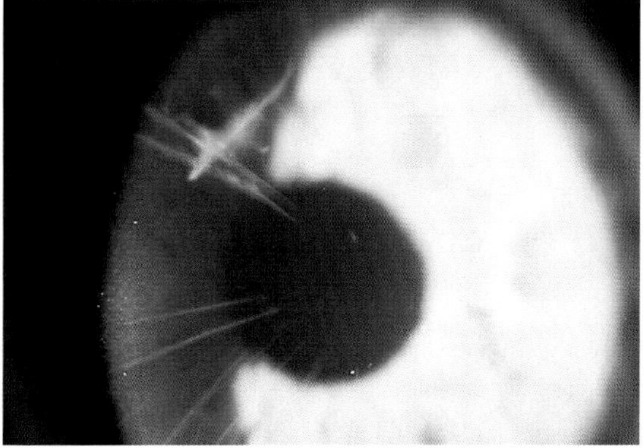

FIGURE 19.2.3 Intersecting incisions with irregular epithelial healing.

Presentation

- Symptoms: foreign-body sensation, pain, and glare.
- Findings: usually noted intraoperatively. There may be a wound gape causing persistent epithelial defect, recurrent erosions, or epithelial plugs or cysts; irregular astigmatism; loss of BCVA.

Management any wound gape can be sutured after thorough irrigation and debridement of surrounding epithelium.

19.2.4 Infectious Keratitis—corneal infection caused by infiltration of the RK incision, usually by bacterial pathogens. Fungal and HSV keratitis are also possible. Incidence is 0.25 to 0.70%. Risk factors include perforation, ocular surface disease, persistent epithelial defect, and contact lens wear.

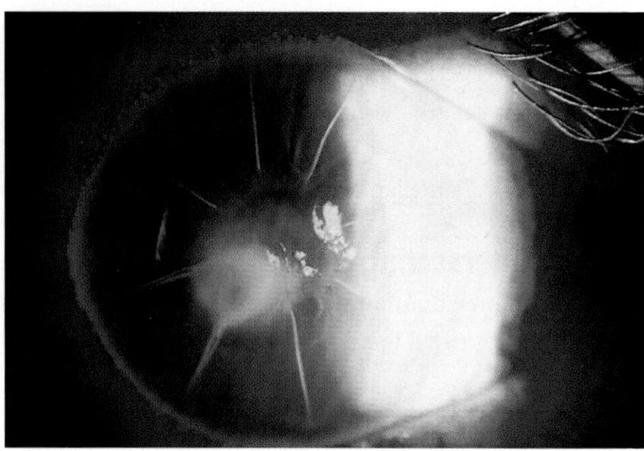

FIGURE 19.2.4 Bacterial keratitis in RK incision.

Differential Diagnosis

sterile infiltrate, deposits of topical drops (e.g., ciprofloxacin), foreign body.

Presentation

- Symptoms: redness, pain, photophobia, decreased vision.
- Findings: stromal infiltrate beginning within an incision, usually spreading quickly along the length and depth of the incision. Advanced cases lead to wound gape, perforation, cataract, and rarely endophthalmitis. Common bacterial isolates include gram positives, especially *Staphylococcus aureus* and *Staphylococcus epidermidis.* Isolates in later-onset infections (sometimes years after the procedure) tend to be gram negatives such as *Pseudomonas aeruginosa* due to an association with contact lens wear. Fungal and viral pathogens have also been reported.

Management

all infiltrates are treated as infectious. The area is scraped and cultured on appropriate media. Prompt antibiotic treatment with a fluoroquinolone for mild infiltrates or broad-spectrum fortified antibiotics (such as vancomycin and tobramycin) for moderate to severe infiltrates is indicated; 70% of patients will obtain 20/40 or better BCVA.

Severe cases may require emergent therapeutic patch graft or elective PK.

19.2.5 Disabling Glare and Haloes—irregular corneal contour or loss of corneal clarity can result in disabling glare, haloes, polyopia, and other visual distortions.

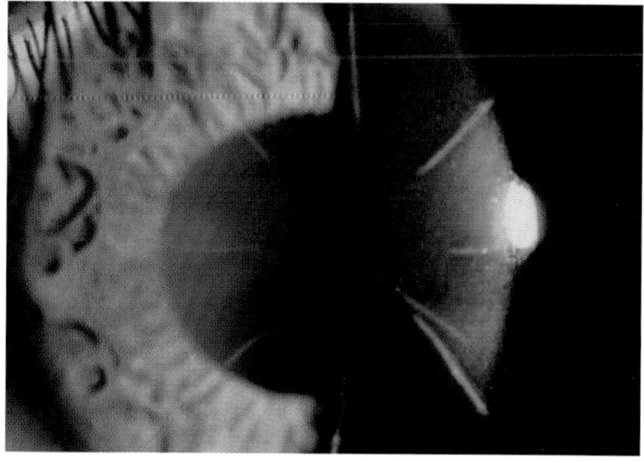

FIGURE 19.2.5 Decentered clear zone.

Presentation

- Symptoms: glare is often seen as a starburst pattern around light sources, especially at night, and is common after RK. Haloes are seen as glowing auras around light sources.
- Findings: there may be invasion of the central optical zone by incisions, central scarring, or incisional debris. Topography may reveal a decentered optical zone or irregular astigmatism. Young myopes may be symptomatic because of large pupils, especially under scotopic conditions.

Management a trial of a weak miotic (pilocarpine, 0.5 to 1% qid); high-quality sunglasses. Scars may respond to topical steroids. Disabling glare may require a rigid contact lens or, in severe cases, lamellar keratoplasty or PK.

19.2.6 Diurnal Refractive Fluctuation—changes in corneal hydration cause changes in corneal curvature in some patients after RK. Fluctuations can also occur due to hypoxia or increased IOP.

Differential Diagnosis inadequate wound healing, underlying keratoconus, dry eye syndrome, fluctuations of IOP.

Presentation

- Symptoms: morning hyperopic change (corneal hydration causes flattening) with myopia increasing throughout the day. This is common after RK but resolves in most patients after a few weeks.
- Findings: stromal edema may be seen, especially around incision sites. Careful cycloplegic refraction and topography at different times of day confirm the diagnosis.

Management in most cases, this phenomenon resolves with time. Rarely, separate sets of glasses may be prescribed.

19.2.7 Hyperopic Drift—a trend toward progressive hyperopia (more central corneal flattening) following RK is well documented. The effect is more pronounced in eyes that have had more surgery (i.e., longer, more, or deeper incisions).

Presentation

- Symptoms: early-onset presbyopia, eye strain, headache. May have excellent distance vision.
- Findings: the average rate of hyperopia was 0.21 D/year for 2 years, and then 0.06 D/year for the next 8 years in a perspective study (PERK). Limiting the use of RK for mild myopia (<4.00 D) and using newer techniques such as mini-RK have reduced hyperopic drift.

Management

- Prevention: most surgeons aim for slight undercorrection to avoid problems of hyperopic shift and to postpone the onset of presbyopic symptoms.
- Hyperopia is treated with spectacles or contact lenses. A trial of miotics (e.g., pilocarpine 2% qid) may be used for hyperopia of 1.5 to 3.0 D, after discussion of the risks of retinal tears. Alternatively, marked hyperopia may be treated with cleaning and suturing of incisions

in the early postoperative period. Holmium–YAG thermokeratoplasty and hyperopic PRK or LASIK may also be options.

19.2.8 Ruptured Globe

—the cornea is weakened after RK, and corneal rupture secondary to blunt trauma has been reported. Risks should be carefully discussed, especially in patients involved in contact sports. Limiting RK to four incisions has been shown to significantly reduce corneal weakening.

Presentation

- Symptoms: sudden loss of vision, pain, and extrusion of intraocular contents after blunt trauma. Trauma may be incidental.
- Findings: full-thickness rupture along RK incisions, sometimes extending across the central clear zone. Median time after surgery was 20 months. Of 26 reported cases, about half of the involved eyes had best-corrected visual acuity of 20/200 or less; after repair, about one-third achieved visual acuity better than 20/40.

Management surgical repair (see Chapter 1, Ruptured Globe).

19.3 Photorefractive Keratectomy (PRK)

an excimer laser technique of central cornea stromal ablation and flattening for the treatment of myopia. Photoastigmatic keratotomy using elliptical ablation zones and hyperopic PRK using ring ablation zones are also possible. The excimer laser generates pulses of ultraviolet light that uncouple chemical bonds at the surface of the cornea without penetration to deeper structures and without significant generation of heat.

- First-generation excimer lasers use broad beams with automated diaphragms and slits to control treatment areas.
- Second-generation excimer lasers include scanning slit and flying spot lasers, which use smaller beams, allowing for more flexible treatments and, theoretically, the potential for better results.

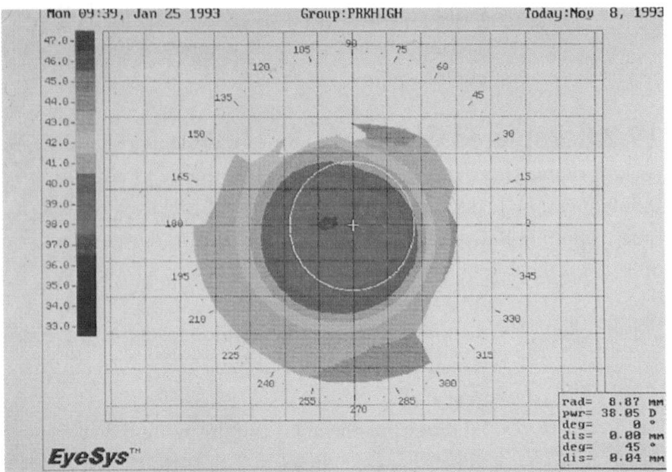

FIGURE 19.3 Normal topography after PRK.

Technique the anesthetized corneal epithelium is debrided or ablated. The computer nomogram determines the number of pulses to achieve a desired ablation depth, given a particular treatment protocol (multipass, multizone, etc.) The surgeon monitors centration over the pupil and stromal hydration. A bandage contact lens and topical NSAIDs are helpful to reduce postoperative pain. Postoperative medication regimens may include topical NSAIDs (usually limited to 1 to 2 days to avoid the development of subepithelial infiltrates), topical corticosteroids (risk of IOP rise, cataract, HSV, ptosis), and antibiotic. The case is followed carefully until the epithelium heals.

19.4 Selected Complications of Photorefractive Keratectomy

19.4.1 Decentered Ablation—eccentric ablation of 1 mm or more with respect to the visual axis is usually clinically significant. Causes include poor globe fixation, incorrect marking of visual axis, and eye movement during the procedure.

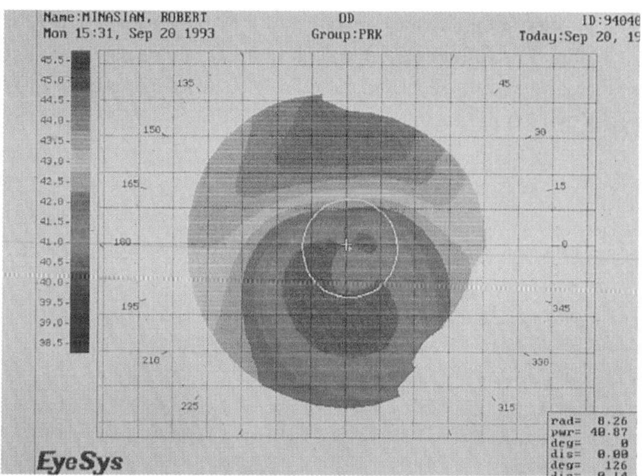

FIGURE 19.4.1 Inferiorly decentered PRK ablation.

Presentation

- Symptoms: monocular diplopia, glare, haloes, decrease in visual acuity, especially at night.
- Findings: undercorrection, irregular astigmatism, loss of BCVA. Patients with large pupils are more symptomatic. Corneal topography establishes the diagnosis.

Differential Diagnosis

asymmetric stromal healing within the ablation zone.

Management

videokeratography should be routinely obtained 1 month after PRK to establish or rule out the diagnosis. Medical treatment options include RGP contact lens wear and weak miotics. Consider retreatment with a larger ablation zone, or a compensatory asymmetric treatment, especially when there is undercorrection. Surgical treatment options are considered after stabilization of refraction, topography, and haze for at least 3 months, which seldom occurs before 6 months after surgery.

19.4.2 Central Islands—a topographic abnormality, usually defined as steepening of at least 1 to 3 D over a diameter of at least 1 to 3 mm in the central or paracentral cornea. A multifactorial etiology is likely, including central fluid collection, inhomogeneous beam profile, and central masking plume of ablated material. May be less frequent with scanning slit or flying spot lasers.

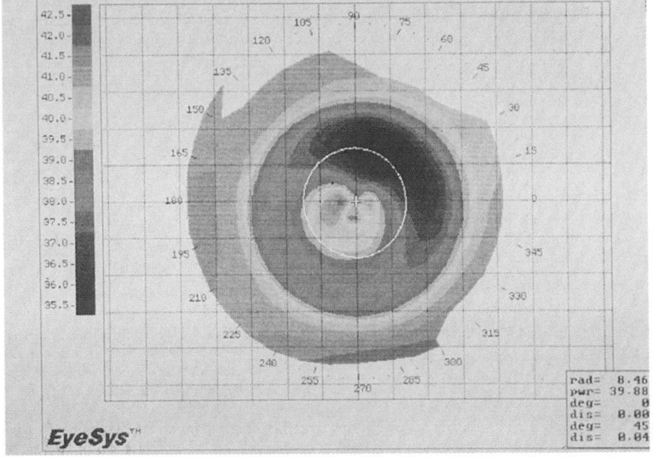

FIGURE 19.4.2 Topography of a central island.

Presentation

- Symptoms: usually transient monocular diplopia, ghost images, loss of BCVA, and prolonged visual recovery.
- Findings: residual myopia may be present; videokeratographic evidence as just noted. The finding is now becoming rare because of software factoring additional central treatment to prevent central islands.

Management the majority regress spontaneously 3 to 12 months after PRK. Retreatment is an option. One method includes transepithelial PRK of 7.0 mm until central and far peripheral epithelium are treated, followed by PRK retreatment for 50 to 100% of the pre-retreatment refraction.

19.4.3 Disabling Glare or Haloes—visual complaints after PRK of starburst effects or halo effects around lights, usually due to edge effects of the ablation zone.

Presentation

- Symptoms: photophobia, glare, difficulty with night vision.
- Findings: may have decentered ablation (see above) or corneal haze. Pupil size is often larger than optical zone ablation. Incidence is as high as 80% with 4.0-mm ablation zone diameters and less than 5% with 6-mm or more ablation zone diameters.

Management pupil size in light and dark should be noted preoperatively to choose ablation diameter and to rule out poor candidates for surgery. Small optical zones (<5.5 mm) may be retreated in some cases with a larger ablation zone diameter. A trial of miotics is possible, after risks of retinal detachment and other side effects are discussed.

19.4.4 Delayed Epithelial Healing—incomplete epithelial healing more than 4 days after PRK. The incidence is 1.5 to 9.4%.

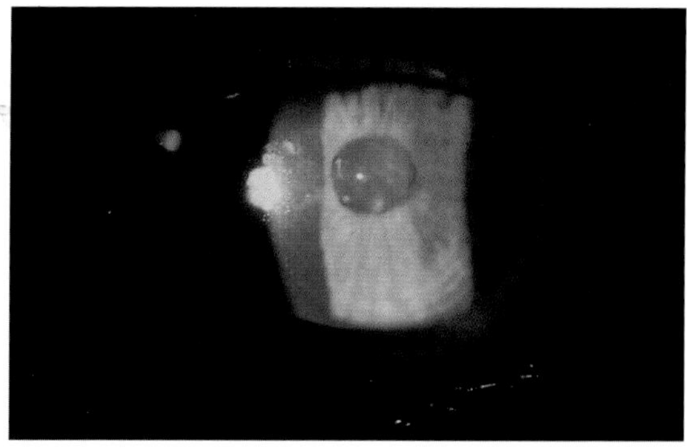

FIGURE 19.4.4 Delayed healing and filamentary keratitis after PRK.

Presentation

- Symptoms: persistent pain or discomfort, redness, photophobia.
- Findings: incomplete epithelialization can be seen at the slit lamp, usually without the aid of fluorescein; associated with increased haze and regression and risk of infection.

Differential Diagnosis poorly fitting contact lens, foreign body, medication toxicity or allergy, recurrent erosion (rare), infectious keratitis (HSV), bacterial, fungal).

Management dry eye and blepharitis should be evaluated and treated thoroughly before PRK. Minimize corticosteroids and NSAIDs. Treat with topical lubricants. Perform daily follow-up to rule out infection, haze.

19.4.5 Infectious Keratitis—a very rare complication of corneal infiltrate or ulcer after PRK. Bandage contact lens probably increases risk.

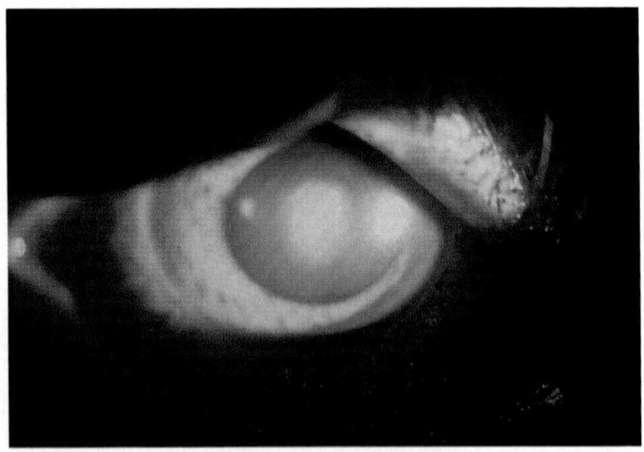

FIGURE 19.4.5 Infectious keratitis after PRK.

Presentation

- Symptoms: blurry vision, redness, photophobia.
- Findings: corneal infiltrate within the epithelial debridement zone.

Differential Diagnosis sterile infiltrate (especially in the presence of a NSAID), HSV (secondary to excimer laser or steroid reactivation), bacterial, fungal, or protozoal keratitis.

Management all infiltrates are treated as infectious with fortified antibiotics and/or fluoroquinolones. Central infiltrates are cultured. Small infiltrates with intact epithelium may be followed closely for resolution. Avoid PRK in patients with a history of HSV keratitis. Consider oral acyclovir, valcyclovir, or famcyclovir prophylaxis for patients with a history of herpetic cold sores.

19.4.6 Haze and Regression

19.4.6 Haze and Regression—scarring due to abnormal production of extracellular matrix components; associated with regression due to corneal steepening and changes in refractive properties of the cornea.

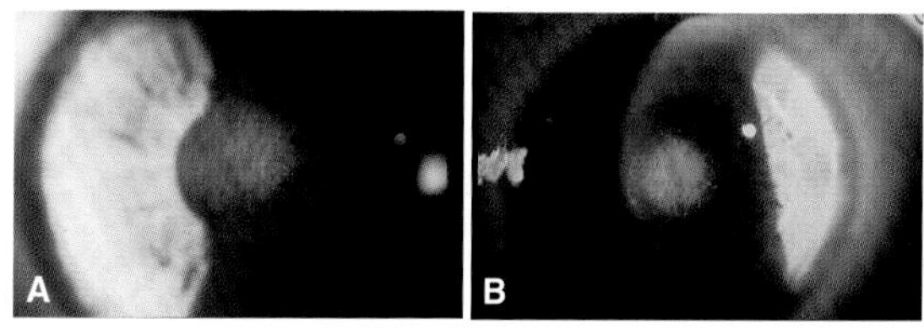

FIGURE 19.4.6a Moderate haze after PRK.
FIGURE 19.4.6b Severe haze and scarring.

Presentation

- Symptoms: gradual decrease in visual acuity, cloudy vision, glare.
- Findings: increased density of haze proportional to degree of myopia treated. Begins in weeks 2 to 4, peaks in months 1 to 3, and resolves in 1 to 2 years after PRK; loss of BCVA; increasingly myopic refraction; may be associated with previous delayed epithelial healing.

Differential Diagnosis

medicamentosa, poorly fitting contact lens, infectious keratitis.

Management

- Topical corticosteroids: the course is prolonged with monitoring for complications, especially increased IOP.
- Repeat excimer ablation: helpful in some cases, especially when regression or undertreatment is present.

However, further scarring may be possible, so retreatment with LASIK may be more appropriate.

19.5 Laser In Situ Keratomileusis (LASIK)

a keratorefractive technique where a corneal lamellar incision is made to raise a corneal lenticule ("flap" or "cap"), followed by an excimer laser ablation of the underlying bare central corneal stroma. Bowman's layer is not ablated, and minimal disturbance of the epithelium minimizes pain, haze, and recovery time. LASIK is used for the treatment of myopia, astigmatism, and hy-

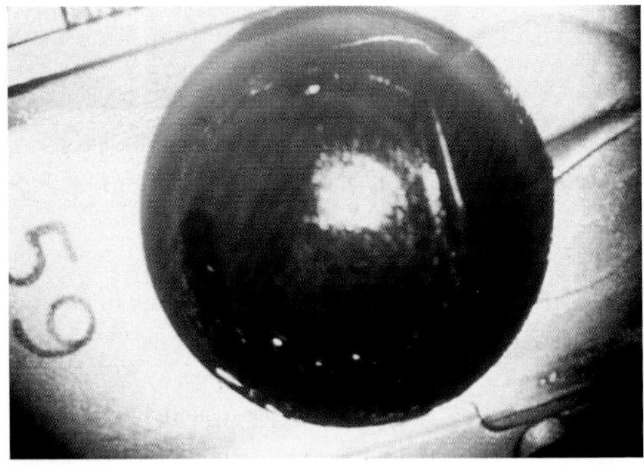

FIGURE 19.5 Intraoperative LASIK during ablation.

peropia.

Technique the microkeratome suction ring is applied to the anesthetized eye. IOP is raised to over 65 mm Hg, and the microkeratome (set at 130 to 180 μm) is advanced and returned, leaving a hinge on the nasal or superior cornea. The flap is flipped over the hinge, and the excimer ablation is performed as for PRK (above). The flap is then placed back, and correct alignment and adherence are ensured with preplaced markings and carefully observed dehydration of the wound edge. Sutures are rarely necessary. Postoperative pain is minimal. Most surgeons do not patch. Medications include topical antibiotics, corticosteroid, and possibly NSAIDs.

Results outcomes are difficult to gauge because no definite nomogram has been developed. Recent published series suggest refractive results similar to those with PRK. There is a growing consensus among refractive surgeons that LASIK is more likely than PRK to achieve good and stable outcomes in patients with moderate to high myopia.

19.6 Selected Complications of Laser in Situ Keratomileusis

19.6.1 Intraoperative Flap Complications—improper microkeratome technique or function may lead to thin, incomplete, eccentric, or free corneal flaps. Rarely, globe perforation with loss of intraocular contents has been reported.

Presentation the microkeratome may have debris in the gears, or the footplate may be malpositioned. Free caps may be associated with flat or small corneas, poor suction, or poorly adjusted microkeratome end stop. Intraocular penetration may damage the iris or lens.

Management

- *Incomplete thin or eccentric flaps:* the flap is replaced and the procedure aborted until a later date.
- *Free cap:* the normal excimer ablation can be continued. After ablation, the cap is placed back as usual. Anchor sutures may be necessary and are removed in 1 week.
- *Lost cap:* for myopic LASIK, the bare stroma can be allowed to epithelialize and heal, and vision may become acceptable. A lamellar corneal graft may be done for a myopic procedure and is necessary for a hyperopic procedure. If severe haze or ectasia ensue, PK is necessary.
- *Intraocular penetration:* this necessitates adequate corneal closure and repair of other damaged structures.

19.6.2 Dislocated Cap—after LASIK, a corneal cap rarely can become dislocated and lost.

Presentation

- Symptoms: decreased vision and pain.
- Findings: a large epithelial defect, which may have begun healing. The flap may be still attached at the hinge or is sometimes found in the fornix. The flap is usually deepithelialized. Later, corneal haze or ectasia may develop.

Management the flap is repositioned and sutured into place with multiple interrupted sutures or a running 8-bite antitorque suture. If the epithelium is not healed after 7 to 10 days, it may be upside-down and should be repositioned. If the flap is lost, the stroma can be allowed to reepithelialize, or a lamellar homograft may be done.

19.6.3 Complications of Acute Rise in Intraocular Pressure—a prolonged application of the suction ring can cause complications due to raised IOP.

Presentation

- Symptoms: acute loss of vision or visual field defects immediately after surgery.
- Findings: ischemic optic neuropathy, retinal vascular occlusions, subretinal hemorrhages, and new lacquer cracks have been reported.

Management experience with the microkeratome and expedience in flap creation are important in avoiding these complications. Careful preoperative screening for retinal vascular and optic nerve diseases is important.

19.6.4 Epithelial Ingrowth—epithelial cell proliferation in the flap interface after LASIK due to incomplete irrigation of epithelial cells.

Presentation

- Symptoms: decreased vision, haze, haloes.
- Findings: nests of migrating epithelial cells as well as local or diffuse haze may be seen at the interface. There

may be shrinkage of the cap and inflammation. Loss of BCVA and irregular astigmatism are possible.

Differential Diagnosis nonepithelial debris (see below), bacterial or fungal keratitis.

Management topical corticosteroids are used to treat inflammation. If debris is seen, early intervention may prevent haze and inflammation; however, waiting 3 months may enable easier rinsing of epithelial cells. If vision is affected, the flap may be raised and the epithelial cells may be scraped from both interface surfaces and thoroughly irrigated. Light ablation of both surfaces with the excimer laser may assist in devitalizing any remaining epithelial cells.

19.6.5 Nonepithelial Debris in Flap Interface—talc, fibers from sponges and drapes, meibomian gland secretions, and debris from the microkeratome may accumulate at the interface if not well irrigated.

Presentation
- Symptoms: rarely, decreased vision, haze, or haloes.
- Findings: scattered debris in the interface may appear crystalline or filamentous. Surrounding inflammation and haze may be incited. Coexistent blepharitis is common.

Differential Diagnosis epithelial ingrowth, bacterial or fungal keratitis.

Management if visually significant, the flap may be raised to irrigate the foreign materials. Topical steroids are used to control inflammation, with the possibility of infection kept in mind.

19.6.6 Corneal Folds in Flap—improper intraoperative flap adherence may cause wrinkles in the corneal cap.

Presentation
- Symptoms: decreased vision.
- Findings: more common in thin flaps. Fine folds are detected better at the slit lamp than at the operating mi-

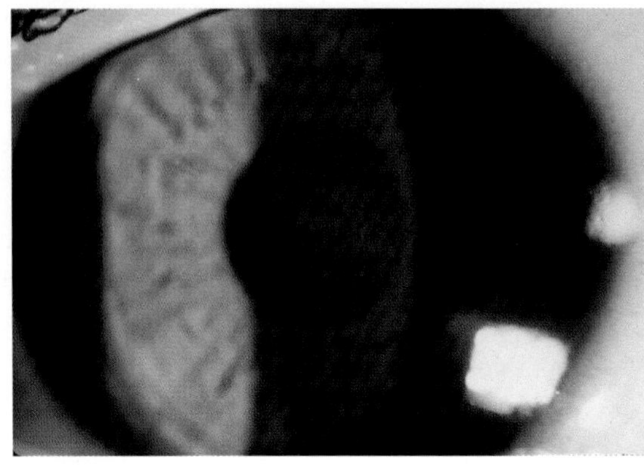

FIGURE 19.6.6 Debris in interface.

croscope. Even minimal folds may cause decreased vision and irregular astigmatism.

Management during the procedure, the flap can be reflected, moistened, and carefully repositioned. If the folds are noted postoperatively (days to a few months), the flap is lifted and stroked to flatten the folds and then replaced with careful attention to the pattern of readherence.

APPENDIX

ABK	aphakic bullous keratopathy
AC	anterior chamber or accomodative convergence
AC/A	accommodative convergence/accomodation ratio
ACh	Acetylcholine
ACL, ACIOL	anterior chamber lens
AION	anterior ischemic optic neuropathy
AK	astigmatic keratotomy
ALT	argon laser trabeculoplasty
AMD	age-related macular degeneration
AMPPE	acute multifocal posterior placoid pigment epitheliopathy
ANA	antinuclear antibodies
ANCA	antineutrophil cytoplasmic antibodies
APD	afferent pupillary defect
ARC	abnormal retinal correspondence
ARN	acute retinal necrosis
ASP	anterior stromal puncture
AV	arteriovenous
AVIT	anterior vitrectomy
BARN	bilateral acute retinal necrosis
BCG	bacillus Calmette-Guérin
BCVA	best corrected visual acuity
BMR	bilateral medical recession
BRAO	branch retinal artery occlusion
BRVO	branch retinal vein occlusion
CA	corneal abrasion
CALT	conjunctiva-associated lymphoid tissue
C/D	cup-to-disc (ratio)
CF	count figures
CHED	congenital hereditary endothelial dystrophy
CHSD	congenital hereditary stromal dystrophy
CLIK	contact lens induced keratoconjunctivitis
CME	cystoid macular edema
CMV	cytomegalovirus
CN	congenital nystagmus
CNV	choroidal neovascularization
CPEO	chronic progressive external ophthalmoplegia
CPSD	corrected pattern standard deviation
CRA	central retinal artery

CRAO	central retinal artery occlusion
CRVO	central retinal vein occlusion
C/S	conjunctiva/sclera
CSC	central serous chorioretinopathy
CSD	cat-scratch disease
CSF	cerebrospinal fluid
CSME	clinically significant macular edema
CSNB	congenitial stationary night blindness
CSR	central serous retinopathy
CT	computed tomography
CU	cornea ulcer
CVA	cerebral vascular accident
CWS	cotton wool spot
CXR	chest x-ray film
D	diopter
DCR	dacryocystorhinostomy
DD	disc diameter
DDT	dye disappearance test
DFE	dilated fundus exam
DM	diabetes mellitus
DTQ	deep and quiet
DVD	dissociated vertical deviation
EBV	Epstein-Barr virus
ECCE	extracapsular cataract extraction
ECG	electrocardiogram
EDTA	disodium ethylene diamine tetracetle acid
EKC	epidemic keratoconjunctivitis
ELISA	enzyme-linked immunosorbent assay
EMG	electromyelogram
EOG	electro-oculogram
EOM	extraocular muscles
ERG	electroretinogram
ERM	epiretinal membrane
ESR	erythrocyte sedimentation rate
5-FU	5-Fluorouracil
ETDRS	early treatment diabetic retinopathy study
FA (NG)	fluoroscein (angiogram)
FAZ	foveal avascular zone
FEVR	familial exudative retinopathy
G6PD	glucose-6-phosphate deficiency
g	gram
GCA	giant cell arteritis
GMS	Gomori's methenamine-silver (stain)

GPC	giant papillary conjunctivitis
h	hour
HSV	herpes simplex virus
HZV	herpes zoster virus
IBD	inflammatory bowel disease
ICE	iridocorneal endothelial (syndrome)
ICCE	intracapsular cataract extraction
IK	insterstitial keratitis
ILM	internal limiting membrane
IM	intramuscular
INO	internuclear ophthalmoplegia
IOL	intraocular lens
IOP	intraocular pressure
IRMA	intraretinal microvascular abnormality
JRA	juvenille rheumatoid arthritis
JXG	juvenille xanthogranuloma
KCS	keratoconjunctivitis sicca
K_{EFF}	effective K value
K	cornea, curvature
KP	keratic precipitates
LASIK	laser in-situ keratomileusis
LP	light perception
LPI	laser peripheral iridotomy
MD	mean defect or mean deviation
MEWDS	multiple evanescent white dot syndrome
MGD	meibomian grand disease
min	minute
ml	milliliter
MLF	medial longitudinal fasciculus
mm Hg	millimeters of mercury
MRA	magnetic resonance angiography
MRI	magnetic resonance imaging
MS	multiple sclerosis
n	number
Nd:YAG	neodymium-YAG
NF	neurofibromatosis
NFL	nerve fiber layer
NLP	no light perception
NPDR	nonproliferative diabetic retinopathy
NS	nuclear sclerosis
NVD	neovascularization of the (optic) disc
NVE	neovascularization elsewhere (in the retina)
NVI	neovascularization of the iris

OCP	ocular cicatricial pemphigoid
OKN	optikinetic nystagmus
PAD	polymorohic amyloid degeneration
PAM	potential acuity meter, primary acquired melanosis
PAS	periodic acid-Schiff (stain), peripheral anterior synechia
PBK	pseudophakic bullous keratopathy
PCL/PCIOL	posterior chamber lens
PCO	posterior capsular opacity
PD	pattern deviation
PDR	proliferative diabetic retinopathy
PED	pigment epithelial detachment, persistent epithelial defect
PEK	punctate epithelial iceratitis
PERG	pattern electoretinogram
PHMB	polyhexamethylene biguanate
PHPV	persistent hyperplastic primary vitreous
PI	peripheral iridectomy/iridotomy
PIC	punctate inner choroiditis
PK (P)	penetrating keratoplasty
PMMA	polymethylmethacrylate (lens)
PMNs	polymorphonuclear leukocytes
PO	per os (oral)
POAG	primary open-angle glaucoma
POHS	presumed ocular histoplasmosis syndrome
PORN	progressive outer retinal necrosis
PPMD	posterior polymorphous dystrophy
PRK	photorefractive keratectomy
PRP	panretinal photocoagulation
PS	posterior synechiae
PSC	posterior subcapsular (cataract)
PSD	pattern standard derivative
PTK	phototherapeutic keratectomy
PVD	posterior vitreous detachment
PVR	proliferative vitreoretinopathy
PXE	pseudoxanthoma elasticum
RA	rheumatoid arthritis
RAPD	relative afferent pupillary defect
RD	retinal detachment
RGP	rigid gas permeable (contact lens)
RI	relaxing incision
RK	radial keratotomy
ROP	retinopathy of prematurity
RP	retinitis pigmentosa
RPE	retinal pigment epithelium

RRD	rhegmatogenous retinal detachment
SC	sickle cell
SEI	subepithelial infiltrate
SLE	systemic lupus erythematosus, slit lamp examination
SLK	superior limbic keratoconjunctivitis
SPK	superficial punctate keratitis
SRN	subretinal neovascularization
SS	Sjögren's syndrome
TFBUT	tear film break-up time
TM	trabecular meshwork
TPPL	trans pars plana lensectomy
TPPV	trans pars plana vitrectomy
TRD	tractional retinal detachment
TRIO	thyroid related immune orbitopathy
U	units
UAIM	unilateral acute idiopathic maculopathy
UGH	uveitis-glaucoma-hyphema (syndrome)
URI	upper respiratory infection
UV	ultraviolet
VA	visual acuity
VEP	visual evoked potential
VF	visual field
VH	vitreous hermorrhage
VKH	Vogt-Koyanagi-Harada (disease)
VZV	varicella-zoster virus
YAG	yttrium aluminum garnet

INDEX